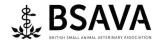

BSAVA Guide to Procedures in Small Animal Practice

3rd edition

T0178682

Editors:

Nick Bexfield BVetMed PhD DSAM DipECVIM-CA PGDipMedSci PGCHE FHEA MRCVS
Queen's Veterinary School Hospital, Department of Veterinary Medicine,
University of Cambridge, Madingley Road, Cambridge CB3 0ES

Julia Riggs MA VetMB AFHEA DipECVS MRCVS
Queen's Veterinary School Hospital, Department of Veterinary Medicine,
University of Cambridge, Madingley Road, Cambridge CB3 0ES

Published by:

British Small Animal Veterinary Association
Woodrow House, 1 Telford Way,
Waterwells Business Park, Quedgeley,
Gloucester GL2 2AB

A Company Limited by Guarantee in England
Registered Company No. 2837793
Registered as a Charity

The drawings in Figures EXOR.1–EXOR.3, A.3, A.4, A.5, A.7, A.9ab, B.3, B.7, B.8, B.13, B.23, B.26, B.27, B.30, B.32, B.33, B.37, C.9, E.1abcd, E.8, E.9a, E.12, E.13, E.15–E.17, I.1, 1.5ab, I.6–I.11, L.2, L.3, L.8–L.16, P.16a, P.16c, P.22, R.3, T.16–T.23, T.26ab, U.5 and V.1–V.5 were drawn by S.J. Elmhurst BA Hons (www.livingart.org.uk) and are printed with her permission.

A catalogue record for this book is available from the British Library.

ISBN: Print: 978-1-913859-13-8 • Online: 978-1-913859-14-5 • ePDF: 978-1-913859-19-0 • EPUB: 978-1-913859-20-6

The publishers, editors and contributors cannot take responsibility for information provided on dosages and methods of application of drugs mentioned or referred to in this publication. Details of this kind must be verified in each case by individual users from up to date literature published by the manufacturers or suppliers of those drugs. Veterinary surgeons are reminded that in each case they must follow all appropriate national legislation and regulations (for example, in the United Kingdom, the prescribing cascade) from time to time in force.

Printed in the UK by Zenith Media, Pontypool NP4 0DQ
Printed on ECF paper made from sustainable forests

18694PUBS24

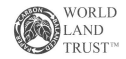

Titles in the BSAVA Manuals series:

Manual of Avian Practice: A Foundation Manual
Manual of Backyard Poultry Medicine and Surgery
Manual of Canine & Feline Abdominal Imaging
Manual of Canine & Feline Abdominal Surgery
Manual of Canine & Feline Advanced Veterinary Nursing
Manual of Canine & Feline Anaesthesia and Analgesia
Manual of Canine & Feline Behavioural Medicine
Manual of Canine & Feline Cardiorespiratory Medicine
Manual of Canine & Feline Clinical Pathology
Manual of Canine & Feline Dentistry and Oral Surgery
Manual of Canine & Feline Dermatology
Manual of Canine & Feline Emergency and Critical Care
Manual of Canine & Feline Endocrinology
Manual of Canine & Feline Endoscopy and Endosurgery
Manual of Canine & Feline Fracture Repair and Management
Manual of Canine & Feline Gastroenterology
Manual of Canine & Feline Haematology and Transfusion Medicine
Manual of Canine & Feline Head, Neck and Thoracic Surgery
Manual of Canine & Feline Musculoskeletal Disorders
Manual of Canine & Feline Musculoskeletal Imaging
Manual of Canine & Feline Nephrology and Urology
Manual of Canine & Feline Neurology
Manual of Canine & Feline Oncology
Manual of Canine & Feline Ophthalmology
Manual of Canine & Feline Radiography and Radiology: A Foundation Manual
Manual of Canine & Feline Rehabilitation, Supportive and Palliative Care
Manual of Canine & Feline Reproduction and Neonatology
Manual of Canine & Feline Shelter Medicine
Manual of Canine & Feline Surgical Principles: A Foundation Manual
Manual of Canine & Feline Thoracic Imaging
Manual of Canine & Feline Ultrasonography
Manual of Canine & Feline Wound Management and Reconstruction
Manual of Canine Practice: A Foundation Manual
Manual of Exotic Pet and Wildlife Nursing
Manual of Exotic Pets: A Foundation Manual
Manual of Feline Practice: A Foundation Manual
Manual of Practical Animal Care
Manual of Practical Veterinary Nursing
Manual of Practical Veterinary Welfare
Manual of Psittacine Birds
Manual of Rabbit Medicine
Manual of Rabbit Surgery, Dentistry and Imaging
Manual of Raptors, Pigeons and Passerine Birds
Manual of Reptiles
Manual of Rodents and Ferrets
Manual of Small Animal Practice Management and Development
Manual of Wildlife Casualties

For further information on these and all BSAVA publications, please visit our website: www.bsava.com

Contents

A series of videos (see Index for further information) to accompany the procedures in this Guide is available from the BSAVA Library. Use the QR code or type the web address **bsavalibrary.com/ proceduresvideos** into a web browser to access these resources.

Foreword

Since the first edition of the *BSAVA Guide to Procedures in Small Animal Practice* was published in 2010, it has become an indispensable resource in practices for recent graduates and experienced clinicians alike. It is an ever-popular member benefit for first year qualified members, whether it is accessed in hard copy or via the BSAVA app. The value to busy vets of such a clear, relevant and trustworthy publication cannot be over-emphasized.

The second edition (2014) developed and improved the guide, with even clearer entries and the use of colour photographs. New procedures were added, the guide was reorganized and fully indexed.

How, then, to improve on a very good reference? Editors Nick Bexfield and Julia Riggs have managed this and a large part of their success is visual. New high-resolution images illustrate a number of the procedures. Photographs and illustrations from other BSAVA Manuals have been incorporated to augment the text. The truly transformative step has been the addition of a suite of quality videos filmed to help explain the techniques. Whether illustrating a neurological examination, bone marrow biopsy or placing an oesophagostomy tube, these videos clearly demonstrate what is described in the text.

In addition, all existing procedures have been updated and new techniques have been added, including how to place a cystotomy tube, endotracheal intubation, point-of-care ultrasound (POCUS) and wet-to-dry dressings.

I am confident that the new edition will soon become the essential daily reference for those in general practice.

Carl Gorman
BVSc MRCVS

BSAVA President 2023–4

Preface

It is our pleasure to introduce to you the third edition of the *BSAVA Guide to Procedures in Small Animal Practice*, which has been written for veterinary surgeons, veterinary nurses and students. We have been delighted by the success of the previous editions, which suggests that this Guide has become the number one reference for step-by-step instructions on diagnostic and therapeutic procedures performed routinely in small animal veterinary practice. The third edition aims to build on this success, to increase the confidence and accuracy with which these procedures are performed, by responding directly to the feedback we have received from the BSAVA readership.

We have reviewed and updated all the procedures in the Guide in line with new editions of BSAVA Manuals and with progress in the field of veterinary medicine. New procedures for this edition include how to place a cystostomy tube, endotracheal intubation, point-of-care ultrasound (POCUS) and wet-to-dry dressings, all of which are being performed in primary care practice. We have added additional colour diagrams and photographs, to clarify and really bring to life the procedures being described.

An exciting innovation for the third edition is the inclusion of high-definition procedure videos. They have been produced to augment the text and will be of particular value to highlight specific steps in procedures that are challenging to explain in words or still images. In addition, we have augmented videos of local anaesthesia nerve blocks and arthrocentesis with still images to show the anatomical landmarks for needle insertion points. We are sure that the videos will become a 'go to' resource for practitioners to refer to prior to performing a procedure.

We are once again indebted to the innumerable contributors who have written procedures within the BSAVA Manuals on which we have drawn. We are also grateful to our colleagues who have reviewed procedures within this edition, including Chiara Adami, Malina Filipas, Chantelle Franklin, Paul Freeman, Charlotte Hodds, Hanna Machin, Jose Novo Matos, Laura Owen, Cat Partington, Fran Silveira and David Williams. In addition, it would have not been possible to include so many high-quality videos without the help of colleagues including Chiara Adami, Sharon Chandler, Robert Dudley, Paul Freeman, Sarah Hodson, Susana Monforte-Monteiro, Matthew Rhodes, Becky Walters and David Williams. It was a real pleasure to work with Ross Welch and Nathan Turner from Perspective Studios Limited, who did an amazing job capturing the videos and selected still images for this edition.

We would also like to thank Samantha Elmhurst for her illustrations, and our numerous colleagues who have contributed images or assisted in acquiring them specifically for this Guide. Finally, we would like to thank the Publishing team at BSAVA for their patience and attention to detail, without which this Guide would not have been possible.

Nick Bexfield
Julia Riggs

January 2024

Cardiorespiratory examination

Indications/Use

- Successful management of the animal with cardiorespiratory disease depends on accurate anatomical localization of disease and efficient diagnostic planning
- Determination of the history of the complaint, assessment of the pattern of breathing, and careful examination and auscultation will assist in determining the differential diagnoses for cardiorespiratory problems
- It will also aid in selecting appropriate complementary examinations, including thoracic radiography, echocardiography, arterial blood gas analysis, **electrocardiography** and **blood pressure measurement**

Equipment

- Stethoscope
- Stopwatch or timer

Patient preparation and positioning

- Assessment should be performed on the conscious animal
- The patient should be standing if possible; this is particularly important for cardiac auscultation
- Animals should be kept calm throughout the examination

Observation

> **WARNING**
>
> - Sternal recumbency, standing with elbows abducted and/or hyper-ventilating with the neck extended may indicate that the animal has dyspnoea.

Body condition and shape

- In general, animals with airway-oriented diseases (tracheal collapse, chronic bronchitis, feline bronchial disease) will be in excellent systemic health and have a stable (or often increased) body condition score
- Animals with parenchymal, pleural or cardiac disease with failure are more likely to be systemically debilitated or cachexic
- Animals with congenital heart disease may have stunted growth
- Obesity may be associated with lower airway disease in small breed dogs
- Animals with chronic hyperpnoea can show barrel-chested changes

Gait

- Cats with myocardial disease are at risk of systemic thromboembolism and may present with limb paresis

Breathing pattern

- A visual appraisal of the respiratory pattern should be made before the patient is stressed by an examination

- Restrictive respiratory diseases, such as pleural effusion and parenchymal disorders (pneumonia or oedema), cause rapid and shallow respiratory motions
- Obstructive disorders, such as bronchitis, result in slow, deep breathing
- Assessment of the phase of respiration that is predominantly affected (inspiratory *versus* expiratory) may help to localize obstructive disease:
  - Increased expiratory effort, prolonged expiratory time and abdominal effort on expiration should be considered suggestive of chronic lower airway disease
  - Increased inspiratory effort is suggestive of upper airway disease

Physical examination

Mucous membrane colour

- The colour of the mucous membranes should be assessed:
  - Normal mucous membrane colour is pink to pale pink
  - Pallor can indicate anaemia, but can also be associated with severe peripheral vasoconstriction in low-output states or conditions of elevated sympathetic tone
  - Cyanosis indicates an increased concentration of desaturated haemoglobin, and ranges from slightly 'dusky' in mild cases to nearly navy blue in patients with severe hypoxaemia. Cyanosis is most often seen with severe hypoxaemia resulting from severe respiratory disease, congestive heart failure with severe pulmonary oedema or pleural effusion and right-to-left congenital shunts
  - Right-to-left (reversed) patent ductus arteriosus may result in differential cyanosis in which the cyanosis is only detected in the caudal half of the body
  - Congested or injected mucous membranes occur with polycythaemia, systemic (toxaemia or septicaemia) or local inflammation, venous congestion, fever or exercise
  - Cherry red mucous membranes are seen in carbon monoxide toxicity

Capillary refill time

- Pressure should be applied to the gum with a clean finger and then released; this will cause blanching of the area, which should return to its normal colour within 1–2 seconds (Figure EXC.1)
- An increased capillary refill time (CRT) (>2 seconds) indicates poor peripheral perfusion. Causes include low cardiac output, shock, dehydration or hypovolaemia
- Patients in pain, with septic shock or with fever may demonstrate a decreased CRT (<1 second)

Jugular veins

- Both jugular veins should be visually inspected for distension and pulsation
- In long-haired animals, it is possible to get an impression of jugular venous distension without clipping the hair if the coat is wetted with spirit
- Jugular pulsation should not extend higher than one-third of the neck in healthy standing dogs

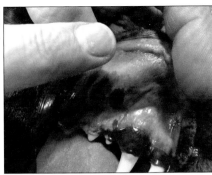

Figure EXC.1: Capillary refill time should be assessed using the oral mucosa.

Distension

- In the absence of a cranial mediastinal mass or obstruction of the cranial vena cava, distension of the jugular veins indicates elevation of right atrial pressures
- For animals with only a mild increase in right-sided pressure, compression of the cranial abdomen may increase venous return to the right heart sufficiently to cause temporary jugular distension ('hepatojugular reflux'). The distension resolves when the abdominal pressure is released

Pulsation

- Jugular pulsation may be prominent with tricuspid regurgitation, pericardial disease, and when atrial contraction occurs against a non-compliant or restricted ventricle or a closed tricuspid valve during rhythm disturbances

Peripheral pulse

Suitable sites for monitoring the pulse include the following:

- Femoral artery (Figure EXC.2a)
- Digital artery (Figure EXC.2b)
- Coccygeal artery (Figure EXC.2c)
- Dorsal pedal artery (Figure EXC.2d)

1 Locate the artery with the fingertips.
2 Assess the pulse character, rate and rhythm.
3 Compare the pulse rate with the heart rate, preferably by simultaneous auscultation, to determine the presence of any pulse deficit.
4 Assess pulse on both sides for asymmetry:
   a Weak pulses may reflect poor stroke volume or increased peripheral resistance
   b Strong pulses reflect an increased difference between diastolic and systolic pressure. Causes include: patent ductus arteriosus, severe aortic insufficiency and hyperthyroidism (cats)
   c Detectable variations of the pulse quality with respiration (pulsus paradoxus) are usually associated with cardiac tamponade
   d Pulses may be absent or asymmetrical in patients with systemic thromboembolism.

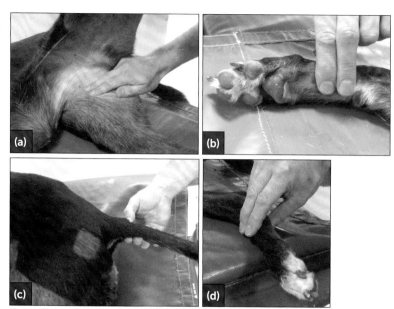

Figure EXC.2: Pulse monitoring sites. (a) Femoral artery on medial aspect of femur. (b) Digital artery on palmar aspect of carpus. (c) Coccygeal artery on ventral aspect of tail base. (d) Dorsal pedal artery just distal to tarsus (between the second and third metatarsals).

Abdominal palpation

1 Assess the size of the liver:
- **a** Liver enlargement will accompany right-sided heart failure in dogs
- **b** The liver may be more palpable than usual in some cats with severe hyperpnoea and air trapping.

2 Assess the size of the kidneys:
- **a** Small, irregularly shaped kidneys may be associated with systemic hypertension
- **b** This should prompt **blood pressure measurement**.

3 Assess for the presence of abdominal effusion:
- **a** Small abdominal effusions may be appreciated as 'slipperiness' of the small intestines
- **b** Larger ascitic effusions are unmistakable on percussion of a fluid thrill.

Cardiac auscultation

Heart rate

- Heart rate can be helpful in differentiating cardiac from respiratory disease in dogs where respiratory disease is associated with elevated vagal tone, leading to an exaggerated respiratory sinus arrhythmia
- Dogs with chronic heart failure are more likely to have increased sympathetic tone and an increased heart rate, although the degree of tachycardia may be modest

- Care should be taken not to place too much reliance on heart rate in brachycephalic dogs with suspected heart failure, as concurrent airway obstruction may cause sufficient elevation in vagal tone that sinus arrhythmia persists despite overt heart failure
- Cats do not always develop a consistent tachycardia with heart failure, and may be more likely than dogs to develop sinus bradycardia with life-threatening congestive failure signs

Heart rhythm

- Normal dogs will have:
  - A regular heart rhythm
  - OR a sinus arrhythmia, where heart rate speeds up with inspiration and then slows with expiration
- Cats normally have a regular heart rhythm
- Bradyarrhythmias can be recognized by a slow heart rate
- Atrial fibrillation sounds characteristically 'chaotic' on auscultation, but can still be confused with frequent atrial or ventricular premature beats

Intensity of heart sounds

- Two heart sounds (S1 and S2) are normally heard in dogs and cats (Figure EXC.3):
  - S1 occurs after closure of the atrioventricular valves, and is heard loudest at the apex of the heart
  - S2 occurs after closure of the aortic and pulmonic valves, and is heard loudest at the base of the heart
- Split S2 heart sounds can be heard if there is a delay between aortic and pulmonic valve closure, often associated with volume or pressure overload of the right-hand side of the heart, including pulmonary hypertension
- High cardiac output states, cardiac enlargement, thin body condition and increased sympathetic tone can increase the intensity of heart sounds
- Pericardial effusion, severe myocardial failure, obesity, space-occupying lesions and pleural effusion may decrease intensity
- Intensity may vary from beat to beat with rhythm disturbances including atrial fibrillation, frequent atrial or ventricular premature beats and irregular ventricular arrhythmia

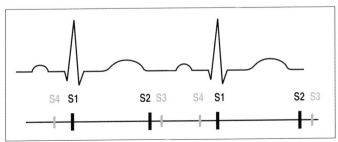

Figure EXC.3: Heart rhythm showing normal (S1 and S2) and abnormal (S3 and S4) heart sounds.

Additional heart sounds

- Additional heart sounds (S3 and S4) are associated with abnormal diastolic ventricular filling. These sounds are called *gallop sounds* and should not be audible in the normal dog or cat
- Impaired ventricular relaxation can also cause an audible gallop, and may account for the presence of a gallop in some geriatric cats without obvious structural heart disease
- In all other cats and dogs, a gallop sound can be considered to be a specific indication of heart disease

Murmurs and clicks

- Murmurs are sounds produced by turbulent blood flow:
  - They are more likely with high blood flow velocity (e.g. in pulmonic stenosis, aortic stenosis, mitral or tricuspid regurgitation)
  - Murmurs are characterized according to their timing (systolic, diastolic, continuous, to-and-fro), character, intensity and location
  - Murmur grades can be divided into soft (1–2), moderate (3), loud (4) and palpable (5–6)

> **NOTES**
>
> - 'Flow' or physiological murmurs tend to be fairly quiet (<grade 2 or 3) and may vary in intensity
> - They may occur with anaemia or can be normal in young animals

- Systolic clicks are high-frequency transient heart sounds, usually associated with degenerative mitral valve disease

Thoracic cavity examination

Thoracic palpation

1 Palpate the thorax for swellings, pain, rib fractures, subcutaneous emphysema and oedema.
2 Assess the strength of the apex beat using the fingers of one hand.
3 Determine the point of maximal intensity of the heartbeat, using a stethoscope or fingers of one hand, to indicate any displacement by intrathoracic masses or effusion, and to detect any thrill (vibration of turbulence in blood flow). *This should preferably be done before auscultation.*
4 Using both hands, gently compress the thoracic cavity to assess for reduced compliance of the cranial thoracic cage (Figure EXC.4), which could indicate a cranial mediastinal mass.

Tracheal palpation

- The full length of the cervical trachea should be palpated with one hand and observed for signs of sensitivity (usually indicated by a cough reflex) (Figure EXC.5)
- Tracheal sensitivity is a non-specific sign of airway irritation and may be present in airway or parenchymal disease
- In dogs and cats with chronic bronchitis, airway collapse or pneumonia, a harsh cough is usually elicited with tracheal palpation
- A *soft cough* is more typical in dogs with pulmonary oedema

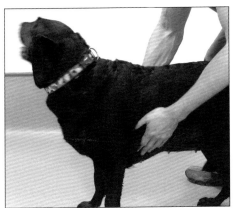

Figure EXC.4: Compression of the thoracic cavity is used to assess reduced compliance of the cranial thoracic cage.

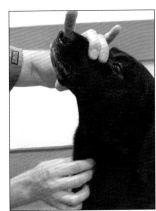

Figure EXC.5: Palpation of the trachea can be used to check for signs of airway sensitivity.

Thoracic auscultation

1 Using a stethoscope, auscultate all lung fields on both sides of the thorax (Figure EXC.6).
2 Note the presence, type and location of any abnormal lung sounds:
   a *Normal* sounds are termed bronchial, vesicular or bronchovesicular
   b *Crackles* and *wheezes* are examples of abnormal noises produced by diseased lungs
   c Determining the specific phase of the respiratory cycle in which abnormal lung sounds occur is important for categorizing the sound and determining the most likely pathology
   d *Absence* of lung sounds is also an important finding:
      i It typically reflects disease of the pleural space
      ii Consolidation of a lung segment can also lead to an absence of lung sounds

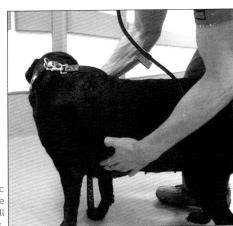

Figure EXC.6: Thoracic auscultation should be performed to evaluate all lung fields.

   iii Loss of lung sounds *dorsally* generally indicates air accumulation
   iv Loss of lung sounds *ventrally* indicates a pleural effusion or space-occupying mass.

Thoracic percussion

1 Place the fingers of one hand flat against the thoracic cage.
2 Curve the fingers of the other hand gently and hold them rigid (Figure EXC.7).
3 Use the curved fingers of the free hand to strike the fingers on the chest wall, causing the production of sounds.
4 Examine all lung fields to detect localized differences in sound transmission:
   a Percussion causes vibration of the chest and intrathoracic structures, and the pitch reflects the underlying air-to-tissue ratio within the thorax
   b Over the heart, a dull percussive sound is heard because of the presence of soft tissue that dampens the transmission of sound
   c When the chest cavity is filled with fluid, or the lung is consolidated by disease, dull sounds are noted in the affected areas; whilst over air-filled lung structures, more resonant sounds are heard
   d In an animal with pneumothorax or air trapping, sounds have increased resonance.

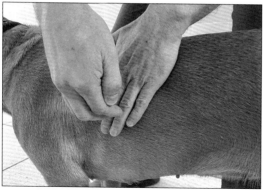

Figure EXC.7: Hand position required for performing thoracic percussion.

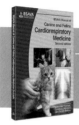

FURTHER INFORMATION

More detail on these procedures and interpretation of the results can be found in the *BSAVA Manual of Canine and Feline Cardiorespiratory Medicine.*

Dermatological examination

Whilst a complete history and thorough clinical examination are essential for dermatological cases, further diagnostic investigations are of paramount importance in reaching a definitive diagnosis. The following procedures can be performed in part, as required, or all together as part of a complete dermatological evaluation. (See also **Fine-needle aspiration** and **Skin biopsy – punch biopsy**.)

Patient preparation and positioning

- The procedures below are usually performed in the conscious animal; a muzzle and/or sedation may be required for fractious patients
- The patient may be positioned standing, sitting or in recumbency, depending on the area to be examined/sampled
- An assistant may be required to hold the animal
- **Adherence to good basic hygiene is required due to the possibility of infectious and zoonotic diseases**

Initial examination

Equipment

- Good lighting
- Otoscope
- Magnifying glass or dermatoscope
- Camera (optional)

Technique

A systematic examination of the animal from nose to tail tip should be performed:

- It is important not to forget to examine the oral cavity, paws, ventrum and hindquarters
- A dermatoscope or magnifying glass allows detailed examination of lesions
- Otoscopy of both ear canals should be performed
- Any deviations from normal skin, coat and mucosa should be noted
- Type and location of any lesions, both primary and secondary, should be noted; photography can aid documentation

> **WARNING**
>
> - It is important to bear in mind that some skin infections can be zoonotic and gloves should be worn. Handling an infected animal can also carry the potential risk of a nosocomial infection; for example, by spreading antibiotic-resistant bacteria from one patient to another. Thus, hygiene routines need to be carefully monitored and this should include both hand hygiene and cleaning of diagnostic instruments (Figure EXD.1).

- A problem list is defined based on the history, physical examination and initial dermatological examination
- A differential diagnosis list for each problem is formulated in order to determine a diagnostic plan. Signalment can help formulate the list of differential diagnoses (e.g. there is a breed predisposition for many diseases that can aid in the diagnostic work-up)

System examinations: DERMATOLOGICAL

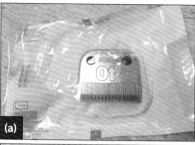

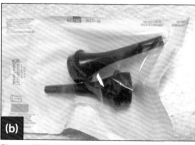

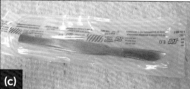

Figure EXD.1: Autoclaved and sterile packed (a) clipper blades, (b) otoscope cones and (c) skin scraping blades for use during a dermatological examination. (Reproduced from the *BSAVA Manual of Canine and Feline Dermatology*)

NOMENCLATURE AND DEFINITIONS OF SKIN LESIONS

Primary lesions:
- Macule – non-palpable area of different colour, <1 cm diameter
- Patch – macule >1 cm diameter
- Papule – solid elevation <1 cm diameter
- Nodule – solid elevation >1 cm diameter
- Plaque – platform-like elevation
- Vesicle – blister <1 cm, filled with clear fluid
- Bulla – blister >1 cm
- Pustule – vesicle filled with pus
- Tumour – large mass
- Wheal – raised, oedematous area (pitting on pressure)

Primary or secondary lesions:
- Alopecia – loss of hair: spontaneous alopecia is primary; self-induced alopecia is secondary
- Scale – flakes of cornified cells
- Crust – dried exudate containing blood/serum/scales/pus
- Follicular casts – accumulation of keratin and follicular material like a sock around the base of the hair shaft
- Comedo – hair follicle plugged with keratin and sebum
- Hyperpigmentation – increased pigmentation
- Hypopigmentation – decreased pigmentation

Secondary lesions:
- Collarette – circular, peeling lesion (often a remnant of a pustule)
- Scar – fibrous tissue replacing damaged dermis/subcutis
- Erosion – epidermal defect, not extending beneath the basement membrane
- Ulcer – skin defect below the level of the basement membrane
- Fissure – deep split
- Lichenification – thickening and hardening of the skin
- Excoriation – mild erosions caused by self-trauma

DIAGNOSTIC TESTS FOR SUSPECTED ORGANISMS

Organism suspected	Diagnostic tests
Bacteria	Cytology; culture and sensitivity testing; response to treatment
Dermatophytes	Wood's lamp; hair pluck; skin scrape; fungal culture
Malassezia yeast	Cytology; tape strip; fungal culture; response to treatment
Fleas	Macroscopic examination; coat brushing; response to treatment
Ticks	Macroscopic examination
Lice	Macroscopic examination; coat brushing
Cheyletiella mites	Tape strip; skin scrape
Demodex mites	Skin scrape (deep); hair pluck; impression smear of pustule; skin biopsy
Sarcoptes/ Notoedres mites	Skin scrape (deep); serology; skin biopsy; response to treatment
Otodectes mites	Cotton swab of ear cerumen
Trombicula mites	Tape strip

Wood's lamp examination

To check for dermatophytosis.

Equipment

- Wood's lamp
- Magnifying glass

Technique

1 Switch on the Wood's lamp and allow it to warm up for 5–10 minutes.
2 Place the animal in a darkened room.
3 Examine the hair coat with the Wood's lamp. A magnifying glass may also be used.
4 Observe for bright apple-green fluorescence of hairs; 5 minutes should be spent looking, as the fluorescence is sometimes delayed. Note that false-positive fluorescence may be observed due to certain topical medications, dead skin scales and some bacteria.

> ### NOTE
>
> - *Microsporum canis*, the most common dermatophyte identified in dogs and cats, generally fluoresces. A World Association of Veterinary Dermatology consensus paper revealed that the typical apple-green fluorescence seen on hairs infected with *M. canis* is positive in 90–100% of cases. Other less common dermatophytes that may also induce fluorescence include *M. distortum*, *M. audouinii*, *M. equinum* and *Trichophyton schoenleinii*

Coat brushing for fleas

Equipment

- Flea comb or stiff plastic hair brush
- White paper
- Container, such as a Petri dish
- Hand lens
- Microscope, slides and coverslips

Technique

1 With the patient standing on a sheet of white paper, brush the coat over several minutes to collect surface debris using a flea comb or stiff plastic hairbrush.
2 Collect the debris into a container, such as a Petri dish, and examine with a hand lens.
3 Transfer the material on to microscope slides and examine.

Wet paper test

The patient can either be brushed while standing on dampened white paper OR debris collected on dry paper can be dampened with damp cotton wool. Black flea faeces give a reddish-brown stain on the damp paper or cotton wool.

Coat brushing for dermatophytes: Mackenzie toothbrush technique

Equipment

- New or sterilized toothbrush
- Fungal culture medium

Technique

1 Brush the **whole coat** of the animal with a new or sterilized toothbrush for several minutes. It is helpful to brush against the natural flow of hairs.
2 Touch the toothbrush head on to a fungal culture plate several times and incubate as per the manufacturer's instructions.

Hair plucking (trichography)

Primarily to assess hair structure and to check for ectoparasites and dermatophytes associated with the hair root.

Equipment

- Haemostats
- Microscope slides or coverslips
- Clear adhesive tape
- Liquid paraffin (mineral oil)
- Microscope
- ± Fungal culture medium

Technique

1   Pluck several hairs, including the roots, using the haemostats (Figure EXD.2). Alternatively, grasp hairs firmly between the finger and thumb and epilate in the direction of hair growth.

2   Place the hairs on to a piece of clear adhesive tape and affix this to a microscope slide, or mount under a coverslip in liquid paraffin.

3   Examine under a microscope:

    a   Examine the tips of the hairs for evidence of breaking and damage, indicated by abrupt, blunt or frayed ends instead of the tapering tips of normal hairs

    b   Examine the roots to assess whether hairs are in anagen (a pronounced bulb present) or telogen (club root with barbs or frayed appearance) phase

    c   The presence of comedones or follicular plugs can also be detected, surrounding the shafts towards the root end of plucked hairs

    d   Examination of the roots of plucked hairs may reveal the presence of *Demodex* or *Cheyletiella* mites, louse eggs or fungal spores (dermatophytosis).

4   Hairs can also be placed on to fungal culture medium and incubated as per the manufacturer's instructions.

5   Where hair plucks are used to identify dermatophytes, infected hairs (*M. canis* only) can be examined with a Wood's lamp, then plucked. Hairs can then be mounted in mineral oil, compounded chlorphenolac, blue–black ink or potassium hydroxide (KOH) 10–20% before microscopic examination to help highlight fungal elements.

System examinations: DERMATOLOGICAL

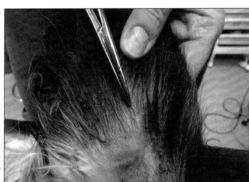

Figure EXD.2: Forceps being used to pluck hair. (Reproduced from the *BSAVA Manual of Canine and Feline Dermatology*)

Adhesive tape impressions of skin

Primarily for cytological examination of the skin surface, but also to check for ectoparasites.

Equipment

- Clippers
- Microscope slides
- Clear adhesive tape, e.g. Scotch® tape
- Stain such as Diff-Quik
- Microscope

System examinations: DERMATOLOGICAL

Technique

1 Repeatedly press the sticky side of the tape against an unhaired (or clipped) region of skin.
2 Gently rub with a thumbnail to ensure good contact of the tape with the skin.
3 Remove the tape from the skin and attach both ends of the tape to a slide, leaving the middle portion free (Figure EXD.3).
4 Stain the tape strip with Diff-Quik or equivalent. Gently rinse off excess stain. Detach one end of the tape and stick the whole strip down flat on to the slide.
5 Blot off excess liquid and perform cytological examination of the tape using a microscope.
6 Alternatively, the tape strip can be examined unstained for ectoparasites.

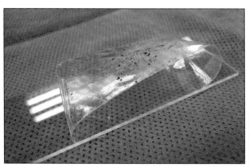

Figure EXD.3: Taped strip from skin, looped on to slide ready for staining. (Reproduced from the *BSAVA Manual of Canine and Feline Dermatology*)

Smears of expressed follicular contents

Primarily to check for ectoparasites.

Equipment

- Microscope slides and coverslips
- Liquid paraffin (mineral oil)
- Scalpel and No.10 scalpel blade
- Microscope

Technique

1 Squeeze the skin to extrude material from hair follicles.
2 Draw a clean microscope slide across the surface to smear this material on to the slide. *Alternatively*, material may be collected on a scalpel blade and then transferred to a slide.
3 No staining is necessary, although a little liquid paraffin may be used for coverslip mounting.
4 Examine the slide with a microscope for ectoparasites, especially *Demodex* mites.

Smears of aural wax/exudate

Primarily for cytological examination and to check for ectoparasites.

Equipment

- Microscope slides and coverslips
- Liquid paraffin (mineral oil)
- Cotton bud
- Microscope
- ± Stain such as Diff-Quik

Technique

1 Collect debris from external ear canal using a cotton bud.
2 Smear debris on to a microscope slide.
3 Liquid paraffin may be used to disperse the sample and for coverslip mounting.
4 Examine the slide unstained with a microscope for ear mites and their eggs.
5 Slides can be stained for cytological examination with a microscope.

Superficial skin scrape

Primarily to check for ectoparasites, but may also identify dermatophytosis. This technique involves the removal of the most superficial levels of the stratum corneum. Site selection will generally depend on the case, but the dorsum is the most common location to identify surface-living parasites.

Equipment

- Clippers
- No. 10 scalpel blade (blunted)
- Microscope slides and coverslips
- Liquid paraffin (mineral oil)
- 10% potassium hydroxide
- Saline
- Blue−black ink or lactophenol cotton blue
- Microscope

Technique

1 If the hair coat is thick, clip it to allow access to the surface of the skin.
2 Moisten the skin with either liquid paraffin (if it is being used as the mounting material) or water (if potassium hydroxide is being used) to ensure that the scraped material remains adherent to the scalpel blade.
3 Hold the scalpel perpendicular to the skin and scrape in the direction of the hair coat to collect material on to the blade.
4 Transfer the collected material into the mounting material (liquid paraffin or 10% potassium hydroxide) on a microscope slide.

> **NOTES**
>
> - Liquid paraffin allows immediate examination of slides and identification of live mites, but has the disadvantage of not clearing debris
> - 10% potassium hydroxide allows good separation of keratinocytes and clearing of material, but is caustic to skin itself and kills mites

System examinations: DERMATOLOGICAL

5   Place a coverslip over the sample and mounting medium, and examine with a microscope under low and then high power.

6   The addition of a drop of blue–black ink or lactophenol cotton blue may permit fungal structures to be seen more easily.

DEEP SKIN SCRAPE

- The technique is identical to that used for superficial skin scraping, only the depth of the scrape differs
- Deep skin scraping removes the full thickness of the epidermis to create capillary ooze (Figure EXD.4)
- Site selection is important for deep skin scraping:
  - Multiple samples should be taken from non-excoriated predilection sites (such as the extensor aspect of the hock and elbow and the periphery of the ear pinnae) to identify *Sarcoptes scabiei*
  - Samples should be taken from non-excoriated areas of comedone formation to identify *Demodex* spp.
- The skin should be gently squeezed to express the mites from the follicles and scraped in the direction of the hair coat

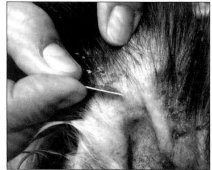

Figure EXD.4: Deep skin scraping from an ear pinna showing capillary ooze.(Reproduced from the *BSAVA Manual of Canine and Feline Dermatology*)

Stained smears from pustules or lesions

Primarily for cytological examination. Occasionally, ectoparasites such as *Demodex* mites may also be seen. (See also **Fine-needle aspiration**)

Equipment

- Hypodermic needles: 21 G
- Microscope slides and coverslips
- Stain such as Diff-Quik
- Microscope

Technique

1   Rupture an intact pustule with a sterile hypodermic needle and smear its contents on to a clean microscope slide.

2   Impression smears can also be made from ulcerated lesions or the cut surface of excised lesions.

3   Air-dry the slide.

4   Stain with Diff-Quik or equivalent, according to the manufacturer's instructions.

5   Perform cytological evaluation using a microscope.

Culture of microorganisms – bacteria

- *Sterile* swabs and bacterial transport medium are required
- Samples for bacterial culture should be taken from new lesions or recently ruptured pustules or vesicles and *not* from old, crusted or excoriated lesions
- **Do not use any aseptic skin preparation or surgical spirit before sampling**
- Rupture an intact pustule with a sterile needle and absorb the contents on to a sterile swab
- Place the swab into transport medium before sending samples to the laboratory
- *Alternatively,* tissue from a **skin biopsy** may be submitted in a sterile container for bacterial culture

Culture of microorganisms – fungi

- Samples can be obtained from coat brushings or hair plucks (see earlier)
- Submission of a sample to an external reference diagnostic laboratory for fungal culture is preferable. Consult the external laboratory for their packaging requirements/recommendations
- Samples can be cultured in-house on Sabouraud's dextrose agar (SDA) in Petri dishes:
    - Incubate in a temperature-controlled environment (or at room temperature in the UK)
    - Examine the plates twice weekly for up to 3–4 weeks
    - SDA encourages the development of typical fungal growth (e.g. characterized by reverse pigmentation and macroconidia)
- Samples can be cultured in-house on dermatophyte test medium (DTM):
    - Incubate at 20–25°C
    - Examine the plates daily
    - DTM incorporates a pH colour indicator, triggered by the production of alkaline metabolites, as early dermatophyte growth uses protein nutrients from the medium
    - A colour change from yellow to red within 10 days is consistent with dermatophyte growth
- Both of these in-house methods are prone to false-positive and false-negative results, so should be interpreted with care
- Refer to the manufacturer's guidance for how to perform, monitor and interpret in-house cultures

System examinations: DERMATOLOGICAL

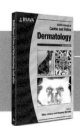

FURTHER INFORMATION

More detail on these procedures and interpretation of the results can be found in the *BSAVA Manual of Canine and Feline Dermatology.*

Neurological examination

System examinations: NEUROLOGICAL

Indications/Use

- To diagnose and localize disorders of the nervous system
- To provide information on the severity of some disorders

Equipment

- Reflex hammer
- A bright light source
- Cotton bud dampened with sterile saline
- Artery forceps
- 70% surgical spirit
- Food (with potent smell)
- Ball of cotton wool

Patient preparation and positioning

- The neurological examination should be performed with the animal conscious and without the administration of any sedation
- Animals should be kept calm throughout the examination
- Positioning will vary, depending on the part of the examination being performed
- Videos of the animal taken in the home environment can be a useful adjunct to the neurological examination, particularly in dogs with nervous or aggressive temperaments, and in cats

Observation

The following parameters should be observed before starting the 'hands-on' part of the examination:

- Mental status and behaviour
- Posture and body position at rest
- Gait (see **Orthopaedic examination**)
- Abnormal involuntary movements

Cranial nerve assessment

Olfactory nerve – CN I

- Smell is assessed by testing the animal's response (sniffing or licking of the nose, aversion of the head) to aromatic substances (e.g. surgical spirit) whilst it is blindfolded or has its eyes covered. Care should be taken not to use irritating substances that could stimulate the trigeminal nerve and cause similar responses. *Alternatively*, the animal's response to food can be observed, again whilst it is blindfolded or has its eyes covered

Optic nerve – CN II

- Vision tests are described in **Ophthalmic examination**

Oculomotor nerve – CN III

- Eye position and movements (a) at rest and (b) by testing for normal physiological nystagmus (vestibulo-ocular reflex), by moving the head from side to side as well as up and down (see Vestibulocochlear nerve – CN VIII, below), should be observed
  - Normal physiological nystagmus (also called 'jerk' nystagmus) is an involuntary rhythmic movement of the eyes, which typically presents with a slow phase in one direction and a quick phase in the other direction
  - Dysfunction of CN III will result in a resting ventrolateral strabismus and inability to move the eyeball medially during physiological nystagmus testing
  - Ptosis of the upper eyelid also occurs with dysfunction of CN III
- The *parasympathetic* function of CN III can be assessed by observation of pupil size and evaluation of the pupillary light reflex (PLR; see **Ophthalmic examination**)
  - Lesions will result in mydriasis of the affected eye
  - The PLR tests the integrity of the retina, optic nerve, optic tract, lateral geniculate nucleus, oculomotor nucleus, CN III and pupillary muscle

Trochlear nerve – CN IV

- Eye position at rest should be observed
- Lesions of the trochlear nerve produce a dorsolateral strabismus (extorsion) of the contralateral eye

Trigeminal nerve – CN V

- The *motor* function of CN V is assessed by evaluating the size and symmetry of the masticatory muscles and testing the resistance of the jaw to opening the mouth (Figure EXN.1)
- The *sensory* function (sensation of the face) can be tested by:
  - The corneal reflex observed on touching the cornea with a damp cotton bud (ophthalmic branch)
  - The palpebral reflex observed on touching the medial or lateral canthus of the eye (ophthalmic or maxillary branch, respectively) (Figure EXN.2)
  - The response to stimulation of the nasal mucosa (ophthalmic branch) (Figure EXN.3)

System examinations: **NEUROLOGICAL**

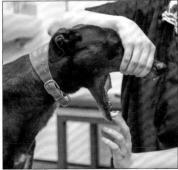

Figure EXN.1: The motor function of CN V can be assessed by testing the resistance of the jaw to opening of the mouth

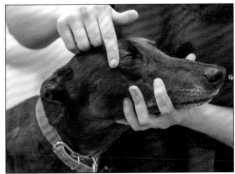

Figure EXN.2: The sensory function of the maxillary branch of CN V can be assessed by the palpebral reflex observed on touching the lateral canthus of the eye.

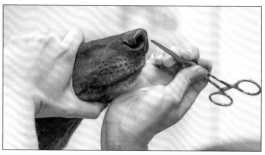

Figure EXN.3: The sensory function of the ophthalmic branch of CN V can be assessed by observing the response to stimulation of the nasal mucosa.

- A reflex response is best distinguished from a conscious response by stimulating the nasal mucosa: the normal animal will pull its head away, while the animal with forebrain disease may blink or show a facial twitch, but not show a conscious reaction

Abducent nerve – CN VI

- Eye position and movement at rest should be observed
- Normal physiological nystagmus should be assessed (see above)
- Eyeball retraction during the corneal reflex should be observed
- Lesions of the abducent nerve result in: an ipsilateral convergent medial strabismus; an inability to move the eyeball laterally when evaluating the horizontal physiological nystagmus; and an inability to retract the eyeball

Facial nerve – CN VII

- The *motor* function of CN VII is primarily assessed by observation of the face for symmetry (position of the ears and lip commissure on each side within the same plane, symmetry of the palpebral fissure), spontaneous blinking and movement of the nostrils (Figure EXN.4). Motor dysfunction produces: ipsilateral drooping of and inability to move the ear and lip; widened palpebral fissure and absent spontaneous and provoked blinking; absent abduction of the nostril during inspiration; and deviation of the nose toward the normal side due to the unopposed muscle tone on the unaffected side

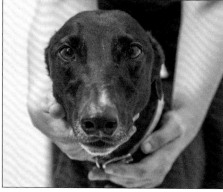

Figure EXN.4: The motor function of CN VII is assessed by observing the face for symmetry, blinking and movement of the nostrils.

System examinations: NEUROLOGICAL

- The Schirmer tear test (see **Ophthalmic examination**) can evaluate the *parasympathetic* supply of the lacrimal gland associated with CN VII. Examining the mouth for moist mucosa can subjectively assess salivation. In addition, the nose should be assessed for dryness (xeromycteria), as this can result from disruption to the parasympathetic supply of the lateral nose glands via CN VII

Vestibulocochlear nerve – CN VIII

- The animal's body and head posture at rest should be observed, and its gait evaluated (see **Orthopaedic examination**). This function can also be more specifically assessed by testing the vestibulo-ocular reflex (see above). Vestibular dysfunction may result in any or all of the following: head tilt; falling; leaning; rolling; circling; abnormal spontaneous and/or positional nystagmus; positional strabismus; and ataxia
- The *auditory* function of CN VIII is difficult to assess. The startle reaction consists of observing the animal's response to noise (e.g. handclap, whistle), but this does not detect unilateral or partial deafness. The best assessment is the animal's response to noise when asleep: most owners can report whether they have to touch their animal in order to wake them. Electrophysiological assessment is necessary to confirm and assess the severity of the hearing loss

Glossopharyngeal and vagus nerves – CN IX and CN X

- The pharyngeal (swallowing or gag) reflex can be evaluated by:
  - Applying external pressure to the hyoid bones to stimulate swallowing
  - Stimulating the pharynx with a finger to elicit a gag reflex
  - Watching the animal eat or drink
  - Opening the animal's mouth wide
- CN IX dysfunction results in dysphagia, absent gag reflex and reduced pharyngeal tone if deficits are bilateral
- CN X dysfunction results in dysphagia, inspiratory dyspnoea (due to laryngeal paralysis), voice changes (dysphonia) and regurgitation (due to megaoesophagus in the case of bilateral vagal disorder)
- The *parasympathetic* portion of CN X can be evaluated by testing the oculocardiac reflex. This is achieved by applying digital pressure to both eyeballs and observing simultaneously a reflex bradycardia (also mediated by CN V)

Accessory nerve – CN XI

- Lesions of this nerve result in atrophy of the trapezius muscle
- The position of the neck should be observed, as this may be deviated toward the affected side in chronic cases
- Isolated lesions of the accessory nerve are an extremely rare finding

Hypoglossal nerve – CN XII

- The tongue should be inspected for atrophy, asymmetry or deviation to one side
- The tone of the tongue should be assessed by manually stretching the tongue and observing a voluntary retraction
- Movement of the tongue should be assessed by applying food paste to the nose and observing the animal licking
- Lesions affecting CN XII can result in problems with prehension, mastication and deglutition

Postural reaction testing

Paw placement

- Sequentially each paw should be placed in an abnormal position (turned over so that the dorsal surface is in contact with the ground) and how quickly the animal corrects it determined (Figure EXN.5). The animal should be standing squarely on all four limbs, with the majority of its weight supported by an assistant
- A piece of paper should be placed under a weight-bearing foot and pulled slowly in a lateral direction. A normal response is to pick up the limb and replace it in the correct position. This should be repeated with the other feet in turn

Hopping reaction

- The hopping reaction is tested by holding the animal so that the majority of its weight is placed on one limb while the animal is moved laterally (Figure EXN.6). Normal animals hop on the tested limb to accommodate a new body position as their centre of gravity is displaced laterally. The hop should be initiated as the shoulder or hip moves lateral to the paw, and the animal then replaces the limb appropriately under the newly positioned body. An equal response should be seen on both sides

Placing response

- Non-visual placing can be tested by:
    - Covering the animal's eyes
    - Lifting the animal until the distal part of the thoracic limb is brought into contact with the edge of a table
    - The normal response is for the animal to place its foot immediately on the table surface

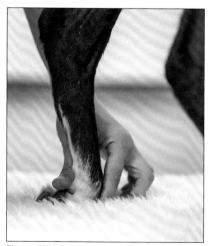

Figure EXN.5: Postural reaction testing can be achieved by placing a paw in an abnormal position and observing how long it takes the animal to return it to the correct position.

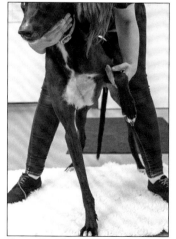

Figure EXN.6: Testing the hopping reaction involves holding the animal so that the majority of its weight is centred over one limb and then moving it laterally.

- Visual placing can be tested by:
  - Allowing the animal to see the table surface
  - Lifting the animal toward the edge of the table
  - Normal animals will reach for the surface before the paw touches the table

Hemi-walking and wheelbarrowing
- Hemi-walking tests the ability of the animal to walk on the thoracic and pelvic limbs of one side of the body, while the limbs on the other side are supported
  - The animal should be pushed away from the side on which its limbs are supported
  - The speed and coordination of movements that restore the appropriate limb position in response to the change in body position should be assessed
- Wheelbarrowing tests the thoracic limbs and highlights subtle weakness and ataxia
  - The pelvic limbs should be lifted off the ground by supporting the animal under the abdomen
  - The animal should be forced to walk forwards

Spinal reflexes: muscle tone and size
Spinal reflex evaluation is performed to classify the neurological disorder as being of lower motor neuron (LMN) or upper motor neuron (UMN) type. This allows the examiner to localize the lesion to specific spinal cord segments or peripheral nerves. Spinal reflexes are best tested with the animal relaxed in lateral recumbency, with the side to be tested uppermost.

- *Lower motor neuron:* If LMNs are damaged, the following clinical signs are characteristically found:
  - Flaccid paresis and/or paralysis
  - Reduced or absent reflexes
  - Reduced or absent muscle tone
  - Early and severe muscle atrophy
- *Upper motor neuron:* If UMNs are damaged, the following clinical signs are characteristically found:
  - Spastic paresis and/or paralysis
  - Normal to increased reflex activity (hyperreflexia)
  - Increased extensor muscle tone (hypertonia) manifested as a resistance to passive manipulation of the limbs
  - Chronic mild to moderate muscle atrophy (disuse atrophy)

Thoracic limbs
Withdrawal (flexor) reflex
The withdrawal (flexor) reflex evaluates the integrity of spinal cord segments C6–T2 (and associated nerve roots) as well as the brachial plexus and peripheral nerves.

> **NOTES**
> - The withdrawal reflex in the thoracic or pelvic limbs does not depend on the animal's conscious perception of noxious stimuli (nociceptive function)
> - The withdrawal reflex is a segmental spinal cord reflex that only depends on the function of the local spinal cord segments

System examinations: NEUROLOGICAL

- The animal should be placed in lateral recumbency and a noxious stimulus applied by pinching the nailbed or digit with the fingers or artery forceps
- This stimulus causes a reflex contraction of the flexor muscles and withdrawal of the tested limb
- If this withdrawal reflex is absent, individual toes should be tested to detect whether specific nerve deficits are present
- When testing the flexor reflex, the contralateral limb for should be observed for extension (crossed-extensor reflex), indicating a UMN lesion cranial to the C6 spinal cord segment

Extensor carpi radialis reflex

The extensor carpi radialis reflex evaluates the integrity of spinal cord segments C7–T2 and associated nerve roots, as well as the radial nerve.

- The extensor carpi radialis muscle belly should be struck with a reflex hammer along the craniolateral aspect of the proximal antebrachium
- The desired reaction is a slight extension of the carpus

Pelvic limbs

Withdrawal (flexor) reflex

The withdrawal (flexor) reflex evaluates the integrity of spinal cord segments L4–S2 (and associated nerve roots) as well as the femoral and sciatic nerves

> **NOTES**
>
> - The withdrawal reflex in the thoracic or pelvic limbs does not depend on the animal's conscious perception of noxious stimuli (nociceptive function)
> - The withdrawal reflex is a segmental spinal cord reflex that depends only on the function of the local spinal cord segments

- The animal should be placed in lateral recumbency and a noxious stimulus applied by pinching the nailbed or digit with the fingers or artery forceps (Figure EXN.7)
- This stimulus causes a reflex contraction of the flexor muscles and withdrawal of the tested limb

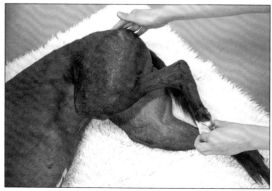

Figure EXN.7: The withdrawal (flexor) reflex can be elicited by pinching the nailbed or digits.

- A normal reflex constitutes flexion of the hip (femoral nerve function), stifle and hock (sciatic nerve function)
- The hock must be extended in order to evaluate sciatic function (i.e. hock flexion)
- When testing the flexor reflex, the contralateral limb should be observed for extension (crossed-extensor reflex), indicating a UMN lesion cranial to the L4 spinal cord segment

Patellar reflex

The patellar reflex evaluates the integrity of spinal cord segments L4–L6 (and associated nerve roots), as well as the femoral nerve.

- The animal should be placed in lateral recumbency, with the stifle slightly flexed and the tested limb supported by placing one hand under the thigh
- Striking the patellar tendon with a reflex hammer induces extension of the limb due to a reflex contraction of the quadriceps femoris muscle (Figure EXN.8)
- A weak or absent reflex indicates a lesion of the L4–L6 spinal cord segments or the femoral nerve

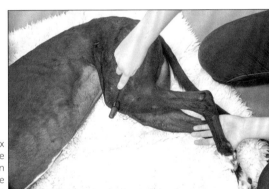

Figure EXN.8: A reflex hammer is used to strike the patellar tendon in order to evaluate the patellar reflex.

Tail and anus

Perineal reflex

- Stimulation of the perineum with artery forceps should result in contraction of the anal sphincter, and flexion of the tail

Sensory evaluation

Cutaneous trunci (panniculus) reflex

- The animal should be placed in sternal recumbency or in a standing position
- The skin of the dorsal trunk should be pinched with artery forceps between vertebral level T2 and L4–L5, and observed for a contraction of the cutaneous trunci muscles bilaterally, producing a twitch of the overlying skin
- The reflex is present in the thoracolumbar region and absent in the neck and sacral region
- Testing is begun at the level of the ilial wings: if the reflex is present at this level the entire pathway is intact and further testing is not necessary

- With spinal cord lesions, this reflex is lost caudal to the spinal cord segment affected, indicating the presence of a transverse myelopathy
- Pinching the skin cranial to the lesion results in a normal reflex, while stimulation of the skin caudal to the lesion does not elicit any reflex

Deep pain perception

- The animal should be placed on its side, ideally with a second person talking to or stroking it to distract attention
- An initial gentle squeeze should be applied to the digits to elicit the withdrawal reflex
- If the animal does not manifest any behavioural response following a gentle squeeze, heavy pressure should be applied to the bones of the digits with artery forceps (Figure EXN.9)
- Only a severe bilateral spinal cord lesion impairs the conscious perception of deep pain; for this reason, testing of deep pain perception is a useful prognostic indicator in cases of spinal cord disease
- Conscious pain perception must be assessed in all limbs and/or the tail that are determined to have no voluntary movements (paralysis/plegia)
- Testing of deep pain perception is not required in limbs for which there is visible voluntary motor function
- The expected reaction is a behavioural response such as turning the head, trying to bite or vocalization, or a physiological response to perception of pain such as an increase in heart rate or pupil dilation
- Withdrawal of the limb is only the flexor reflex and should not be taken as evidence of pain sensation

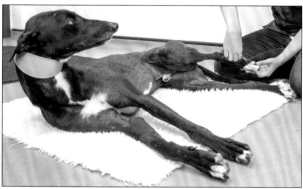

Figure EXN.9: Deep pain perception is tested by applying heavy pressure to digits using artery forceps.

Spinal palpation and neck manipulation

Spinal palpation and neck manipulation to assess for pain should only be performed at the end of the neurological examination.

- The fingers of one hand should be used to apply firm pressure to the thoracic and lumbar spine whilst observing for a pain response (Figure EXN.10)
- The neck should be manipulated in dorsal, ventral and both lateral directions, whilst observing for a pain response (Figure EXN.11)

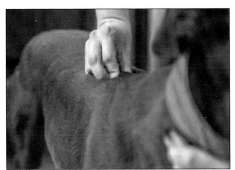

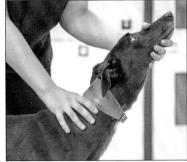

Figure EXN.10: Palpation can be used to assess for pain in the thoracic and lumbar spine.

Figure EXN.11: Neck manipulation should be performed in a dorsal, ventral and lateral direction to assess for pain.

System examinations: **NEUROLOGICAL**

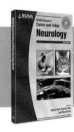

FURTHER INFORMATION

More detail on these procedures and interpretation of the results can be found in the *BSAVA Manual of Canine and Feline Neurology.*

Ophthalmic examination

Indications/Use

- Suspected primary ocular disease
- As part of investigations for suspected or confirmed neurological disease
- As part of investigations for suspected or confirmed systemic diseases with possible ocular involvement (e.g. hypertension, diabetes mellitus, lymphoma)

Equipment

- Bright focal light source, such as a Finoff transilluminator
- Schirmer tear test strips
- Stopwatch
- Direct ophthalmoscope
- Mydriatic – 1% tropicamide
- Ophthalmic lens – 28–30 dioptres (D)
- Topical local anaesthetic – 0.5% proxymetacaine eyedrops
- A goniolens and sterile lubricant (viscous tears, e.g. 1% Celluvisc or sterile K-Y Jelly)
- Applanation or rebound tonometer (e.g. Tonopen, TONOVET)
- Fluorescein test strips (or Minims fluorescein vials; NB these should only be used once) and cobalt blue light source
- 0.9% sterile saline and 5 ml syringe
- Soft paper towel
- Cytobrush and glass slides

Patient preparation and position

- The ophthalmic examination can be performed on the conscious animal without sedation. A muzzle should be used if required
- The animal should be positioned in a standing or sitting position, on a table if possible
- An assistant may be required for restraint and should support the head in a fixed position by holding the animal underneath the chin

The ophthalmic examination

Initial examination

1. Assess for evidence of pain: tears, increased blinking, blepharospasm, photophobia.
2. Assess orbital and periocular conformation, globe size and position. Check for asymmetry or strabismus.
3. Check the following reflexes:
   a. Vestibulo-ocular reflex: reflex eye movements normally allow stabilization of an image on the retina, resulting in slow eye movements opposite to the direction of head movement.
   b. Menace response: direction of a splayed hand towards the eye should elicit a blink or retraction of the head. Avoid creating a draught of air directed towards the cornea.
4. Examine the conformation of the upper and lower eyelids and the position of the nictitating membrane.

5 Note the presence and nature of any ocular discharge.

6 An **obstacle course** may be improvised from chairs, waste bins, etc. Assess the animal's performance: for both eyes; with one eye covered; and in bright and dim lighting conditions.

Schirmer tear test I (STT I)

The STT I measures *aqueous production* in the un-anaesthetized eye and is an indicator of basal and reflex tear production.

> **NOTE**
>
> - Perform STT I before manipulation of the eyelids or direct application of light sources to the eyes, as these may falsely elevate test results

Technique

1 The test strips are notched near one end: identify the notched end of the test strip while it is still in its packet.

2 Bend the test strip transversely at the level of the notch.

3 Remove the test strip from the packet, only handling the end away from the notch.

4 Evert the lateral lower eyelid and place the notched end of the strip in the lateral half of the lower conjunctival sac, so that the notch is at the level of the lid margin and the strip is in contact with the lower lid and cornea (Figure EXOP.1).

5 Release the test strip and the eyelid and hold the lids closed, retaining the test strip securely in position.

6 After 1 minute remove the test strip from the eye.

7 Record the distance aqueous tears have travelled from the notch, indicated by the blue dye in strips where this is provided, otherwise see where the tears have travelled to on the strip.

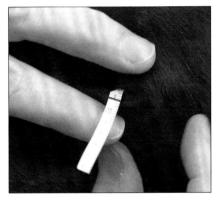

Figure EXOP.1: Positioning of the strip for a Schirmer tear test.

Test results

- Dogs: mean reference value = 15–20 mm/min; <15 mm/min is suggestive of keratoconjunctivitis sicca (KCS)
- Cats: mean reference value = 15–20 mm/min; however, cats with healthy eyes may have STT values that in dogs would suggest KCS
- In every case, the STT value should be correlated with the appearance of the eye and not be taken on its own; a light beam that reflects as a clear reflection suggests a normal tear film, whilst one that reflects as a broken-up reflection suggests a tear film insufficiency

System examinations: OPHTHALMIC

Pupillary light reflexes

1 Note pupil size in a normally lit room.
2 Continue the examination in a dimly lit room.
3 Direct a bright light axially through the pupil in each eye.
4 Look for constriction of the pupil in response to direct light and light directed at the contralateral eye.
5 In the 'swinging flashlight test', the light is directed at each eye alternately, with the observer noting the direct (in the same eye) and indirect (in the other eye) responses. A positive swinging flashlight test is one where the pupil dilates as the light swings into it. This shows a relative afferent pupillary defect, i.e. one where the visual capability of that eye is reduced through, for instance, unilateral retinal detachment or optic neuritis.

Eyelids and conjunctiva

1 Retract the upper eyelid and examine the dorsal bulbar conjunctiva; evert the lid margin and check the upper palpebral conjunctiva and upper lacrimal punctum.
2 Apply light pressure to the globe through the upper lid and protrude the nictitating membrane; check its leading edge, its alignment and its outer surface.
3 Retract the lower lid and assess the conjunctiva and the lower lacrimal punctum as it enters the fornix.

Cornea

1 Check the corneal (Purkinje) reflex (the smoothness and sharpness of the reflection of a light on the corneal surface). A broken or irregular image suggests a defective tear film or a corneal ulcer.
2 Examine the cornea; check for irregularities, opacities, vascularization and pigmentation.

Anterior chamber

1 Direct a bright focal light source into the anterior chamber from various angles and observe from various angles.
2 Note the depth of the anterior chamber and any abnormal contents. Aqueous flare occurs where cells or fibrin are seen in the anterior chamber (hazy appearance between cornea and lens); this is best appreciated with the narrow beam of a Finoff transilluminator or the slit beam from a direct ophthalmoscope.
3 Examine the iris, pupil margin and lens.

Distant direct ophthalmoscopy

The room should be darkened, but mydriatic drops are not required. The examination is conducted at arm's length.

1 Set the ophthalmoscope to zero.
2 Find the tapetal reflex (the green or yellow light reflected from the tapetum) by looking into the pupil horizontally or slightly upwards (Figure EXOP.2).
   a Any genuine opacity, such as cataracts, corneal and vitreous opacities, in the path of the tapetal reflex will obscure it and appear black.

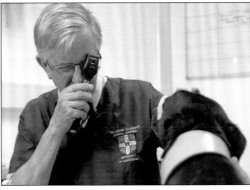

Figure EXOP.2: Distant direct ophthalmoscopy is used to identify ocular opacities.

b A key differential diagnosis for a hazy-looking pupil in an elderly animal is nuclear sclerosis. In these cases, a tapetal reflex is still obvious on distant direct ophthalmoscopy with a ring of black marking the edge of the lens nucleus. In comparison, with a cataract the tapetal reflex is absent or appears as a 'spider's web' of opacity.

3 Lesions can be roughly *localized* in an anteroposterior direction by taking advantage of the effect of parallax: as the observer moves to one side, the opacity also appears to move. The direction of this movement shows the location of the opacity.

a Opacities posterior to the centre of the lens (i.e. posterior polar subcapsular cataracts) move in the same direction as the observer's eye, whilst those in the anterior lens move in the opposite direction.

Close direct ophthalmoscopy

The direct ophthalmoscope is used to examine the fundus. The image is upright and highly magnified, but the field of view is very narrow.

1 Ideally, dilate the pupils with 1–2 drops of 1% tropicamide solution per eye. Mydriasis occurs in 15–20 minutes and lasts for 6 hours. However, it should be noted that using a low light intensity in a dark room allows direct ophthalmoscopy without mydriasis in most cases.

2 Set the ophthalmoscope to zero.

3 Hold the ophthalmoscope vertically, with it touching your own orbital margin. Be close to the patient's eye, so as to maximize the field of view and eliminate distractions such as the iris (Figure EXOP.3).

4 The first structure seen is the tapetum. Assess whether this is hyper-reflective (suggesting retinal detachment), hypo-reflective (suggesting oedema or detachment) or of the correct reflectivity.

5 Assess the retinal vessels (these 'swing' past as the animal moves its eye) and note whether they appear thin (seen with retinal degeneration), thick (seen with haemorrhage associated with hypertension) or of normal calibre.

6 Locate the optic disc by finding the dorsal blood vessel and following it down to the nerve head at the posterior pole. Identify whether the nerve head is 'fuzzy' and 'fluffy' with engorged vessels (suggesting optic neuritis), pale white and flat (suggesting retinal degeneration) or of normal pink colouration.

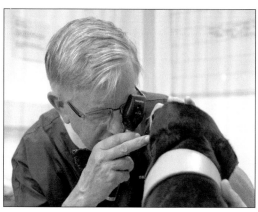

Figure EXOP.3: The ophthalmoscope should be held near the eye of the patient for close direct ophthalmoscopy.

7 Make a systematic examination of the fundus by examining it in quarters. Evaluate the retina for normal variation or changes in colour, reflectivity, pigment, haemorrhage, oedema and detachment.

8 Focus through to the anterior eye.

   a +10 D brings the lens into focus with the ophthalmoscope held at 10 cm from the eye.

   b +20 D is required to examine the cornea and adnexa with the ophthalmoscope held at 5 cm from the eye.

   c Note that negative dioptre settings with red numbers are used to examine the retina when the patient's (not the observer's) eyes are myopic (short-sighted).

Indirect ophthalmoscopy

When compared with direct ophthalmoscopy, indirect methods give an inverted, reversed image, which is less highly magnified but covers a much wider angle of view.

1 Dilate the pupils with 1–2 drops of 1% tropicamide solution per eye. Mydriasis occurs in 15–20 minutes and lasts for 6 hours.

2 Hold an ophthalmic lens (28–30 D) between your index finger and thumb, with the more convex side of the lens facing you.

3 Rest your hand on the patient's head, to allow you to position the lens stably in front of the patient's eye, but initially hold the lens away from the patient's eye.

4 Hold a bright light source (Finoff transilluminator) against your temple and align your eye, the light source and the patient's pupil along the same axis (Figure EXOP.4). Correct alignment will result in visualization of a tapetal reflection. (Note: it may be easier to view the tapetal reflection using a direct ophthalmoscope (see above), which perfectly aligns the light and the direction of viewing.)

5 Bring the lens in front of the patient's eye to examine the fundus. If the image of the fundus is lost, repeat Steps 2–4.

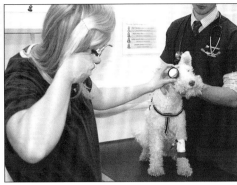

Figure EXOP.4: Indirect ophthalmoscopy involves aligning the patient's eye, light source and clinician's eye along the same axis.

Ancillary tests

These are performed as required for the individual case.

Gonioscopy

Gonioscopy is the examination of the iridocorneal angle and ciliary cleft. It is indicated for cases of suspected glaucoma.

> **NOTE**
>
> - Gonioscopy should be performed prior to pharmacological dilation of the pupil

1   Apply 1–2 drops of 0.5% proxymetacaine to the cornea. This will be effective in 1 minute and the effect will last for 10–20 minutes.
2   If using a Barken lens, sterile water is applied to the concave side of the inverted goniolens using a short tube with an attached syringe. If using a Koeppe lens, sterile lubricant is added to the concave side of the inverted goniolens, directly from the packaging. Air bubbles should be avoided, because they will distort light and prevent adequate visualization.
3   Place the goniolens on to the cornea in one quick motion so as not to lose the water/lubricant.
4   Using a bright light source, such as a direct ophthalmoscope, examine the entire iridocorneal angle and ciliary cleft systematically.

Tonometry

Tonometry is the indirect measurement of intraocular pressure (IOP). Where possible, this should be performed as part of the routine ophthalmic examination. It is specifically indicated for cases of suspected glaucoma (where the IOP will be higher), or uveitis (where the IOP will be lower). Various methods can be used, including rebound and applanation techniques.

Applanation tonometry using a Tonopen

1   Apply 1–2 drops of 0.5% proxymetacaine to the cornea. This will be effective in 1 minute and the effect will last 10–20 minutes.

2   Restrain the patient with its head and eyes directed forwards and its eyelids held open against the orbital rim. *Care must be taken not to press against the globe, because this might falsely elevate the IOP.*

3   Place a disposable sterile protective sheath over the tip of the Tonopen.

4   Using the probe tip, gently and repeatedly contact the central area of the cornea (Figure EXOP.5).

5   Record the IOP measurement from the digital screen at the sound of the longer beep.

Rebound tonometry using a TONOVET

1   Topical anaesthesia is not required.

2   Restrain the patient with its head and eyes directed forwards and its eyelids held open against the orbital rim. *Care must be taken not to press against the globe, because this might falsely elevate the IOP.*

3   Hold the device so that the probe travels horizontally and is close to the eye but not touching.

4   Press the button, at which point the probe will exit the machine and touch the cornea, before rebounding back (Figure EXOP.6). After this has been performed 6 times, and following a long beep, the reading will be displayed and this should be recorded.

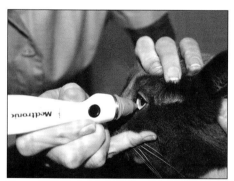

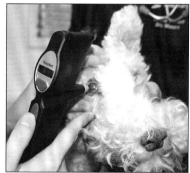

Figure EXOP.5: Applanation tonometry can be performed using a Tonopen.

Figure EXOP.6: Rebound tonometry can be performed using a TONOVET.

Fluorescein test

The fluorescein test is indicated for the diagnosis of corneal ulcers, where epithelium is absent and the stroma is exposed. Note that fluorescein will not stain ulcers that have healed and re-epithelialized, or those that have progressed deep enough to reach the Descemet's membrane.

1   If using a test strip, use a 5 ml syringe to wet the test strip thoroughly with sterile saline (Figure EXOP.7). Touch the test strip on to the dorsal bulbar conjunctiva. Never touch the cornea directly.

2   If using a fluorescein vial, apply 1–2 drops onto the dorsal lateral aspect of the cornea (Figure EXOP.8).

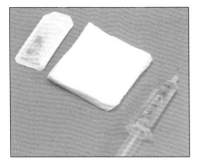

Figure EXOP.7: Equipment for the fluorescein test.

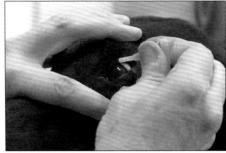

Figure EXOP.8: Fluorescein should be applied to the dorsal lateral aspect of the cornea.

3 Irrigate the eye with saline to flush excess fluorescein from the ocular surface. This helps to avoid false-negative effects (e.g. fluorescein pooling in a healed ulcer) and just leaves an epithelialized facet.

4 Examine the eye using a blue light source. Positive staining indicates a defect in the epithelium and, hence, an ulcer.

System examinations: OPHTHALMIC

Orthopaedic examination

Indications/Use

- Lameness
- Abnormal gait
- Non-ambulatory
- Pyrexia of unknown origin

Observation

Note should be taken of the following:

- Difficulty and/or reluctance in getting up or walking
- Failure to bear full weight on one or more limbs
- Shifting weight from one leg to the next while standing or sitting
- Posture
- Body shape abnormalities:
  - Focal muscle loss
  - Medial/lateral deviation of distal limbs
  - Limb hyperflexion or hyperextension
  - Angular or rotational deformities
- Evidence of old injuries; in particular, the feet, nails, pads and interdigital skin should be checked

Gait examination

- The animal should be observed walking at a moderate pace, both toward and away from the veterinary surgeon, on a firm level surface, as well as in front of or around the veterinary surgeon:
  - For most dogs, this is best accomplished outdoors with the animal on a lead
  - Cats and very small dogs are best observed walking around the consulting room
  - Assessment walking up and down stairs can be helpful in some circumstances
  - Videos of the animal taken in the home environment can be a useful adjunct to the orthopaedic examination, particularly in dogs with nervous or aggressive temperaments, and in cats
- Animals should be assessed for:
  - Thoracic limb lameness:
    - A downward nod of the head as the 'sound' limb is placed to the ground
    - Lifting of the head as the lame limb strikes the ground
  - Pelvic limb lameness:
    - 'Hiking up' of the gluteal region on the lame side during weight bearing
    - 'Bunny hopping' gait in bilaterally affected animals
  - Swinging leg lameness:
    - Seen while the affected limb is in flight
    - Characteristic pattern of movement, depending upon the injury. For example:
      - Pelvic limb: contracture of the gracilis muscle results in outward rotation of the tarsus, with inward rotation of the foot
      - Thoracic limb: contracture of infraspinatus muscle will cause the foot to swing in a lateral arc during protraction

- A shortened gait or reluctance to move a joint or joints through the full range of motion
- Abnormal flicking forward of the feet during protraction, e.g. due to reluctance to flex the elbows
- Neurological problems leading to paresis (weakness), ataxia (incoordination), spasticity (stiffness) or hypermetria. *These should be distinguished from lameness due to orthopaedic disorders by performing a full **neurological examination***

Palpation

- Palpation of the axial and appendicular skeleton should follow a set sequence:
  - Palpation of the spine, starting at the head and finishing at the tail
  - Palpation of each limb from top to toe, comparing each leg with its opposite
- Note should be taken of the following:
  - Changes in muscles: asymmetry of shape due to swelling, atrophy, spasm, contracture or weakness should be noted
  - Anatomical deformities: the spatial relationship of normal anatomical structures, particularly bony prominences, should be checked. For example, craniodorsal hip luxation results in dorsal displacement of the greater trochanter and increased distance between the greater trochanter and ischiatic tuberosity
  - Swellings (may involve bones, joints or soft tissues)
  - Joint effusions: best appreciated where the joint capsule is least supported by the periarticular structures:
    - Elbow effusions – caudolateral aspect
    - Carpal effusions – dorsal aspect
    - Interphalangeal effusions – dorsal aspect
    - Stifle effusions – either side of the patellar ligament
    - Tarsal effusions – just in front of the calcaneus
  - Joint thickening
  - Pain from bone, muscle, tendons, neural tissue or joints

Manipulation

- Manipulation of the axial and appendicular skeleton should follow a routine sequence:
  - The lower cervical spine should be flexed and extended in the axial plane and to the left and right
  - The lumbar spine should be flexed, extended and rotated
  - Each limb should be manipulated proximally to distally
- Animals should be assessed for:
  - Anatomical deformity or displacement (e.g. luxation, subluxation)
  - Pain
  - Range of movement of entire limb and each joint
  - Crepitus
  - The integrity of the supporting structures of each joint (collateral, dorsal, palmar, plantar ligaments, plus specialized structures such as cruciate ligaments and patella)

System examinations: ORTHOPAEDIC

Shoulder

- Combined shoulder flexion and elbow extension, whilst placing direct pressure on the biceps tendon within the intertubercular groove, can identify bicipital tendon pain
- To assess for medial instability, the animal is placed in lateral recumbency and the thoracic limb is extended and maintained perpendicular to the spine. The forelimb is then abducted, whilst applying firm downward pressure over the acromion process. An increase in the angle of abduction compared with the contralateral limb is suggestive of medial instability

Elbow

- Medial compartment pain can be detected by simultaneous flexion of the elbow and supination of the distal limb

Carpus

- Extension is normally limited at 10 degrees of hyperextension

Hip

- 110 degrees is the normal range of flexion and extension in a dog. (See also **Ortolani test**, below)

Stifle

- Stability of the patella should be assessed in full extension and mild flexion to detect medial and lateral luxation, respectively. (See also **cranial draw test** and **tibial compression test**, below)

Tarsus

- Collateral stability should be checked in both flexion and extension
- To assess the tibiotarsal joint, the base of the metatarsals should be grasped in one hand, whilst the lateral and medial malleoli are stabilized with the other
- To assess the tarsometatarsal and calcaneoquartal joints, the base of the metatarsals should be grasped in one hand, whilst the calcaneus is stabilized with the other

Examination of the anaesthetized or sedated animal

- Once an area of lameness has been identified in the conscious animal, additional information may be obtained under sedation or anaesthesia:
  - Some manipulations may be uncomfortable whether or not structures are abnormal (e.g. **Ortolani test**)
  - A joint may be too painful to allow full assessment (e.g. **cranial draw test**, **tibial compression test**)
  - Muscle tension in the conscious dog may mask instability
  - Instability may be subtle

Cranial draw test

Indications/Use

- To diagnose partial or complete rupture of the cranial cruciate ligament (CCL)
- Often used in association with the **tibial compression test** (see below)

Contraindications

- Periarticular fibrosis and meniscal injury, with the caudal horn of the medial meniscus wedged between the femoral condyle and tibial plateau, may prevent cranial draw in a CCL-deficient stifle

Patient preparation and positioning

- This can be performed in the conscious animal; however, if the patient is tense (due to pain or temperament) or if the CCL is only partially torn, sedation or general anaesthesia may be required
- A conscious patient may be restrained in a standing position on three legs, with the affected limb held off the ground
- Sedated or anaesthetized patients may be positioned in lateral recumbency, with the affected limb uppermost

Technique

1 Grasp the distal femur in one hand, placing the thumb over the lateral fabella and the index finger on the patella.
2 Use the other hand to grasp the proximal tibia, placing the thumb over the head of the fibula and the index finger on the tibial crest.
3 Apply a cranial force to the tibia while the stifle joint is held in nearly full extension, and then while the joint is held in 30–60 degrees of flexion (Figure EXOR.1).

Results

- Complete rupture of the CCL is associated with cranial displacement of the tibia relative to the femur, in both *extension and flexion*
- Isolated rupture of the craniomedial band of the CCL is associated with cranial displacement of the tibia relative to the femur, in *flexion* only
- Isolated rupture of the caudolateral band of the CCL will *not* result in cranial displacement of the tibia relative to the femur
- A short cranial draw motion, with a distinct end point, may be detected in young animals and is normal

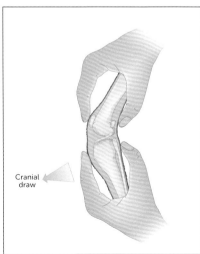

Cranial
draw

Figure EXOR.1: Technique for performing the cranial draw test.

Tibial compression test

Indications/Use

- To diagnose partial or complete rupture of the cranial CCL
- Note: not all dogs with CCL disease have femorotibial instability that can be detected by this test
- Often used in association with the **cranial draw test** (see above)

Patient preparation and positioning

- This can be performed in the conscious animal; however, if the patient is tense (due to pain or temperament) or if the CCL is only partially torn, sedation or general anaesthesia is required
- A conscious patient should be restrained in a standing position on three legs, with the affected limb held off the ground
- Sedated or anaesthetized patients may be positioned in lateral recumbency, with the affected limb uppermost

Technique

1 Grasp and maintain the distal femur in a fixed position with one hand, placing the thumb over the lateral fabella and the index finger lightly on the tibial crest.
2 Use the other hand to grasp the metatarsal region.
3 Maintain the stifle joint in slight flexion, while slowly flexing the hock (Figure EXOR.2).

Results

- Cranial displacement (tibial thrust) of the tibial crest relative to the femur is suggestive of CCL injury

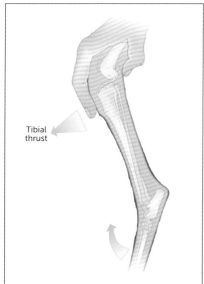

Tibial thrust

Figure EXOR.2: Technique for performing the tibial compression test.

Ortolani test

Indications/Use

■ To detect hip laxity in the young dog (to support a diagnosis of hip dysplasia)

> **NOTE**
>
> ■ Not all dogs with hip dysplasia show a positive Ortolani sign. For example, dogs with gross subluxation or luxation of the femoral head, and dogs in which capsular fibrosis has stabilized the hip joint will not show the sign

Patient preparation and positioning

■ May be attempted in the conscious animal but is potentially painful and therefore best performed with the dog heavily sedated or under general anaesthesia

■ The animal may be positioned in lateral or dorsal recumbency. The description below applies to lateral recumbency

Technique

1 Position the stifle in mild flexion and grasp it with one hand, with the other hand placed on the dorsal aspect of the pelvis to stabilize it.

2 Apply firm pressure to the stifle in a dorsal direction in an attempt to subluxate the hip joint.

3 Whilst maintaining dorsal pressure on the stifle, gently abduct the limb until a 'click' or 'clunk' is detected (Figure EXOR.3).

   a If the dorsal acetabular rim is intact, the femoral head falls abruptly into the acetabulum

   b In dogs with a poor dorsal acetabular rim, the femoral head appears to slide back into the acetabulum

4 Whilst maintaining dorsal pressure on the stifle, if the limb is now adducted, re-luxation of the hip will occur.

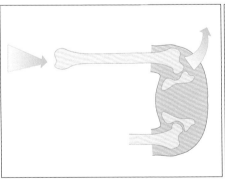
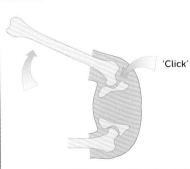

'Click'

Figure EXOR.3: Ortolani test technique.

Results

- The 'click' or 'clunk' (see Step 3) represents the relocation of the femoral head within the acetabulum. This is the positive Ortolani sign, consistent with hip joint laxity

Assessment of the nervous system

- An orthopaedic examination should *routinely* include assessment of deep and superficial pain perception, proprioception in all four limbs and spinal reflexes in the limbs (see **Neurological examination**).

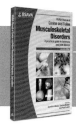

FURTHER INFORMATION

More detail on disorders of the musculoskeletal system can be found in the *BSAVA Manual of Canine and Feline Musculoskeletal Disorders*.

Abdominocentesis

Indications/Use

- To obtain abdominal fluid for analysis in cases of abdominal effusion (diagnostic abdominocentesis)
- To remove abdominal fluid in animals that have clinical signs associated with a large volume of fluid, e.g. respiratory distress due to the pressure on the diaphragm (therapeutic abdominocentesis)

Contraindications

- Coagulopathy
- Marked distension of an abdominal viscus
- Marked organomegaly

Equipment

- As required for **Aseptic preparation – (a) non-surgical procedures**
- **For diagnostic abdominocentesis:**
  - Hypodermic needles:
    - Cats: 23 G; ¾ inch
    - Dogs: 21 G; ¾ inch to 1.5 inches
  - 5 ml syringe
- **For therapeutic abdominocentesis:**
  - 21 G, 1 inch butterfly catheter or 21–23 G hypodermic needle attached to a 3-way tap
  - 10–20 ml syringe, depending on volume of fluid to be removed
- EDTA, plain and sterile collection tubes
- Microscope slides

Patient preparation and positioning

- Depending on the temperament of the patient, sedation may be required
- The patient should be restrained in lateral recumbency, with its feet towards the clinician
- It may be necessary to empty the patient's bladder by manual expression or **urethral catheterization** to reduce the risk of accidental cystocentesis
- **Aseptic preparation – (a) non-surgical procedures** should be carried out on an area approximately 10 cm x 10 cm, centred on the umbilicus, and a fenestrated drape placed

Technique

- Diagnostic abdominocentesis should be performed using either a single-site centesis or a four-quadrant approach. In patients with smaller effusions, the chances of fluid retrieval can be increased by using ultrasound guidance
- Therapeutic abdominocentesis should be performed using a single-site centesis
- For single-site centesis, the needle or butterfly catheter should be inserted at right angles to the skin, 1–2 cm caudal to the umbilicus and 1 cm ventral to the midline (linea alba) (Figure A.1)
- For centesis using the four-quadrant approach, approximate needle insertion sites are indicated in Figure A.2

A

1 Insert the needle through the skin and abdominal wall and twist it slightly to encourage fluid flow.

   a The needle should be inserted without a syringe attached. An open needle is more likely to result in fluid flow, as suction with a syringe will draw the omentum or viscera on to the needle.

   b If using a butterfly catheter, this can be connected to a 3-way tap and syringe as it is inserted.

2 If using a needle, allow fluid to drip into a sampling tube (Figure A.2).

3 If no fluid is obtained, apply slight negative pressure with a 5 ml syringe.

4 If fluid is still not obtained, the needle can be reinserted in different locations using the four-quadrant approach (see above).

5 If there is still a suspicion of abdominal fluid, diagnostic peritoneal lavage can be performed.

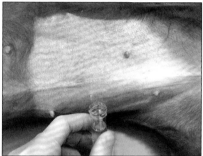

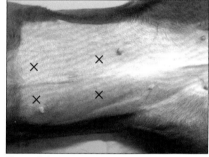

Figure A.1: The approximate sampling site for single-site centesis is 1–2 cm caudal to the umbilicus and 1 cm ventral to the midline.

Figure A.2: The approximate sampling sites for a four-quadrant centesis approach are indicated by the black crosses (head is to the left; umbilicus is central).

Sample handling

- Fluid should be placed in an EDTA tube for total nucleated cell count and cytology
- Direct smears can also be prepared for cytology by applying a drop of fluid to a microscope slide
- Fluid should be placed in a plain tube for total protein and any other biochemical (e.g. creatinine, potassium, amylase, lipase, glucose, bilirubin) or serological tests
- A sample in a sterile plain tube can be submitted for bacteriological culture, if necessary

Potential complications

- If blood is aspirated: stop the aspiration, place the blood in a glass tube and observe for clot formation. Blood from the abdominal cavity (i.e. haemorrhagic effusion) will usually not clot, whereas blood from a vessel or organ will clot within 5–15 minutes (unless the animal has a coagulopathy). If bleeding persists, abdominal pressure should be applied by way of manual compression or a pressure bandage

- Puncture of the gastrointestinal (GI) tract: if fluid suggestive of GI contents is obtained, indicating that the GI tract has been punctured, any hole should seal when the needle is removed. The patient should, however, be monitored for developing peritonitis
- Continued drainage after needle removal: in some animals with large abdominal effusions, the centesis hole may continue to drain fluid. If this occurs, a pressure dressing may be applied

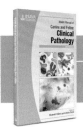

FURTHER INFORMATION

For interpretation of the results of fluid analysis, see the *BSAVA Manual of Canine and Feline Clinical Pathology.*

Anaphylaxis – emergency treatment

Identification

Anaphylaxis is an acute severe allergic reaction characterized by venous and arteriolar dilatation and increased capillary permeability, which, in severe cases, result in decreased venous return to the heart, hypotension and hypoperfusion. Signs of anaphylaxis include:

- Angioedema: this commonly results in swelling of the face and distal limbs, but can include swelling of the pharynx and larynx
- Bronchospasm
- Pruritus
- Urticaria: raised red skin wheals or hives
- Vomiting
- Anaphylactic shock

Procedure

1 Perform a rapid assessment of the airway, respiration and circulation.
2 If an upper airway obstruction is evident with spontaneous respiration:
    a Perform endotracheal (ET) intubation with sedation as required (see **Endotracheal intubation**)
    b Administer supplemental oxygen as required: if measurements of oxygen are unavailable administer 100% oxygen.
3 Remove any known triggers.
4 Establish vascular access.
5 **For a mild reaction, administer antihistamines/corticosteroids:**
    a Chlorphenamine:
       i Cats: 2–5 mg/cat i.m. or slow i.v.
       ii Dogs: 2.5–10 mg/dog i.m. or slow i.v.
    b Consider dexamethasone at 0.5 mg/kg i.v. once

A

6 For a severe reaction, administer adrenergic agents:

a Adrenaline at 10 µg/kg of a 1:1000 solution (1000 µg/ml) preferably i.v., although the i.m. route can also be used. (Alternatively, adrenaline can be given into the trachea if intravenous access is difficult, although this is considered less effective. To do this, insert a dog urinary catheter via the ET tube to the level of the carina and administer the adrenaline diluted 1:10 with saline or sterile water)

b Chlorphenamine:

    i Cats: 2–5 mg/cat i.m. or slow i.v.

    ii Dogs: 2.5–10 mg/dog i.m. or slow i.v.

c Salbutamol inhaler 100 µg per metered inhalation ('puff'):

    i Cats: 1 puff q4–6h or as needed

    ii Dogs: 1–3 puffs q4–6h or as needed.

7 If available, initiate monitoring of S_pO_2, ETCO$_2$, blood pressure, venous blood gas, acid–base and electrolyte status, as well as **electrocardiography**.

a Monitor for adrenaline-induced arrhythmias and hypertension.

8 Treat hypoperfusion with intravenous fluid therapy and vasopressors as required.

a Crystalloids should be administered in boluses, as required, to achieve normotension (mean arterial pressure of 80–120 mmHg, systolic arterial pressure of 100–200 mmHg) and good perfusion (lactate <2.5 mmol/l).

b Vasopressors should be considered if hypotension is unresponsive to fluid therapy:

    i Dobutamine:

        1 Cats: 1–5 µg/kg/min i.v. by constant rate infusion. Start at the lower end of the dose range and increase slowly until the desired effect is observed

        2 Dogs: 2.5–5 µg/kg/min i.v. by constant rate infusion. Start at the lower end of the dose range and increase slowly until the desired effect is observed.

    ii Dopamine:

        1 Cats: 1–5 µg/kg/min i.v. by constant rate infusion

        2 Dogs: 2–10 µg/kg/min i.v. by constant rate infusion.

9 Following initial emergency treatment, if bronchospasm and angioedema persist, consider dexamethasone (at 0.5 mg/kg i.v. once).

10 Long-term prophylaxis requires identification and avoidance of the causative agent.

Arthrocentesis

Indications/Use

- Joint disease of unknown aetiology
- Pain on manipulation of a joint
- Joint effusion
- Joint heat
- Periarticular thickening
- Suspected immune-mediated joint disease

- Suspected infective arthritis
- Monitoring response to therapy in infective arthritis and immune-mediated polyarthritis

Contraindications
- Severe coagulopathy

Equipment
- As required for **Aseptic preparation – (a) non-surgical procedures**

GLOVES

Sterile gloves should be worn if the clinician wishes to palpate bony landmarks and the needle insertion site. As experience is gained, such palpation may not be necessary and gloves may not be required, provided the needle insertion point is not touched.

- Hypodermic needles: 21–23 G; ⅝ to 1.5 inches, depending on joint size
- 2–10 ml syringes (larger syringe sizes allow better negative pressure, especially if joint fluid is expected to be of normal viscosity. A 10 ml syringe can be used if there is a palpable effusion and a large volume of fluid is expected)
- Microscope slides
- EDTA and heparin collection tubes
- Blood culture bottle/bacteriology swab in transport medium

Patient preparation and positioning
- Heavy sedation or general anaesthesia is required
- The patient should be placed in lateral recumbency, with the affected joint uppermost. The exception to this would be if using a medial approach for arthrocentesis of the elbow, whereby the patient would be positioned with affected limb on the table
- The joint for aspiration will often be dictated by the findings on clinical examination (e.g. pain on joint manipulation, palpable effusion); see **Orthopaedic examination**
- An assistant may be required to hold the limb and flex or extend the joint as required
- **Aseptic preparation – (a) non-surgical procedures** is performed on an area approximately 5 cm x 5 cm over the site for arthrocentesis

Technique
1 **a. Carpus:** The antebrachiocarpal (radiocarpal) joint is generally the most accessible.
   i   Partially to fully flex the carpus to locate the antebrachiocarpal joint, which is palpable as a depression just distal to the radius.
   ii Insert the needle medial to the common digital extensor tendon and cephalic vein, which pass over the centre of the joint space (Figure A.3). The needle insertion site is just lateral to the tendon of extensor carpi radialis. The antebrachiocarpal joint does not communicate with the other carpal joints.

iii If no fluid is obtained, or blood contamination occurs, try tapping the intercarpal joint to obtain a sample. The intercarpal and carpometacarpal joints communicate.

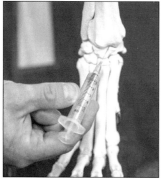
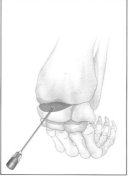
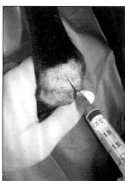

Figure A.3: Position of the needle for arthrocentesis of the antebrachiocarpal joint. Arthrocentesis is best performed with the carpus partially to fully flexed.

1 **b. Elbow:** The caudolateral approach is the easiest and most atraumatic.
   i Flex the elbow to approximately 45 degrees and palpate the lateral condyle of the humerus and olecranon.
   ii Advance the needle parallel to the long axis of the ulna, midway between these two landmarks. The needle should slide between the lateral epicondylar crest of the humerus and the anconeal process of the ulna (Figure A.4).
   iii Once the needle is through the skin, apply slight downward (medial) pressure on the shaft of the needle with the thumb while it is advanced towards the joint space. This is necessary in order to maintain the caudal-to-cranial orientation of the needle parallel to the olecranon and straight into the joint. In most cases, the needle needs to be inserted deep into the joint before fluid is aspirated.

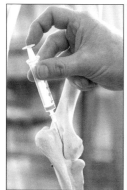
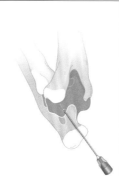
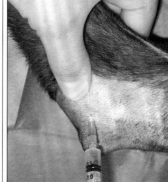

Figure A.4: Position of the needle for arthrocentesis of the elbow joint. Arthrocentesis is best performed with the elbow flexed to approximately 45 degrees.

Alternative:

A

i   Position the patient with the affected leg on the recumbent side and flex the elbow to approximately 45 degrees.

ii   Insert a needle 1—2 cm distal to the medial humeral epicondyle; a subtle depression at the level of the joint space can sometimes be palpated.

iii Direct the needle very slightly proximally (as opposed to truly perpendicular to the surface of the skin), so that it is inserted parallel to the articular surfaces of the trochlea and ulna.

1   c. Tarsus (hock): The talocrural joint space is most readily aspirated.

i   Flex and extend the talocrural joint to locate its position.

ii   With the joint in a neutral position, insert the needle on the dorsolateral aspect of the talocrural joint, just medial to the palpable lateral malleolus of the fibula.

iii Advance the needle towards the plantaromedial aspect of the joint (Figure A.5).

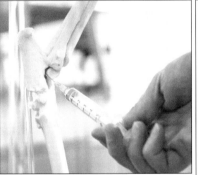
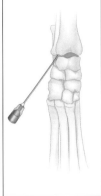
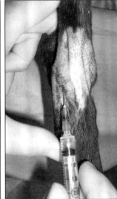

Figure A.5: Position of the needle for arthrocentesis of the talocrural joint.

Alternative:

i   Aspirate the plantarolateral joint space by inserting the needle parallel to the calcaneus, just medial to the lateral malleolus (Figure A.6).

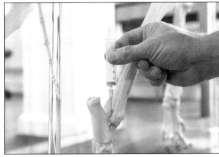

Figure A.6: Position of the needle for arthrocentesis of the plantarolateral joint.

A

1   d. Stifle: The joint capsule of the stifle has three sacs, all of which communicate.

i   With the joint partially flexed, apply digital pressure to the joint capsule on the medial side of the patellar ligament.

ii   Introduce the needle just lateral to the straight patellar ligament, midway between the femur and tibia.

iii Direct the needle into the joint space, through the fat pad, towards the intercondylar space in the centre of the joint (Figure A.7).

iv   If no synovial fluid is aspirated, the needle should be moved inwards or outwards and re-aspiration attempted, as the needle tip may be located in the fat pad.

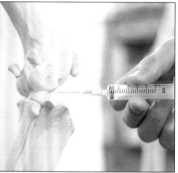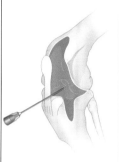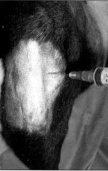

Figure A.7: Position of the needle for arthrocentesis of the stifle joint using a lateral approach to the straight patella ligament.

Alternative:

i   Insert the needle parallel to the straight patellar ligament, midway between the tibial tuberosity and patella.

ii   Direct the tip of the needle lateral to the patella in the lateral parapatellar joint pouch (Figure A.8).

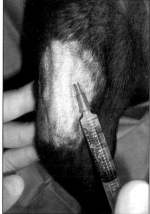

Figure A.8: Position of the needle for arthrocentesis of the stifle joint using a parallel approach to the straight patella ligament.

2 Attach a syringe to the needle and gently aspirate until synovial fluid appears in the hub of the needle.

3 Once sufficient fluid has entered the syringe (which may only be a hubful), release the suction to minimize inadvertent aspiration of blood, before withdrawing the needle and syringe. To reduce the chance of blood contamination further, the syringe can be removed from the needle prior to needle removal from the joint space.

Sample handling

- To maximize preservation of cell morphology, smears should be made immediately and allowed to air dry. The 'squash' technique should be used (Figure A.9a; see also **Fine-needle aspiration**). However, if the synovial fluid is of poor viscosity, a 'blood smear' technique may be possible (Figure A.9b; see also **Blood smear preparation**)
- If more than approximately 0.2–0.3 ml of fluid is obtained, this can be placed in an EDTA tube for cytological evaluation and total nucleated cell count
- If bacterial infective arthritis is suspected, synovial fluid should be placed in blood culture media. Alternatively, a few drops of fluid can be added to a sterile bacteriology swab and placed in a commercial transport medium (e.g. Amies charcoal)

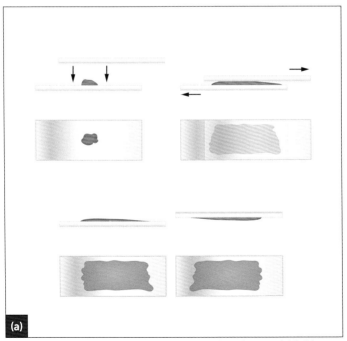

(a)

Figure A.9: Routine techniques for the preparation of a synovial fluid smear. **(a)** 'Squash' technique. (Reproduced from the *BSAVA Manual of Canine and Feline Musculoskeletal Disorders*). (continues) ▶

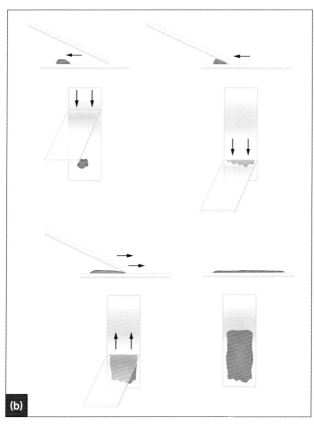

Figure A.9: (continued) Routine techniques for the preparation of a synovial fluid smear. (b) 'Blood-smear' technique for synovial fluid with poor viscosity. (Reproduced from the *BSAVA Manual of Canine and Feline Musculoskeletal Disorders*).

(b)

Potential complications

- Iatrogenic articular cartilage damage
- Iatrogenic septic arthritis
- Haemorrhage

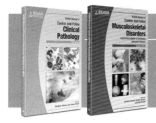

FURTHER INFORMATION

Details of the evaluation of synovial fluid are given in the *BSAVA Manual of Canine and Feline Clinical Pathology* and in the *BSAVA Manual of Canine and Feline Musculoskeletal Disorders*.

Aseptic preparation – (a) non-surgical procedures

Indications/Use

- Skin preparation for any veterinary procedure requiring aseptic technique, where there is a risk of iatrogenic contamination leading to infection

Equipment

- Surgical gloves (non-sterile are usually sufficient for non-surgical procedures)
- Regularly maintained, clean and sharp electric clippers
- Vacuum cleaner
- Cotton wool or soft swabs
- Container to hold used cotton wool or soft swabs
- Tap water
- Appropriate antiseptic:
  - For routine preparation of healthy skin, 4% chlorhexidine gluconate or 10% povidone–iodine, used in combination with 70% surgical spirit, is appropriate
  - Chlorhexidine gluconate and povidone–iodine should be avoided in animals with known skin sensitivities to either of these antiseptics
  - Chlorhexidine gluconate is specifically toxic to the conjunctiva, cornea, meninges and middle and inner ear
    - 0.2% povidone–iodine solution without alcohol is therefore recommended for preparation of the periocular area but must not be allowed to contact the cornea
    - 1% povidone–iodine solution without alcohol is recommended for preparation of the external ear canal for surgery
  - Alcohol has a desiccating effect when applied to mucous membranes and therefore should not be used for procedures close to, or involving, the mucous membranes (e.g. intraoral surgery)
  - The application of antiseptics directly to open wounds is not recommended

---

NOTE

- Sterile applicators containing 2% chlorhexidine gluconate and 70% isopropyl alcohol, designed specifically for skin antisepsis are now available. They should be used according to the manufacturer's recommendations, rather than following the technique below

---

- Appropriate sterile skin drapes; these may be:
  - Well maintained and laundered cloth drapes
  - Disposable semi-impermeable synthetic drapes
  - Sterile fenestrated drapes (one may be appropriate for non-surgical procedures)

A

Technique

> **NOTE**
>
> - Non-sterile surgical gloves should be worn

1 Hair removal:
   a Remove hair from the procedure site with electric clippers
   b Include margins up to 15 cm around the proposed procedural site. Clip sufficient hair to avoid contamination of the veterinary surgeon, the procedural site and sterile equipment
   c Remove clipped hair from the procedural site. A vacuum cleaner may be used with anaesthetized animals, but using a vacuum cleaner around a conscious or sedated animal may cause undue distress to the patient.

2 Skin preparation:
   a Apply antiseptic of an appropriate concentration to balls of damp cotton wool or swabs
   b Clean the clipped area by applying gentle pressure in a circular motion, beginning at the proposed procedural site (e.g. site of needle insertion) and working outwards in concentric circles. Use a fresh cotton wool ball or swab each time cleaning is returned to the centre of the procedural site
   c Continue cleaning for at least 3 minutes until no dirt can be seen grossly on the cotton wool balls or swabs
   d Dampen the hair around the clipped area to flatten it away from the procedural site
   e Squirt or gently spray surgical spirit on to the procedural site. **NB Do NOT use surgical spirit to prepare sites that include the eyes, ears or mucous membranes.**

3 Draping:
   a Draping may not be required for short minor procedures where the risk of contamination of the procedural site and sterile equipment is negligible (e.g. fine-needle aspiration of skin masses, arthrocentesis)
   b Draping should always be used if in doubt. A simple fenestrated drape laid over the site may be sufficient to prevent contamination of a procedural site. For short procedures and procedures performed in non-anaesthetized patients, towel clamps are, respectively, not required and not advised.

> **NOTE**
>
> - Draping should be performed by a veterinary surgeon or nurse who has scrubbed hands and is wearing sterile gloves and gown

Potential complications

- Clipper rash
- Dermatitis due to idiosyncratic reaction to antiseptic
- Break in asepsis

Aseptic preparation – (b) surgical procedures

A

Indications/Use

- Skin preparation for all surgical procedures

Equipment

- Surgical gloves – non-sterile and sterile
- Regularly maintained, clean and sharp electric clippers
- Vacuum cleaner
- Cotton wool or soft swabs
- Container to hold used cotton wool or soft swabs
- Tap water
- Appropriate antiseptic:
  - For routine preparation of healthy skin, 4% chlorhexidine gluconate or 10% povidone–iodine, used in combination with 70% surgical spirit, is appropriate
  - Chlorhexidine gluconate or povidone–iodine should be avoided in animals with known skin sensitivities to either of these antiseptics
  - Chlorhexidine gluconate is specifically toxic to the conjunctiva, cornea, meninges and middle and inner ear
    - 0.2% povidone–iodine solution without alcohol is therefore recommended for preparation of the periocular area but must not be allowed to contact the cornea
    - 1% povidone–iodine solution without alcohol is recommended for preparation of the external ear canal for surgery
  - Alcohol has a desiccating effect when applied to mucous membranes and should not be used for procedures close to, or involving, the mucous membranes (e.g. intraoral surgery)
  - The application of antiseptics directly to open wounds is not recommended

---

NOTE

- Sterile applicators containing 2% chlorhexidine gluconate and 70% isopropyl alcohol, designed specifically for skin antisepsis are now available. They should be used according to the manufacturer's recommendations, rather than following the technique below. For surgical procedures, these applicators are generally used for final skin preparation in the operating theatre, following appropriate preparation of the skin

---

- Appropriate sterile skin drapes: these may be well maintained and laundered cloth drapes, or disposable semi-impermeable synthetic drapes
  - Four sterile field drapes are appropriate for most surgical procedures
  - Sterile transparent adherent plastic drapes and sterile skin towels may be used at the veterinary surgeon's discretion
- Sterile towel clamps

A

Technique

> **NOTE**
>
> - Non-sterile surgical gloves should be worn for the hair clip and initial skin preparation. Sterile gloves are preferred for final skin preparation in the operating theatre

1 Hair removal:
   a Remove hair from the surgical site with electric clippers
   b Include margins of at least 15 cm around the proposed surgical incision
   c Remove clipped hair immediately with a vacuum cleaner
   d For operations on the limbs, clip the entire limb apart from the phalanges. Phalanges should only be clipped when they are included in the surgical field. Wrap the unclipped phalanges and as much of the paw as the surgical site permits in a semi-impermeable, self-adhesive, non-adherent outer bandage material.

2 Skin preparation outside the operating room:
   a Apply antiseptic of an appropriate concentration to balls of damp cotton wool or soft cotton swabs
   b Clean the clipped area by applying gentle pressure in a circular motion, beginning at the proposed incision site and working outwards in concentric circles. Use a fresh cotton wool ball or swab each time cleaning is returned to the incision site
   c Continue cleaning until no dirt can be seen grossly on the cotton wool balls or swabs
   d For operations including the phalanges, soak the paw in a dilute solution of antiseptic for 3 minutes or until all gross dirt has been removed
   e Dampen the hair around the clipped area to flatten it away from the surgical site.

3 Patient transfer to the operating room:
   a Transfer the patient to the operating room
   b Position the patient appropriately for surgery, using sandbags and ties
   c For limb operations, suspend the limb from the toes or paw. This is carried out using ropes tied to vertical stands, with top horizontal crossbars that can be raised and lowered.

4 Skin preparation inside the operating room:
   a Apply antiseptic of an appropriate concentration to sterile swabs
   b Wearing sterile gloves, clean the clipped area by applying gentle pressure in a circular motion, beginning at the proposed incision site and working outwards in concentric circles. Use a fresh swab each time cleaning is returned to the incision site
   c Continue this scrubbing for at least 3 minutes
   d Squirt or gently spray surgical spirit on to the surgical site. **NB Do NOT use surgical spirit to prepare surgical sites that include the eyes, ears or mucous membranes.**

5 Draping:

   a Sterile surgical drapes are placed around the surgical field. Draping should leave only the aseptically prepared skin exposed and cover all hair. Drapes are secured in place with towel clamps placed at each of the four corners of the surgical field and then along the sides of the surgical field as necessary

   b Sterile surgical skin towels may be attached to the edges of the skin incision using towel clamps following the initial skin incision. Such skin draping has not been shown to decrease the incidence of surgical site infection, but is preferred by some surgeons

   c A sterile transparent adherent plastic drape may be used to cover skin that is exposed following routine draping. This may decrease the incidence of surgical site infection and is preferred by many surgeons, especially for orthopaedic procedures

   d For limb operations, a non-scrubbed assistant wearing non-sterile gloves passes the foot to the surgeon. The surgeon covers the foot with an appropriately sized sterile surgical drape, which is wrapped around the distal limb and secured with a towel clamp. The surgeon avoids contacting the foot directly, so as to remain sterile. The entire distal limb including the towel clamp and drape are wrapped in a semi-impermeable, self-adhesive, non-adherent outer bandage material, which has been sterilized specifically for this purpose. The limb is then held by a sterile surgical assistant, while it is draped using four sterile surgical drapes as above.

NOTE

- Draping should be performed by a veterinary surgeon or nurse who has scrubbed their lower arms and hands and is wearing a mask, hat, sterile gloves and gown

---

Potential complications

- Clipper rash
- Dermatitis due to idiosyncratic reaction to antiseptic
- Break in asepsis

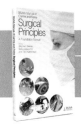

FURTHER INFORMATION

For more interpretation on aseptic technique, see the *BSAVA Manual of Canine and Feline Surgical Principles*.

Bandaging

Indications/Use
- To control limb oedema and swelling
- To support the limb following surgery

Equipment
- Adhesive tape (2.5 cm wide)
- Tongue depressor (optional)
- Cast padding or cotton roll
- Conforming gauze bandage
- Outer protective bandage material (e.g. self-adhesive non-adherent bandage)

Patient preparation and positioning
- Sedation or general anaesthesia may be required where the limb is painful or the animal is non-compliant
- The animal should be placed in lateral recumbency with the affected limb uppermost
- The affected limb should be supported in a weight-bearing position and an appropriate dressing placed directly over any wounds or surgical incisions

Technique
1 Place two strips of adhesive tape (stirrups) on the distal limb, on either the dorsal and palmar/plantar surfaces or the medial and lateral surfaces. These tape strips should extend beyond the tip of the toes and are stuck to each other or to a tongue depressor.
2 Beginning distally, apply cast padding material or cotton roll up the limb, in a spiral fashion, overlapping the layers by 50%. The bottom of the bandage should be at the level of the nailbeds of digits III and IV.
3 Place conforming gauze snugly over the cotton layer, again overlapping layers by 50%. The conforming gauze should compress the cotton but not create venous stasis. It should not extend proximally beyond the level of the cotton.
4 Separate the tape stirrups, rotate them through 180 degrees, and apply them proximally to the bandage to limit slippage. The pads and nails of the axial digits should remain exposed.
5 Apply an outer protective bandage material to the bandage. This should not be applied tightly: it should be pulled free from the roll, the tension released from the material, and the material simply placed over the gauze. When complete, it should be possible to insert two fingers between the top of the bandage and the patient's skin.

Robert Jones technique
- The Robert Jones bandage is a heavily padded modification, which provides effective support for the first aid management of distal limb fractures (Figure B.1)
- It is only suitable for fractures distal to the elbow in the forelimb and distal to the stifle in the hindlimb

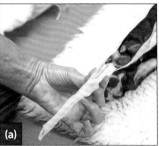
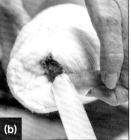
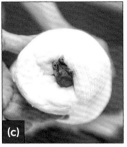

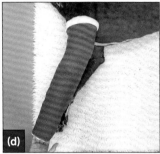

Figure B.1: Robert Jones bandage technique. **(a)** Two strips of adhesive tape should be placed on the distal limb and stuck to a wooden tongue depressor. **(b)** Following the application of padding material and conforming gauze, the adhesive strips should be separated and rotated through 180 degrees before being applied to the bandage. **(c)** The toes should remain exposed. **(d)** An outer protective bandage material should be applied. Note the padding material extends more proximally than the outer cohesive layer.

- For fractures of the humerus or femur, the distal edge of the Robert Jones bandage acts as a fulcrum, across which the fracture pivots, with the possibility of exacerbating soft tissue injury and further fracture displacement
- One version of the Robert Jones bandage can be achieved by applying four layers of cast padding material or cotton roll prior to conforming gauze and an outer protective bandage layer. Bandage materials should be applied to the limb as for the soft padded bandage. Care should be taken to minimize wrinkles during the application of the padding material, and to ensure the distal limb is not rotated as the padding is applied. It should be possible to insert two fingers between the top of the bandage and the patient's skin when complete

Bandage care and maintenance

- Soft padded bandages should be checked every 4 hours for the first 24 hours and at least twice daily thereafter for complications
- Written instructions should always be given to clients at discharge; owners must understand their responsibility regarding bandage maintenance
- Exercise restriction is generally indicated
- The bandaged limb should be monitored for swollen toes, cold toes, wetness, soiling or slippage and changed if necessary
- The bandage must be kept clean and dry. A plastic bag may be placed over the foot while the animal is walking outside and then removed when it is indoors
- If no open wounds are present, the bandage may be changed every 7–10 days. If open wounds are present, the bandage should be changed as needed, sometimes several times daily
- In young, rapidly growing animals the bandage should be changed every 4–5 days

Potential complications

- Venous stasis
- Limb oedema
- Moist dermatitis
- Maceration of skin underlying a wet bandage
- Contamination of wounds
- Pressure necrosis, particularly around the olecranon and calcaneus
- Skin irritation at the site of the tape stirrups

Barium contrast media

Barium contrast media appear radiopaque on a radiograph due to barium sulphate having a higher atomic number than soft tissues. Barium sulphate is inert with no osmotic potential and is not absorbed or acted upon by alimentary secretions. There is a wide variety of barium sulphate preparations used in veterinary radiography and some of the preparations available at the time of writing are shown in Figure B.2. None of these preparations is authorized for veterinary use and most are POM.

> **OPTIONS**
>
> - Barium paste is primarily used to highlight abnormalities of oesophageal mucosa
> - A barium meal (barium paste added to food) is best for identifying functional abnormalities

Formulation	Trade name	Package sizes
94% w/w granules to reconstitute as suspension	Baritop plus	200 g pack 1000 g pack
100% w/v suspension	Baritop 100	300 ml can
95% w/w cherry flavoured powder to reconstitute as a suspension	Tonopaque	180 g bottle 1200 g bottle
98% w/w vanilla flavoured powder to reconstitute as a suspension	HD 200 plus	312 g bottle
100% w/v liquid barium suspension 105% w/v liquid barium suspension	Liquid Polibar plus	1900 ml
60% w/v liquid barium suspension	Liquid E-ZPaque	1900 ml
40% w/v liquid barium suspension	Varibar	148 g
Barium-impregnated polyethylene spheres	BIPS	Large (5 mm diameter) and small (1.5 mm diameter) combined in capsules
Barium sulphate powder	Barium sulphate BP	Various

Figure B.2: Preparations of barium sulphate used in veterinary radiography.

Use

- Barium contrast media are used for studies of the gastrointestinal (GI) tract
- Barium-impregnated polyethylene spheres (BIPS) may be used to assess intestinal transit times and gastric emptying rate, as well as to detect obstructions
- As with all contrast studies, plain radiographs should be obtained prior to the administration of barium
- Barium paste is used for oesophageal studies as it adheres to the mucosa. Barium can also be mixed with food to evaluate the oesophagus and may demonstrate strictures or dilatations not seen with liquid barium or paste
- Liquid barium may be used to evaluate any part of the GI tract and is used alone for evaluation of the stomach and intestines. Flavoured preparations designed for human use may be unpalatable for some animals

Safety and handling

- Skin irritation may occur with skin contact
- Take care not to spill barium on the patient's coat; any spills should be carefully cleaned off

Contraindications and complications

- Barium is insoluble and should not be used outside the GI tract
- A barium study should not be performed <24 hours before endoscopy
- Leakage of barium into body cavities may lead to granulomatous reactions or adhesions
- If perforation of the GI tract is suspected, low-osmolar water-soluble contrast media, rather than barium media, should be used
- Care should be taken when administering barium to dysphagic animals, distressed patients, or those with swallowing disorders or laryngeal paralysis, as aspiration of barium into the bronchi and lungs may occur and can result in aspiration pneumonia
- If inappropriately sized BIPS are used, mechanical obstruction of the GI tract can occur (seen primarily in cats and very small dogs)
- May cause constipation, transient diarrhoea and abdominal pain

Barium studies of the gastrointestinal tract – (a) oesophagus

Indications/Use

- Regurgitation
- Retching
- Haematemesis
- Dysphagia
- Hypersalivation and pain associated with suspected ulceration/oesophagitis
- Aspiration/recurrent bronchopneumonia
- A suspected oesophageal foreign body (i.e. one not evident on survey radiographs and where there is no evidence of oesophageal perforation) can be considered as an indication for a contrast study of the oesophagus. However, endoscopy is considered the preferred diagnostic technique where available
- There is no justification for the use of barium in the investigation of suspected pharyngeal stick injuries

> **WARNING**
>
> - Care should be taken when administering barium to dysphagic animals, distressed patients, those with swallowing disorders or laryngeal paralysis, or those with severe oesophageal disease, as aspiration of barium into the bronchi and lungs may occur and may result in aspiration pneumonia.

Contraindications

- Suspected or confirmed oesophageal perforation: non-ionic iodinated contrast media should be used instead
- There is no justification for the use of barium in the investigation of suspected pharyngeal stick injuries
- Suspected gastrointestinal (GI) tract perforation
- Suspected oesophageal foreign body

Equipment

- Barium sulphate (see **Barium contrast media**)
- Lukewarm water for dilution
- Soft tinned food
- Food bowl
- 20–60 ml syringe with catheter tip
- Radiographic or fluoroscopic equipment

Patient preparation and positioning

- Studies of the GI tract are usually performed with the patient conscious. Sedation may occasionally be necessary in some patients, but the risk of regurgitation and/or aspiration should be considered. Barium should never be administered orally to an anaesthetized animal
- Contrast medium should be administered orally with the patient in a sitting or standing position
- The animal is subsequently positioned for radiography (see below)
- Alternatively, horizontal beam fluoroscopy can be performed with the patient in a standing position

Technique

1. Obtain plain left lateral and dorsoventral radiographs of the thorax and cranial abdomen. This is important, as significant findings such as foreign material may be masked by contrast medium. These views also allow for the detection of any pre-existing aspiration pneumonia.

> **WARNING**
>
> - If gross megaoesophagus is diagnosed on plain radiography, administration of barium is not required and is contraindicated because of the risk of aspiration pneumonia.

2. Barium can be administered as a suspension, paste or with food. It is usually difficult to administer a sufficiently large volume of barium liquid by syringe into the buccal fold and to position the patient for radiography

before the barium is propelled into the stomach. Thick barium paste placed on the tongue or hard palate usually persists long enough for radiographs to be obtained. However, paste is not appropriate for demonstrating the presence or extent of oesophageal dilatation. It is usually more convenient to mix a soft or semi-liquid food with 30 ml of barium liquid and allow the patient to eat most of the mixture before positioning and obtaining the required views.

3   Immediately obtain either a left (preferred) or right lateral radiograph of the cervical and thoracic oesophagus. Additional information may be gained from a dorsoventral view, especially if a vascular ring anomaly is suspected.

4   Where patient cooperation permits, repeat the oesophageal study 2–3 times as abnormalities can be dynamic and changes may only be evident on one image.

5   If necessary, encourage the patient to eat a mixture of soft tinned food to which approximately 20–30 ml of 100% w/v barium sulphate suspension has been added, and repeat radiography.

Potential complications

■ A barium study should not be performed <24 hours before endoscopy
■ Leakage of barium into body cavities may lead to granulomatous reactions or adhesions
■ If perforation of the GI tract is suspected, low-osmolar water-soluble contrast media should be used
■ Care should be taken when administering barium to dysphagic animals, distressed patients, or those with swallowing disorders or laryngeal paralysis, as aspiration of barium into the bronchi and lungs may occur and can result in aspiration pneumonia
■ May cause constipation, transient diarrhoea and abdominal pain

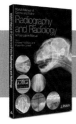

FURTHER INFORMATION

For information on barium studies, see the *BSAVA Manual of Canine and Feline Radiography and Radiology.*

Barium studies of the gastrointestinal tract – (b) stomach and small intestine

Indications/Use

- Persistent vomiting
- Haematemesis or melaena
- Assessment of the location of the stomach in relation to the liver, diaphragm or cranial abdominal masses
- Assessment of gastrointestinal (GI) tract displacement by changes in size or position of adjacent organs
- Abdominal discomfort or swelling
- To assess a palpable abdominal mass associated with the GI tract
- Chronic diarrhoea

ULTRASONOGRAPHY AND ENDOSCOPY

Ultrasonography and endoscopy have superseded contrast radiographic studies as the techniques of choice for evaluation of the GI tract. However, radiographic and fluoroscopic (dynamic) studies using barium as a positive-contrast agent remain important diagnostic tools for examination of the oropharynx, oesophagus and stomach. Fluoroscopy is the modality of choice for assessing swallowing disorders and is used when a functional disorder is suspected.

WARNING

- Care should be taken when administering barium to dysphagic animals, distressed patients and those with swallowing disorders or laryngeal paralysis, as aspiration of barium into the bronchi and lungs may occur and may result in aspiration pneumonia.

Contraindications

- Swallowing disorders predisposing to the aspiration of barium
- Suspected GI tract perforation
- Suspected oesophageal foreign body
- Obvious foreign body (lucent or opaque) or convincing signs of obstruction on survey films
- Suspected linear foreign body

Equipment

- Barium sulphate suspension (see **Barium contrast media**)
- Lukewarm water for dilution
- Soft tinned food
- Food bowl
- 20–60 ml syringe with catheter tip
- Radiographic equipment

Patient preparation and positioning

- For an elective examination, food should be withheld for 24 hours prior to the procedure
- Ideally, the study is performed with the patient conscious, but where necessary neuroleptanalgesia (acepromazine and/or butorphanol/ buprenorphine) may be used to facilitate patient cooperation. The effect on intestinal motility is usually minimal and may be less than the delay caused by anxiety in a nervous patient
- A satisfactory study usually requires 8–10 exposures (orthogonal views). Thus, such studies are unsuitable for all but the most relaxed and cooperative of cats
- Contrast medium should be administered orally with the patient in a sitting or standing position
- The animal is subsequently positioned for radiography (see below)

Technique

1   Obtain survey radiographs, including the thorax to rule out the presence of an oesophageal foreign body or other oesophageal disease. These should include both left and right lateral, ventrodorsal (VD) and dorsoventral (DV) views, centred on the cranial abdomen. If necessary, an enema should be administered.

2   For examination of the stomach and small intestine, use a volume of 5–10 ml/kg of a 30–50% w/v barium sulphate liquid suspension. This can be mixed with warm water and semi-liquid food to improve palatability, but the consistency should be liquid. The use of barium–food mixtures (chunks or biscuit) is usually limited to oesophageal studies.

3   The liquid barium mixture is usually administered into the buccal pouch via syringe. In cooperative patients, the use of a gag and stomach tube is usually efficient and well tolerated. However, it should be noted that as this procedure is performed less frequently, clinicians may be less experienced at placing a stomach tube in the conscious patient.

4   Following administration of the contrast medium, immediately obtain four radiographic views (as used for the survey films).

5   Repeat these views at 10–15 minute intervals, depending on the rate at which gastric emptying is observed. In most patients, gastric emptying starts immediately and is advanced by 30 minutes. In patients with delayed emptying due to structural disease, functional disease (pylorospasm) or in nervous animals, this can take up to 2–3 hours, and the need for further exposures should be adapted accordingly.

6   A barium study of the small intestine ('barium follow-through study') follows the positive-contrast gastrogram, either as the principal purpose of the study or as a continuation of the study if no lesion is identified in the stomach. For the small intestine, lateral and VD views suffice. Obtain films every 15 minutes until the barium has reached the colon.

7   Obtain a radiograph 24 hours after the administration of barium to demonstrate that all the contrast medium has reached the colon and that no barium has been retained in the stomach or small intestine, which could represent a foreign body or retention in damaged mucosa.

B

> **NOTE**
>
> - If the barium study is performed to demonstrate displacement of the GI tract during the investigation of an abdominal mass or diaphragmatic rupture, it is more economical to omit the initial films and take radiographs 30–45 minutes after administration of the contrast medium. By this time, the stomach and most of the small intestine should contain contrast medium

Potential complications

- A barium study should not be performed <24 hours before endoscopy
- Leakage of barium into body cavities may lead to granulomatous reactions or adhesions
- If perforation of the GI tract is suspected, low-osmolar water-soluble contrast media should be used
- Care should be taken when administering barium to dysphagic animals, distressed patients, or those with swallowing disorders or laryngeal paralysis, as aspiration of barium into the bronchi and lungs may occur and can result in aspiration pneumonia
- May cause constipation, transient diarrhoea and abdominal pain

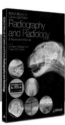

FURTHER INFORMATION

For information on barium studies, see the *BSAVA Manual of Canine and Feline Radiography and Radiology.*

Barium studies of the gastrointestinal tract – (c) large intestine

Indications/Use

- Tenesmus
- Haematochezia or melaena
- Chronic diarrhoea
- Identification of the position of the large intestine in relation to caudal abdominal/intrapelvic masses
- To rule out stricture of the colon

> **ENDOSCOPY**
>
> Endoscopy has generally superseded contrast radiographic studies as the technique of choice for evaluation of the lower gastrointestinal (GI) tract. However, radiographic studies using barium as a positive contrast agent may have a place for the investigation of selected large intestinal diseases.

Contraindications

- Perianal fistulae
- Large rectal or colonic mass that would preclude the passage of the tube for administering barium sulphate
- Suspected rupture of the lower GI tract

Equipment

- Barium sulphate suspension (see **Barium contrast media**)
- Equipment for giving an enema and administering contrast medium: 20–60 ml syringe; lukewarm water or 0.9% sterile saline; enema pump or tubing and funnel; sterile aqueous lubricant (e.g. K-Y jelly)
- Radiographic equipment
- Foley catheter (with a 'Christmas tree' adapter for a Luer syringe)
- Suture material

Patient preparation and positioning

- For an elective examination, food should be withheld for 24 hours prior to the procedure
- A rectal examination is required to ensure that it is safe to administer the enema and barium sulphate
- At least one non-irritant cleansing enema (e.g. warm water) should be given 2–3 hours prior to the procedure, to evacuate the large intestine. This can be performed with the patient in lateral recumbency or standing and is usually best performed outside. If survey radiographs indicate that patient preparation is inadequate, then a further 2–3 warm water enemas should be administered
- The patient should be heavily sedated or anaesthetized. This will not interfere with the results of the contrast study

Technique

1 Obtain plain lateral and ventrodorsal (VD) radiographs of the abdomen to assess patient preparation and whether further enemas are required.
2 Insert a Foley catheter into the rectum.
3 Gently inflate the bulb of the Foley catheter. If there is an air leak, use a purse-string suture or manually occlude the anus to make an airtight seal.
4 Slowly insufflate the colon using 5–10 ml/kg of air.
5 Obtain lateral and VD radiographs. Oblique views can also be useful to assess intrapelvic structures obscured by the pelvic bones. Palpate the colon and add more air, if needed, based on the radiographs obtained.
6 Perform a positive-contrast study if required.
7 Slowly instill the colon with 5–15 ml/kg of a 15–20% w/v barium solution. This solution can be made by diluting a 100% suspension with water. The barium suspension should be warmed to body temperature to avoid artefacts caused by spasm of the colon. Colloidal suspensions rather than barium powder should be used to avoid clumping, which could be misinterpreted as pathology.
8 Obtain lateral and VD radiographs.

Potential complications

- Rupture of the colon
- Trauma to the colon
- Haematochezia
- Diarrhoea

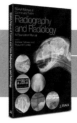

FURTHER INFORMATION

For information on barium studies, see the *BSAVA Manual of Canine and Feline Radiography and Radiology.*

Blood pressure measurement – (a) direct

Invasive blood pressure measurement by means of an arterial catheter is considered the 'gold standard' technique but requires specialized equipment and is technically demanding in terms of placement of the catheter, maintaining patency of the arterial catheter and ensuring accurate 'zeroing' of the apparatus to ambient air at the level of the right atrium.

Indications/Use

- Monitoring arterial blood pressure in critically ill patients
- Monitoring arterial blood pressure during anaesthesia
- Arterial catheters can also be used for serial collection of arterial blood samples in critically ill patients, particularly for blood gas analysis in patients with pulmonary disease

Contraindications

- Coagulopathy
- Arterial catheters should not be placed at sites where risk of bacterial contamination and infection are high (e.g. due to local tissue damage, local skin infection, diarrhoea, urinary incontinence)

Equipment

- Scalpel and No.11 scalpel blade
- 20–22 G peripheral venous over-the-needle catheter
- T-connector or extension set containing heparinized saline (1 IU of heparin per ml of 0.9% sterile saline)
- 70% surgical spirit
- Adhesive tape
- Soft padded bandage and outer protective bandage
- Non-compliant manometer tubing

- Pressure transducer: must be 'zeroed' to ambient air at the level of the right atrium
- Display monitor
- Pressurized continuous flush system

Patient preparation and positioning

- The patient should be positioned in lateral recumbency
- The patient's limb must be held still; this can be achieved by manual restraint
- For monitoring of the anaesthetized patient, arterial catheters should be placed soon after anaesthetic induction and before the animal's blood pressure falls, as low blood pressure makes palpation of a peripheral arterial pulse more challenging

Sites

The dorsal pedal artery in the hind paw is most commonly used (Figure B.3). Other arteries that may be used include: the femoral artery; the auricular artery; the palmar metacarpal artery in the forepaw; and the median caudal artery

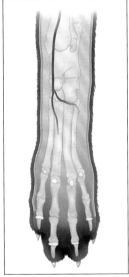

Figure B.3: The dorsal pedal artery in the hind paw is most commonly used for catheter placement.

Technique

1   Place a catheter into a peripheral artery.
   a   Palpate the arterial pulse. The artery is palpated just distal to the tarsus (hock), between the second and third metatarsal bones, on the dorsal aspect.
   b   Clip the skin overlying the artery and then spray or lightly wipe with surgical spirit. Excessive scrubbing/wiping of the skin should be avoided, as this may result in spasm of the artery.
   c   Make a small stab incision in the skin overlying the arterial pulse.
   d   Place a peripheral venous catheter through the skin incision and insert it into the artery using short, firm, purposeful movements to push the stylet and catheter through the muscular wall of the artery. For entry into the artery, the catheter should be positioned at a slight angle to the artery – approximately 10–30 degrees.
   e   The dorsal pedal artery runs at about 30 degrees to the long axis of the metatarsus from medial to lateral. During catheter placement, palpate the arterial pulse constantly, proximal to the site of entry of the catheter into the artery. This allows the operator to guide the catheter tip towards the artery, which cannot be seen.
   f   As soon as arterial blood is seen in the flash chamber of the catheter, lower the stylet and catheter to a position parallel to the artery and advance together a little further into the artery, before advancing the catheter over the stylet and completely into the artery.

B

g Withdraw the catheter stylet and attach a T-connector or extension set containing heparinized saline to the catheter. Arterial blood should be seen to pulsate within the hub of the catheter or T-connector.

h Secure the catheter firmly in place with adhesive tape and cover with a bandage.

WARNING

- The bandage over an arterial catheter must be labelled clearly to avoid inadvertent administration of fluids or drugs into an artery.

---

2 Connect the T-connector to a pressure transducer via non-compliant tubing filled with heparinized saline. Alternatively, collect an arterial blood sample.

3 To allow trouble-free continuous monitoring (avoiding clotting in the arterial line), combine the set-up with a pressurized continuous flush system. If this is not available, flush the arterial catheter hourly.

4 The transducer–monitor combination gives a continuous reading of blood pressure and shows the pressure waveform. Systolic and diastolic pressures are taken as the cyclic maximum and minimum pressures, respectively. Mean pressure is calculated automatically. Direct arterial blood pressure monitoring is usually continuous. Specialized monitoring systems can be used to provide information on cardiac output from the analysis of the arterial waveform (pulse wave analysis).

5 On removal of the catheter, apply direct pressure to the artery for 5 minutes, then wrap with a light pressure dressing (e.g. folded gauze swab secured in place over the artery with adhesive tape). Always inspect the catheter to ensure all components have been removed.

Potential complications

- Excessive arterial bleeding/exsanguination following a failed attempt at catheterization or accidental removal of the catheter
- Vascular damage and subsequent tissue necrosis distal to the catheter, particularly in feline patients. The risk of this complication can be minimized by:
  - Avoiding placing adhesive tape too tightly around the paw
  - Never using arterial catheters for administering drugs or fluids
  - Regular monitoring of the catheter and paw; arterial catheters should be checked every hour
  - Prompt removal of arterial catheters when they are no longer required
- Infection
- Thrombosis/thromboembolism
- Embolism of a piece of catheter due to accidental transection of the catheter with a blade or scissors
- Air embolism
- Accidental intra-arterial drug administration leading to chronic pain, tissue necrosis or even amputation

Blood pressure measurement – (b) indirect

Non-invasive blood pressure measurements are technically less demanding than invasive measurements and can be rapidly applied in the emergency situation, although they might not be as reliable or accurate. There are two non-invasive methods in general use: the oscillometric method and the Doppler method. Both require a cuff.

Indications/Use

- Monitoring arterial blood pressure in critically ill patients
- Monitoring arterial blood pressure during anaesthesia

Equipment

- Doppler ultrasound probe
- Coupling gel
- Adhesive tape
- Inflatable cuff attached to a manometer
  OR
- Oscillometric blood pressure monitor with cuffs

CUFF SIZE

The proper cuff width is 40% of the circumference of the site where the cuff will be placed (Figure B.4). Cuffs that are too wide lead to falsely low readings; those that are too narrow lead to falsely high readings.

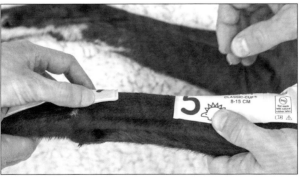

Figure B.4: The cuff should be 40% of the circumference of the site where it is to be placed. Here, the cuff with red writing is appropriate, whereas the cuff with blue writing is too small.

Patient preparation and positioning

- Can be performed on conscious, sedated or anaesthetized animals
- For conscious animals, it is important that they are relaxed. A quiet, stress-free environment is ideal. Allow the animal a period of at least 5–10 minutes to relax

■ The limb used should not be weight-bearing and the animal should be positioned such that the cuff is at the level of the right atrium

B

■ For the Doppler technique, it is necessary to prepare the skin overlying the artery to be used for blood pressure measurement. Normally the fur should be removed by shaving. However, in cats with short fur, wiping down the fur with surgical spirit may be adequate. Common sites for the detection of an arterial pulse using the Doppler technique are:
  - The palmar arterial arch on the palmar aspect of the proximal metacarpal region
  - The plantar arterial arch on the plantar aspect of the proximal metatarsal region
  - The dorsal pedal artery on the dorsal aspect of the proximal metatarsal region
  - The median caudal artery on the ventral aspect of the tail

Technique

Doppler ultrasonography

An inflatable cuff attached to a manometer occludes an artery and a piezoelectric crystal placed over the artery distal to the cuff detects flow. The re-entry of blood into the artery as the cuff is released causes a frequency change (Doppler shift) in the sound waves. This is detected by the piezoelectric crystal and converted to a sound that is detected by the operator. **This method primarily measures systolic pressure. Recording of diastolic pressure may be inaccurate.**

1 Attach the cuff to a handheld sphygmomanometer. Place the cuff around the limb or tail, proximal to the probe, avoiding the joints. In dogs, the cuff should be applied snugly enough to allow insertion of only a small finger between the cuff and the leg or tail. Most cuffs have a mark that should be placed directly over the artery.

> **PRACTICAL TIP**
>
> If the cuff is applied too tightly, the measurement will be erroneously low because the cuff partly occludes the artery; if applied too loosely, the measurement will be erroneously high because excessive cuff pressure will be required to occlude the artery.

2 Apply coupling gel directly to the transducer with the machine switched off.
3 Turn the machine on. Gently position the Doppler ultrasound probe over the prepared skin. Listen carefully for a pulse signal, moving the probe gently until a clear signal can be heard (Figure B.5). If required, secure the probe to the prepared area with adhesive tape.
4 If no signal is heard, consider:
  a Applying more coupling gel
  b Gently moving the probe
  c Securing the probe to the prepared skin before hearing a signal. Excessive digital pressure on the probe may occlude the artery, whereas the pressure from the tape alone may be less, allowing the pulse signal to be heard.

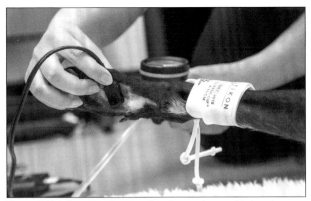

Figure B.5: A Doppler ultrasound probe can be used to locate a pulse signal for blood pressure measurement.

5 Gently inflate the cuff using the sphygmomanometer. Inflate the cuff an additional 10–20 mmHg beyond the point at which the pulse can no longer be heard.

6 Slowly deflate the cuff and listen carefully for a return of the pulse signal. The systolic blood pressure reading is the pressure at which the pulse can first be clearly heard.

7 Continue deflating the cuff and listen for the point (diastolic pressure) at which the audio signal of the pulse returns to pre-inflation quality. Thereafter completely deflate the cuff.

8 In a conscious animal, take 6–8 blood pressure measurements to ensure reliability. Discard the first measurement if it is very different from the others. Variability in systolic readings should be <20%. Record the mean systolic and diastolic pressures.

Oscillometric technique

This uses a cuff to occlude the artery and detects oscillations of the underlying artery when it is partly occluded. **This system determines systolic, diastolic and mean arterial pressures.** This method is less accurate in very small patients, patients with low blood pressure and patients with dysrhythmias. Muscle contractions also create oscillations and are a source of potential error.

1 Place the cuff snugly (see Step 1, above) over one of the following:
  a The radial artery proximal to the carpus
  b The saphenous artery proximal to the tarsus
  c The brachial artery proximal to the elbow
  d The median caudal artery at the base of the tail.

2 Attach the cuff to a control unit that continually senses arterial pressure and inflates to a pressure greater than the systolic, and then automatically deflates the cuff.

3 The heart rate is displayed. Verify that this matches the patient's heart rate by manually counting the rate using direct heart auscultation or palpation of an artery.

4 Record the values for 3–5 cycles and report the averages for systolic, diastolic and mean pressures.

B

Potential false readings

Incorrect blood pressure readings may be obtained due to:

- Inappropriate cuff size
- Inappropriate placement of the cuff
- Excessive motion of the limb or tail
- Low blood pressure
- Severe vasoconstriction (e.g. following alpha-2 agonist drug administration)
- Dysrhythmias
- Obesity
- Peripheral oedema
- Limb conformation that does not permit snug placement of the cuff
- Stress

Blood sampling – (a) arterial

Indications/Use

- To obtain a sample of arterial blood for assessment of:
  - Respiratory function
  - Arterial oxygen concentration
  - Acid–base status

Contraindications

- Coagulopathy
- Sampling should not be performed at sites where the risk of bacterial contamination and infection is high (e.g. due to local tissue damage, local skin infection, diarrhoea, urinary incontinence)

Equipment

- A pre-heparinized arterial blood gas syringe with a ⁵/₈ inch needle attached (typically 25 G for cats and small dogs, or 22 G for larger dogs) (Figure B.6)
- 70% surgical spirit
- Cotton wool or gauze swabs
- 25 mm wide self-adhesive non-adherent bandage (e.g. Vetrap)

Patient preparation and positioning

- Arterial blood sampling is performed in the conscious animal
- Sedation should be avoided as it will affect test results
- Animals should be positioned appropriately for the blood collection site (see below)

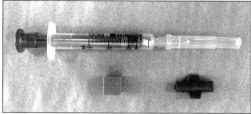

Figure B.6: A pre-heparinized arterial blood gas syringe is used for obtaining samples.

Sites

Most commonly, the dorsal pedal (metatarsal) artery is used, but in cats and small dogs it is sometimes easier to use the femoral artery.

Dorsal pedal (metatarsal) artery

- The animal is placed in lateral recumbency, either on a table (cats and small dogs) or on the floor (large dogs), with the leg to be sampled placed closest to the table or floor
- An assistant restrains the patient's head with one hand and the uppermost hindlimb with the other
- The artery is palpated just distal to the tarsus (hock), between the second and third metatarsal bones, on the dorsal aspect (Figure B.7)

Femoral artery

- The animal is placed in lateral recumbency, either on a table (cats and small dogs) or on the floor (large dogs), with the leg to be sampled placed closest to the table or floor
- The animal is restrained manually and the upper limb abducted so that the femoral artery can be palpated
- The femoral artery pulse is palpable on the medial thigh, ventral to the inguinal region and proximal to the stifle (Figure B.8)

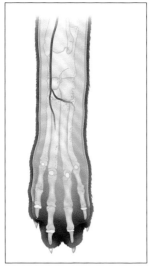

Figure B.7: The dorsal pedal artery is most commonly used to obtain arterial blood samples.

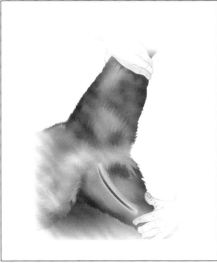

Figure B.8: The femoral artery can be used in cats and small dogs to obtain arterial blood samples.

Technique

1 Stretch the skin over the artery.
2 Palpate the artery.
3 Gently clip the skin overlying the artery and then spray or lightly wipe with surgical spirit. Excessive scrubbing/wiping of the skin should be avoided, as this may result in spasm of the artery.
4 Gently rest two fingertips of one hand against the artery, so that the arterial pulse can be felt.
5 With the other hand, direct the needle, with the syringe attached, towards the artery, at an angle of about 30–60 degrees. Point the needle bevel upwards.
6 Penetrate the artery in one quick firm purposeful movement.
7 When the artery has been penetrated, a flash of blood will be seen in the hub of the needle.
8 Collect approximately 1 ml of blood. Proprietary arterial sampling syringes have a plunger that allows air to be displaced; the syringe is prefilled with air to the volume of blood required and once the artery is punctured the syringe fills directly under arterial pressure with no need for further manipulation of the plunger.
9 Remove the syringe and needle from the artery.
10 On removal of the needle, apply direct pressure to the site for 5 minutes, then cover with cotton wool or a gauze swab and cohesive bandage.
11 Hold the syringe upright and tap it to cause air bubbles to rise. Eject any air from the syringe.
12 Cap the sample with an airtight seal to prevent exposure to room air. Rubber bungs or plastic caps are available with pre-heparinized blood gas syringes.
13 Analyse the blood sample as soon as possible, ideally **within 5 minutes**.

Blood gas values

Figure B.9 details arterial blood gas values for dogs and cats.

Potential complications

- Significant haemorrhage is very uncommon, provided direct pressure is applied to the artery (see above)
- Bruising and the formation of a small haematoma will occur in some patients, but can be minimized by good technique and by the application of direct pressure to the artery
- Arterial thrombosis and thrombophlebitis are uncommon, but are more likely if repeated attempts are made to collect blood from an artery

Parameter	Dogs	Cats
pH	7.35–7.46	7.31–7.46
PCO_2	30.8–42.8 mmHg (4.10–5.69 kPa)	25.2–36.8 mmHg (3.35–4.89 kPa)
PO_2	80.9–103.3 mmHg (10.76–13.74 kPa)	95.4–118.2 mmHg (12.69–15.72 kPa)
[HCO_3^-]	18.8–25.6 mmol/l	14.4–21.6 mmol/l
Base excess	0 ± 4	0 ± 4

Figure B.9: Approximate normal arterial blood gas values for dogs and cats breathing room air.

Blood sampling – (b) venous

Indications/Use

- To obtain a sample of venous blood for clinical pathology

Contraindications

- Coagulopathy
- Sampling should not be performed at sites where risk of bacterial contamination and infection are high (e.g. due to local tissue damage, local skin infection, diarrhoea, urinary incontinence)

Equipment

- Clippers
- Hypodermic needles:
  - Cats: 21–23 G; $^5/_8$ inch
  - Dogs: 21 G; $^5/_8$ or 1 inch
- 2–10 ml syringes
- 70% surgical spirit
- 4% chlorhexidine gluconate or 10% povidone–iodine
- Cotton wool or gauze swabs
- 25 mm wide self-adhesive non-adherent bandage (e.g. Vetrap)
- Appropriate blood tubes for tests required (Figure B.10)

Patient preparation and positioning

- Venous blood sampling is performed in the conscious animal, although sedation may be required in fractious animals
- Cats can be wrapped in a large towel to control their limbs when sampling from the jugular vein; for sampling a peripheral vein, the target limb can be excluded from the towel
- The animal should be positioned appropriately for the blood collection site (see below)
- A generous area over the target vein should be clipped, sufficient to allow identification of the vein and the direction in which it runs
- Using cotton wool or gauze swabs, the skin over the vein should be cleaned with 4% chlorhexidine or 10% povidone–iodine, followed by spraying or wiping with surgical spirit

---

REDUCING STRESS

- Many cats and some dogs are frightened by the noise of clippers
  - Battery-operated models often make less noise and some are specifically designed to be quiet
  - Switch the clippers on at a distance from the animal while talking to it, to mask the initial noise
  - If the animal is fear-aggressive or particularly nervous, using a peripheral vein, which can be clipped with curved scissors, should be considered
- Applying a local anaesthetic cream (e.g. EMLA) or spray (e.g. Intubeaze) to the skin may help to reduce resistance from the animal

---

Additives	Universal *	Vacutainer *	Sample	Tests	Comments
EDTA	Pink / Red	Lavender or Pink	Whole blood	Haematology	Fill tube precisely to level indicated. Underfilling may cause artefacts; overfilling may lead to clotting
None	White / Clear	Red	Serum	Biochemistry; bile acids; serology	
Serum gel	Brown	Gold	Serum	Biochemistry; bile acids; serology	
Lithium heparin	Orange or Green	Green or Orange	Plasma	Biochemistry; electrolytes	Do not use blood that has been mixed with EDTA
Sodium fluoride and potassium oxalate	Yellow	Grey	Whole blood	Blood glucose	Fluoride/oxalate inhibits red blood cells oxidizing glucose
Sodium citrate	Lilac	Light blue	Whole blood	Coagulation tests; platelet counts	

Figure B.10: Blood tubes used for collecting samples. *Always check cap colour codes, as they may vary with manufacturer.

Sites

- The jugular vein is usually preferred, as it is large enough to allow a sample to be withdrawn rapidly without requiring excessive negative pressure. This minimizes haemolysis and blood clot formation within the sample
- The cephalic vein and the lateral saphenous vein may be used in certain situations:
  - If the jugular vein is not accessible
  - If the animal resents being restrained for jugular sampling
  - If there is a planned procedure that may be compromised by jugular vein haematoma or haemorrhage (e.g. jugular catheter placement or thyroid surgery)

Jugular vein

- The animal is placed in a sitting position, either on a table (cats and small dogs) or on the floor (large dogs)
- An assistant positions themselves to one side of the patient
- The assistant places their arm over the patient's back and round the front of the patient, to encircle and control the forelimbs
- The assistant's other arm is used to extend the animal's neck by grasping its muzzle and directing the nostrils towards the ceiling
- Fear-aggressive cats, or those that are especially fractious, can be restrained for jugular sampling by placing them on their side or on their back, controlling the limbs with the hands and body, or wrapping the cat in a towel
- With one hand, the vein should be raised by applying gently pressure to the jugular groove at around the level of the jugular inlet (Figure B.11)

Cephalic vein

- The animal is placed in a sitting position or in sternal recumbency, either on a table (cats and small dogs) or on the floor (large dogs)
- An assistant positions themselves to one side of the patient
- The assistant passes their hand under the patient's neck and holds the head turned away from the clinician
- The assistant's other arm is used to extend the patient's forelimb
- The assistant holding the animal raises the vein by wrapping a thumb around the forelimb just distal to the elbow, and then gently rotating their wrist to encourage the vein on to the cranial aspect of the forelimb (Figure B.12)

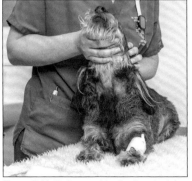

Figure B.11: Patient positioning for obtaining blood samples from the jugular vein.

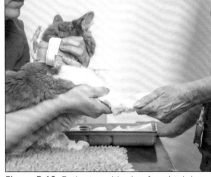

Figure B.12: Patient positioning for obtaining blood samples from the cephalic vein.

Lateral saphenous vein

- The animal is placed in lateral recumbency, either on a table (cats and small dogs) or on the floor (large dogs)
- An assistant restrains the animal's head with one hand
- With the other hand, the assistant extends the uppermost hindlimb, at the same time stretching out the body
- The assistant raises the vein by encircling the caudal aspect of the upper hindlimb, applying pressure at the level of the stifle (Figure B.13)

Technique

1 Insert the needle into the vein with syringe attached and the bevel pointing upwards, at an angle of approximately 30 degrees.
2 Follow the line of the vein with the needle tip (Figure B.14).

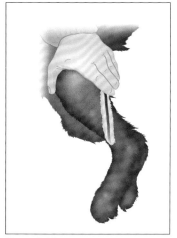

Figure B.13: Patient positioning for obtaining blood samples from the lateral saphenous vein.

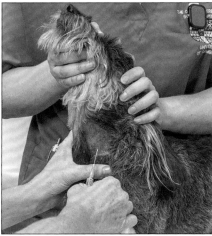

Figure B.14: The line of the vein should be followed with the needle tip.

3 Aspirate blood by applying gentle negative pressure to the syringe plunger. Avoid excessive suction on the syringe, as this may collapse the vein. If no blood is present in the hub, try gently redirecting the needle to enter the vein, but avoid large sweeping movements. If necessary, withdraw the needle and start again with a fresh one.
4 Release the pressure on the vein.
5 Remove the needle. If the sample was obtained from the jugular vein, apply gentle pressure to the venepuncture site for 30–60 seconds. If the cephalic or saphenous vein was used, apply a light bandage of gauze swab or cotton wool held by cohesive bandage for 30–60 minutes.
6 Place the blood sample into the appropriate tube(s).

EDTA TUBES

Blood should be placed in the tube containing EDTA anticoagulant last, as inadvertent contamination of other sample collection tubes with EDTA can adversely affect the results of several biochemical parameters including potassium, calcium and alkaline phosphatase.

---

7 Gently invert the sample tube(s) several times to ensure adequate distribution of any additive. Do NOT shake the tube, as this may cause haemolysis.

Potential complications

These are very uncommon but may include:

- Minor haemorrhage
- Subcutaneous haematoma formation
- Thrombophlebitis

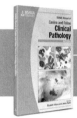

FURTHER INFORMATION

For information on the interpretation of blood samples, see the *BSAVA Manual of Canine and Feline Clinical Pathology.*

Blood smear preparation

Indications/Use

- Assessment of:
  - White blood cell differential count
  - Leucocyte abnormalities (e.g. toxic neutrophils, left shift, blast cells)
  - Red blood cell morphology (e.g. polychromasia, anisocytosis, fragmented cells, spherocytes, Heinz bodies, parasites)
  - Platelet count
  - Platelet abnormalities (e.g. macroplatelets, platelet clumps)

Equipment

- Fresh blood collected in an EDTA anticoagulant tube (see **Blood sampling – (b) venous**)
- Microhaematocrit tube
- Microscope slides
- A 'spreader' slide: this is narrower than the smear slide to avoid spreading the cells over the edge of the slide. 'Spreaders' can be made by breaking the corner off a normal slide, having first scored it with a blade or diamond writer

- Hairdryer
- Suitable stain (e.g. Diff Quik)
- Microscope
- Immersion oil

Technique

1 Invert the EDTA tube several times to make sure the blood is well mixed. Remove a small amount of blood using a microhaemocrit tube held at a near horizontal angle.

2 Place a small drop of blood on the midline of a microscope slide, towards one end (Figure B.15a).

3 Hold the 'spreader' between the thumb and middle finger, placing the index finger on top of the 'spreader' (Figure B.15b).

4 Place the 'spreader' in front of the blood spot, at an angle of about 30 degrees, and draw it backwards until it comes into contact with the blood, allowing the blood to spread out rapidly along the edge of the 'spreader' (Figure B.15c).

5 The moment this occurs, while keeping the 'spreader' slide at the same angle, move it rapidly yet smoothly away from you to create a blood smear (Figure B.15d).

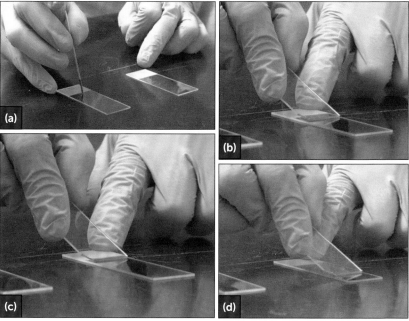

Figure B.15: (a) A small amount of blood should be placed on a microscope slide. (b) The 'spreader' slide should be held between the thumb and middle finger with the index finger placed on top of the 'spreader'. (c) The 'spreader' should be placed in front of the blood spot and drawn backwards until it comes into contact with the blood. (d) The 'spreader' slide should be kept at the same angle and moved rapidly yet smoothly away to create a blood smear.

6   As the smear is made, a 'feathered edge' forms. Do not lift the 'spreader' slide until the feathered edge is complete.
7   Ideally, the smear should extend approximately two-thirds of the length of the slide.
8   Rapidly air-dry the blood smear by waving it in the air or using a hairdryer.
9   The smear can be sent to an external laboratory or stained in house with Romanowsky-type stains (e.g. Diff-Quik) for routine examination.

PRACTICAL TIP

Figure B.16 details the common faults encountered when making blood smears and how to avoid them.

Fault	How to avoid
Film too thick	Use a smaller drop of blood
Film too thin	Use a larger drop of blood and/or faster spreading motion
Alternating thick and thin bands	Ensure spreading motion is smooth and avoid hesitation
Streaks along length of the smear	Ensure edge of 'spreader' is not irregular or coated with dried blood Ensure no dust on slide or in blood
'Holes' in smear	Ensure slide is free of grease
Narrow, thick smear	Allow blood to spread right across 'spreader' slide before making smear

Figure B.16: Faults and how to avoid them.

Examination

The stained smear is examined using a microscope:

1   Scan the whole smear at low power (X100 total magnification).
2   Examine areas of interest under higher power (X1000, using oil immersion).
3   Focus on the section of the smear (typically just behind the feathered edge) that is composed of a monolayer of cells.
4   Evaluate, in turn: red blood cells, white blood cells and platelets (see also **Platelet count**).

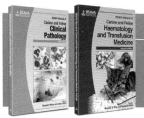

FURTHER INFORMATION

For information on the interpretation of blood smears see the *BSAVA Manual of Canine and Feline Clinical Pathology* and in the *BSAVA Manual of Canine and Feline Haematology and Transfusion Medicine*.

Blood transfusion – (a) collection

Donor selection

The Royal College of Veterinary Surgeons Code of Professional Conduct for Veterinary Surgeons (guidance note 25.22) states that 'Taking blood from healthy donors with the permission of the owner and with the intention of administering the blood or its products to a recipient is routine veterinary practice where there is an immediate or anticipated clinical indication for the transfusion. Such a clinical procedure would be acceptable on the scale of an individual veterinary practice or between other practices in the locality. However, the collection of blood for the preparation of blood products on a larger commercial scale for general therapeutic use in animals may require licences under the Animals (Scientific Procedures) Act 1986 (ASPA); this larger commercial scale activity would also need to be licensed under the Veterinary Medicines Regulations.'

Dogs

- Healthy and vaccinated (not within the last 14 days)
- Regularly receives prophylactic endo- and ectoparasitic treatments
- Suitable temperament
- >25 kg lean bodyweight
- 1–8 years of age
- Full haematology and biochemistry analysis, or as a minimum a packed cell volume (PCV) >35% and a normal total solids
- Ideally dog erythrocyte antigen (DEA) 1.1-negative
- No history of a previous blood transfusion
- Born and having lived in the UK its entire life

Cats

- Healthy and vaccinated (not within the last 14 days)
- Regularly receives prophylactic endo- and ectoparasitic treatments
- Suitable temperament
- Preferably indoor only (but not essential)
- Preferably 5 kg, but a minimum of 4 kg lean bodyweight
- 1–8 years of age
- Full haematology and biochemistry analysis, or as a minimum PCV >30% and a normal total solids
- Blood typed (A, B or AB)
- Ideally having undergone an echocardiogram to rule out the presence of occult cardiac disease
- Born and having lived in the UK its entire life
- Negative for feline leukaemia virus (FeLV) and feline immunodeficiency virus (FIV). These tests must be repeated prior to every donation for outdoor cats. If time permits, negative for *Mycoplasma haemofelis* evaluated by polymerase chain reaction (PCR)

Equipment

- As required for **Aseptic preparation – (a) non-surgical procedures**
- Blood collection containers:
  - **Dogs:** 250 ml or 450 ml single commercial blood collection bag containing an anticoagulant, such as citrate phosphate dextrose (CPD) or

citrate phosphate dextrose adenine-1 (CPDA-1), attached to an extension tube and a swaged-on 16 G phlebotomy needle. These closed systems are much preferred to open systems due to the reduced potential for bacterial contamination and thus prolonged shelf-life. The collection bag should be removed from its plastic storage bag and prepared according to the manufacturer's instructions
  - **Cats:** Three 20 ml syringes prefilled with anticoagulant (1 ml CPD or CPDA-1 per 7 ml whole blood), a 19 or 21 G butterfly catheter or needle, 3-way tap, short extension tubing and capped needles or syringe caps. Alternatively, a small animal single bag syringe collection system can be used; this comes with a butterfly catheter and 3-way tap
- Topical local anaesthetic cream (e.g. EMLA cream)
- Electronic scales (for weighing blood collection bags)
- Artery forceps
- Gauze swabs
- Clamping device and clamps
- Materials for a light neck bandage

Patient preparation and positioning
- Ensure that the donor meets the criteria listed above
- Most dogs are able to donate blood without being sedated
- Cats typically require sedation

EXAMPLES OF FELINE DONOR SEDATION PROTOCOLS

- Medetomidine 0.015–0.02 mg/kg i.v., butorphanol 0.3 mg/kg i.v. and midazolam 0.2 mg/kg i.v. Repeat doses of medetomidine can be administered if required. Atipamezole may be given to antagonize the medetomidine if required
- Ketamine 5 mg/kg i.m. and midazolam 0.25 mg/kg i.m. given together in the same syringe. Two separate doses of this sedative combination are prepared in advance; the second dose can be given as a 'top-up' intravenously (in 0.05–0.1 ml increments) as required

---

- If time allows, topical local anaesthetic cream should be applied at least 45 minutes prior to the procedure
- Dogs should be restrained in lateral recumbency (Figure B.17a) or in a sitting position on a table or on the floor
- Cats should be restrained in sternal recumbency with their neck extended, on their back with the neck extended (Figure B.17b) or in lateral recumbency with the neck outstretched
- In cats, an intravenous catheter should be pre-placed in a cephalic vein for the purpose of administering intravenous fluids following blood donation
- **Aseptic preparation – (a) non-surgical procedures** is carried out on the skin overlying the jugular groove

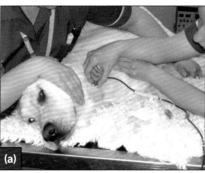
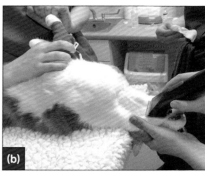

(a)   (b)

Figure B.17: Patient positioning for blood collection in **(a)** dogs and **(b)** cats.

Collection procedure

Dogs

Contamination of the venepuncture site should be avoided once it has been aseptically prepared. The phlebotomist and assistant should wear sterile gloves.

1   An assistant applies gentle pressure at the thoracic inlet to raise the jugular vein.
2   Remove the needle cap and perform venepuncture using the 16 G phlebotomy needle attached to the collection bag. If no flashback of blood is seen in the tubing, check needle placement and tubing for occlusion. The needle may need to be repositioned, but should not be fully withdrawn from the patient.
3   Place the electronic scales on a hard flat surface and zero the scale with the blood bag on it. Position the bag lower than the donor to aid in gravitational flow.
4   Mix the anticoagulant in the collection bag with the incoming blood using a gentle rocking motion at 15-second intervals.
5   Weigh the blood bag periodically. The maximum canine donation volume is approximately 16–18 ml/kg. The volume of blood that should be collected into a commercial blood bag is 450 ml, with an allowable 10% variance (405–495 ml). The weight of 1 ml of canine blood is approximately 1.053 g; therefore, the weight of an acceptable unit using one of these bags is approximately 426–521 g. However, always refer to the manufacturer's instructions.
6   When the bag is full, clamp the tubing with a pair of artery forceps and remove the needle from the jugular vein.
7   Using a gauze swab, apply pressure over the venepuncture site for 5 minutes. A light neck bandage should be applied for several hours.
8   Strip any blood remaining in the tubing into the bag, using fingers, inverting the bag several times to ensure adequate mixing. Allow the tubing to refill with anticoagulant blood and clamp the distal (needle) end with a hand sealer clip or heat sealer. If these are not available, a knot can be tied in the line, although this is less desirable.
9   Clamp the entire length of the tubing into 10 cm segments to be used for cross-matching.
10 Label the bag with the product type, donor identification, date of collection, date of expiration, donor blood type, donor PCV and phlebotomist identification prior to use or storage.

11   Following donation, food and water can be offered. Activity should be restricted to lead walks only for the next 24 hours, and it is advised that a harness or lead passed under the chest is used instead of a neck collar and lead, to avoid pressure on the jugular venepuncture site.

Cats

Contamination of the venepuncture site should be avoided once it has been aseptically prepared. The phlebotomist and assistant should wear sterile gloves.

1   Attach a syringe prefilled with anticoagulant to one port of the 3-way tap and a butterfly catheter or 21 G needle to another port. A short extension tube can be attached between the 3-way tap and the butterfly catheter.

2   Flush the tubing with anticoagulant solution.

3   If using a small animal single bag syringe collection system, prime this with anticoagulant before use.

4   An assistant applies pressure at the thoracic inlet to raise the jugular vein.

5   Perform venepuncture using the butterfly catheter or needle (bevel directed upwards). Without removing the butterfly catheter or needle, fill each syringe in turn. Rock the syringes throughout to ensure adequate mixing of blood and anticoagulant.

6   When each syringe (or the bag of the small animal single bag syringe collection system) has been filled, close the 3-way tap, remove the syringe and place a capped needle or syringe cap on the end.

7   The maximum volume of blood drawn should never exceed 18% of the total blood volume. Based on a 5 kg cat, 18% blood volume would be 60 ml. When the required amount of blood has been collected, stop raising the jugular vein and remove the butterfly catheter or needle from the vein.

8   Using a gauze swab, apply pressure over the venepuncture site for 5 minutes. A light neck bandage can be applied for several hours.

9   Label each syringe (or blood collection system bag) with the donor identification, blood type, time of collection and phlebotomist identification.

10   Immediately after blood collection, administer warmed isotonic crystalloids at a dose double the volume of blood collected, over 1–2 hours.

11   Monitor the donor's vital signs closely during recovery. Once fully awake, a light meal and water can be offered. The donor can usually be discharged after 8–12 hours. Remove the neck bandage before sending the cat home and check the venepuncture site for bleeding.

Potential complications

- Haematoma
- Hypovolaemic shock

Storage

- Whole blood collected in a bag should be stored in a refrigerator maintained at 1–6°C with the bag in an upright position. Positioning the bag in this manner maximizes gas exchange with the red cell solution to help preserve the viability of the red blood cells during storage and following transfusion
- Whole blood collected in a bag can be stored for a period of 21 days if CPD or CPDA-1 was used and the collection was performed in a sterile manner
- Blood collected using an open system (e.g. into syringes) should be administered within 4 hours, or refrigerated and used within 24 hours

Blood transfusion – (b) cross-matching

Indications/Use

- To determine serological compatibility between a patient and donor blood

Dogs

Dogs do not have naturally occurring alloantibodies to foreign red blood cells, so cross-matching prior to a first transfusion is not required. However, cross-matching should be performed whenever:

- The recipient has received a blood transfusion >4 days previously, even if a dog erythrocyte antigen (DEA) 1.1-negative donor was used
- There is a history of transfusion reactions
- The recipient's transfusion history is unknown
- The recipient has had puppies

Cats

Cats have naturally occurring alloantibodies to foreign red blood cells. Blood typing should always be performed, but as this does not detect all known blood groups, it may be best practice to perform a cross-match even prior to the first transfusion.

Equipment

- Approximately 5 ml of blood collected in an EDTA anticoagulant tube from both the donor and recipient
- Centrifuge
- 5 ml plain plastic tubes
- 0.9% sterile saline
- Pipette
- Microscope slides
- Cover slips
- Microscope

NOTE

- Commercially available cross-matching kits are available for use in dogs and cats (e.g. Alvedia Cross Match Kit, Woodley Cross Match Kit). These should be used according to the manufacturer's instructions

---

Patient preparation and positioning

See **Blood sampling – (b) venous**

Technique

1   Collect blood from the jugular veins of the donor *and* recipient. Approximately 2 ml of blood from each should be placed into separate EDTA tubes (see **Blood sampling – (b) venous**). Alternatively, a sample of anticoagulated blood from the clamped sections of tubing of the blood collection bag or collection syringes can be used.

---

2 Centrifuge the tubes (usually at 3000 RPM for 2 minutes), remove the supernatants (plasma) and transfer them to clean labelled 5 ml plain tubes (donor and recipient) for later use.

3 If a centrifuge is not available, allow the EDTA tubes to stand for ≥1 hour until the red blood cells have settled before using the supernatant.

Standard cross-match procedure

1 Wash the red blood cells three times by filling the tube with 0.9% sterile saline to resuspend the cells before centrifuging at 3000 RPM for 2 minutes. Discard the supernatant after each wash.

2 Resuspend the washed red blood cells to create a 3–5% solution by adding 0.2 ml of red blood cells to 4.8 ml of saline (1 drop of red blood cells to 20 drops of saline).

3 For each donor, prepare three tubes labelled as major, minor and recipient control.

4 To each tube add 1 drop of the appropriate 3–5% red blood cells and 2 drops of plasma according to the following:

   a Major cross-match = donor red blood cells and recipient plasma

   b Minor cross-match = recipient red blood cells and donor plasma

   c Recipient control = recipient red blood cells and recipient plasma.

5 Incubate the tubes for 15 minutes at room temperature. Note: some clinicians also recommend incubating samples at 4°C and 37°C.

6 Centrifuge the tubes at 1000 RPM for approximately 15 seconds to allow the cells to settle. Examine the samples for haemolysis (reddening of the supernatant).

7 Gently tap the tubes to resuspend the cells. Examine and score the tubes for agglutination.

8 If macroscopic agglutination is not observed, transfer one drop of the tube contents to a labelled glass slide, add a coverslip and examine for microscopic agglutination. This should not be confused with rouleaux formation (see **Haemagglutination**).

9 For the recipient control:

   a If there is no haemolysis or agglutination in the recipient control tube, the results are valid and incompatibilities can be interpreted

   b If there is haemolysis or agglutination present in the recipient control tube, then the compatibility and suitability of the donor cannot be accurately assessed.

Rapid slide cross-match procedure

An alternative and more rapid, but potentially less accurate, procedure for cross-match analysis involves visualizing the presence of agglutination on a slide rather than in a tube.

1 For each donor prepare three slides labelled as major, minor and recipient control.

2 Place 1 drop of red blood cells and 2 drops of plasma on to each slide according to the following:

   a Major cross-match = donor red blood cells and recipient plasma

   b Minor cross-match = recipient red blood cells and donor plasma

   c Recipient control = recipient red blood cells and recipient plasma.

3 Gently rock the slides, or stir with a microhematocrit tube, to mix the plasma and red blood cells. Add a coverslip and examine for agglutination after 1–5 minutes.

4 For the recipient control: agglutination will invalidate results.

Results of cross-matching

- Any agglutination and/or haemolysis is a 'positive' result
- A positive **recipient control** indicates that the patient is autoagglutinating. This makes interpretation of the test difficult, although it may be possible to repeat the test with additional washing of the recipient's red blood cells
- A positive **major cross-match** indicates a significant antibody titre in the recipient against the donor red blood cells and **precludes the use of that donor for transfusions**

WARNING

- Despite using blood products from a cross-match-compatible donor, it is still possible for a patient to experience a haemolytic or non-haemolytic transfusion reaction. Recipient monitoring during and following the administration of blood products is essential.

- A positive **minor cross-match** indicates the presence of antibodies in the donor against the recipient red blood cells. If this reaction is strong, even small volumes of donor plasma may cause a significant transfusion reaction and precludes the use of the donor (unless the red blood cells can be washed). With a weaker reaction, packed red blood cells from the donor may be transfused

Blood transfusion – (c) typing

Indications/Use

- **Dogs:** As dog erythrocyte antigen (DEA) 1.1 is the most antigenic blood type, it is strongly advised that the DEA 1.1 status of both the donor and recipient is determined prior to transfusion. However, in an emergency, DEA 1.1 blood can be given to any dog
- **Cats: All donor and recipient cats must be blood typed** prior to transfusion, even in an emergency situation

Equipment

- Approximately 2 ml of blood collected into an EDTA tube (see **Blood sampling – (b) venous**)
- Blood can be submitted to a commercial laboratory for typing
- Alternatively, commercial kits are available for in-house typing (two examples are given below)

Dogs

- Quick Test DEA 1.1 (preferred method): This immunochromatographic test uses monoclonal antibodies to determine whether a dog is DEA 1.1 positive or negative. A line adjacent to the DEA 1.1 line and the control line indicates that the dog is positive for this blood group

- Rapid Vet-H test: This is a test card with three test 'wells' used for determining whether a dog is DEA 1.1 positive or negative (Figure B.18). Two wells contain anti-DEA 1.1 antibodies and there is also a 'control' well that contains no anti-DEA 1.1 reagent. Interpretation is based on looking for the presence or absence of agglutination in the patient test well; this should also be compared with the control well

Cats

- Quick Test A+B (preferred method): This immunochromatographic test uses monoclonal antibodies to differentiate blood types. A line adjacent to the relevant blood group (A or B) and the control line (C) indicates the cat's blood group (Figure B.19a)

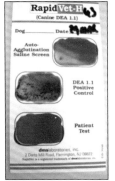

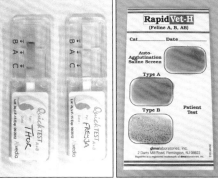

Figure B.18: Rapid Vet-H test for blood typing in dogs.

Figure B.19: (a) Quick Test A+B and **(b)** Rapid Vet-H test for blood typing in cats.

- Rapid Vet-H test: This is a test card with three test 'wells' (Figure B.19b). The type A well contains anti-type A reagent, whilst the type B well contains anti-type B reagent. There is also a 'control' well containing no anti-A or anti-B reagents. Interpretation is based on looking for an agglutination reaction in either or both test wells; this should also be compared with the control well

WARNING

- Care should be taken when blood typing severely anaemic dogs and cats. The *prozone effect* (due to the low number of red blood cells, the quantity of antigen is reduced compared with the amount of antibody in the reagent) may prevent proper agglutination of blood with the reagent. It may be helpful to centrifuge the whole blood sample and remove one drop of the plasma, to therefore increase the relative concentration of red blood cells. The red blood cells and plasma are then remixed prior to performing the blood typing test.
- Despite using blood products from a blood-typed donor, it is still possible for a patient to experience a haemolytic or non-haemolytic transfusion reaction. Recipient monitoring during and following administration of blood products is essential.

Patient preparation and positioning

See **Blood sampling – (b) venous**

Technique

Use a commercial blood typing test kit and follow the manufacturer's instructions.

Blood transfusion – (d) giving

Indications/Use

- Anaemia
- Coagulopathies, although consideration should be given to the use of fresh frozen plasma or cryoprecipitate. Stored whole blood will be severely depleted in several clotting factors and platelets
- Preparation for anticipated blood loss during surgery

Contraindications

- Administration of non-typed blood to a cat or non-cross-matched blood to a dog that has previously received a blood transfusion (see **Blood transfusion – cross-matching** and **Blood transfusion – typing**)
- Administration of non-typed or non-cross-matched blood to a cat

Equipment

- As required for **Intravenous catheter placement (a) - peripheral veins**. The largest diameter catheter possible should be placed to avoid red cell haemolysis during blood administration
- Whole blood:
  - **Dogs:** As dogs do not have naturally occurring alloantibodies to foreign red blood cells, they can receive any blood type in an emergency situation. However, it is good practice, even on first transfusion, that:
    - Dog erythrocyte antigen (DEA) 1.1-negative dogs should *only* receive DEA 1.1-negative blood
    - DEA 1.1-positive dogs may receive *either* DEA 1.1-negative or -positive blood. As the majority of dogs are DEA 1.1-positive, DEA 1.1-negative blood should ideally be reserved for those dogs that really require it (i.e. DEA 1.1-negative dogs)
  - **Cats:**
    - Type A cats must *only* receive type A blood
    - Type B cats must *only* receive type B blood
    - The rarer type AB cats do not possess either alloantibody; they should ideally receive type AB blood, but when this is not available type A blood is the next best choice, followed by type B blood

---

INSPECTION OF BLOOD

Visual inspection of the blood is necessary prior to administration. Discoloration (brown, purple), the presence of clots or haemolysis may indicate bacterial contamination and the blood should not be used.

- **Dogs:** Blood infusion set incorporating an in-line filter (170–260 μm) and suitable for connecting to a 250 ml or 450 ml commercial blood collection bag
- **Cats:** Blood collected into a small animal single bag syringe collection system and a blood giving set with an in-line filter (170–260 μm) (Figure B.20a). Alternatively, blood collected into syringes can be administered via an extension set using a syringe driver (Figure B.20b). A filter should be used, such as a paediatric filter with reduced dead space or microaggregate filters of 18–40 μm (e.g. SA150 filter available from the Pet Blood Bank UK)
- Zip lock bag
- Clean bowl/tray to be used as a water bath
- Thermometer
- Drip stand
- Transfusion recording chart
- Adhesive tape

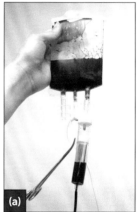
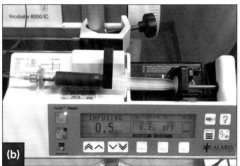

(b)

(a)

Figure B.20: Blood transfusions in cats can be administered either **(a)** using a small animal single bag syringe collection system with a giving set or **(b)** using a syringe driver and extension set.

Patient preparation and positioning

- The patient should ideally be conscious. However, it is sometimes necessary to give blood to an anaesthetized patient intraoperatively
- The patient should be placed on comfortable bedding (Figure B.21)
- Patients should not receive food or medication during a transfusion and the only fluid that may be administered through the same catheter is 0.9% sterile saline
- An **intravenous catheter** should be placed in a peripheral vein. *Alternatively*, blood can be given via an **intraosseous cannula** if venous access cannot be obtained

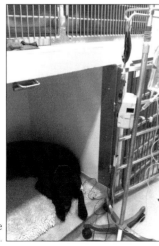

Figure B.21: The patient should be placed on comfortable bedding for the administration of a blood transfusion.

Technique

A

B

> ### NOTES
>
> - Blood is usually administered intravenously via an intravenous catheter, but it may also be given via the intraosseous route if venous access cannot be obtained (e.g. kittens, puppies). It should *not* be given intraperitoneally
> - If time allows, blood should be warmed gently to room temperature. However, if preferred, it can be warmed to body temperature (37°C) using a warm water bath. The temperature of the water bath must be monitored using a thermometer, as it must not exceed 37°C. Blood bags should be placed in plastic zip lock bags to prevent contamination of the ports. Incorrect warming may lead to haemolysis of red cells, as well as provide favourable conditions for the proliferation of any microbial contaminants
> - Care should be taken if blood is administered to patients with an increased risk of volume overload (e.g. cardiovascular disease, impaired renal function)
> - Blood should not be given through a catheter that contains, or has contained without flushing, calcium-containing fluids (e.g. Hartmann's (lactated Ringer's) solution, Ringer's solution, some colloids)
> - Gloves should be worn when handling blood products, as it is critical to try to maintain sterility as much as possible

Volume

The amount of whole blood to be administered can be calculated as follows:

- As a 'rule of thumb':
  - 2 ml whole blood/kg bodyweight raises the packed cell volume (PCV) by 1%
- Suggested formulae for calculating the amount of whole blood required for transfusion are:

CATS

Volume of donor blood required =

recipient's bodyweight (kg) x **60** x $\dfrac{\text{desired PCV} - \text{recipient's PCV}}{\text{PCV of donated blood}}$

DOGS

Volume of donor blood required =

recipient's bodyweight (kg) x **85** x $\dfrac{\text{desired PCV} - \text{recipient's PCV}}{\text{PCV of donated blood}}$

- **Total volume given should not exceed 22 ml/kg unless there are severe ongoing losses**

Rate

The rate of whole blood administration depends on the cardiovascular status of the recipient:

- In general, the rate should be only 0.25−0.5 ml/kg/h for the first 20−30 minutes
- If the transfusion is well tolerated, the rate may then be increased to around 5−10 ml/kg/h, aiming to deliver the remaining product within 4 hours. *Blood should not be administered over a period longer than 4 hours owing to the increased risk of bacterial proliferation within the product*
- In an animal with an increased risk of volume overload (cardiovascular disease, impaired renal function), the rate of administration should not exceed 3−4 ml/kg/h
- In an emergency (e.g. severe acute haemorrhage), red cells can be given at a much faster rate with care

---

WARNING

- Fluid pumps should NOT be used for red blood cell transfusions unless they have been validated appropriately for such use by the manufacturer because they could induce red cell haemolysis.

Monitoring

- Continuous monitoring during the transfusion is required for signs of a reaction
- The following parameters should be recorded prior to the transfusion ('baseline'), every 5 minutes during the first 30 minutes of the transfusion, and then every 15 minutes for the remainder of the transfusion:
  - Demeanour
  - Rectal temperature
  - Pulse rate and quality
  - Respiratory rate and character (see **Cardiorespiratory examination**)
  - Mucous membrane colour and capillary refill time
  - Plasma and urine colour
- PCV and total protein should also be monitored prior to, upon completion of, and at 12 and 24 hours after transfusion
- Transfusion records should be kept for future reference

Adverse reactions and action required

Acute haemolytic reaction with intravascular haemolysis

- Seen in type B cats receiving type A blood, as well as in DEA 1.1-negative dogs sensitized to DEA 1.1 upon repeated exposure
- Clinical signs may include fever, tachycardia, dyspnoea, muscle tremors, vomiting, weakness, collapse, haemoglobinaemia and haemoglobinuria
- May lead to shock, disseminated intravascular coagulation, renal damage and, potentially, death
- **Treatment involves immediate discontinuation of the transfusion** and treatment of the clinical signs of shock

Non-haemolytic immunological reactions

- Acute type I hypersensitivity reactions (allergic or anaphylactic), most often mediated by immunoglobulin E and mast cells
- Clinical signs including urticaria, pruritus, erythema, oedema, vomiting and dyspnoea secondary to pulmonary oedema
- **Treatment involves immediate discontinuation of the transfusion** and evaluation of the patient for evidence of haemolysis and shock. Steroids (dexamethasone 0.5–1.0 mg/kg i.v.) and antihistamines (chlorphenamine 4–8 mg q8h for dogs; 2–4 mg q8–12h for cats) may be required

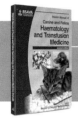

FURTHER INFORMATION

For information on blood collection, cross-matching, typing and giving, see the *BSAVA Manual of Canine and Feline Haematology and Transfusion Medicine.*

Bone biopsy – needle core

Indications/Use

- To obtain a sample of bone in suspected cases of:
  - Primary bone tumours
  - Metastatic bone tumour
  - Bacterial osteomyelitis
  - Mycosis
- To obtain a bone marrow core biopsy sample

Contraindications

- Coagulopathy
- Fracture in the region to be sampled
- Significant skin or soft tissue infection over the site of collection

Equipment

- Jamshidi bone biopsy needle (Figure B.22a):
  - 12 G for dogs >5 kg
  - 14 G for dogs <5 kg and cats
- *Alternatively*, an Arrow® OnControl® Powered Bone Access System (Figure B.22bc):
  - Power driver
  - Bone marrow biopsy tray containing connector and sterile sleeve
  - Biopsy needle
    - 11 G, 152 mm
    - 11 G, 102 mm
- As required for **Aseptic preparation – (a) non-surgical procedures**

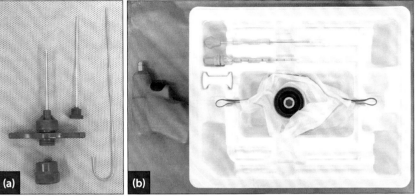

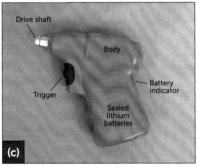

Figure B.22: A bone biopsy can be performed using **(a)** a Jamshidi needle or **(b)** the Arrow® OnControl® Powered Bone Access System. The plastic tray contains the connector and sterile sheath along with a biopsy needle. **(c)** The power driver (drill) is orange.

- Scalpel and No.10 scalpel blade
- Tissue glue or suture materials for skin closure
- Container of 10% neutral buffered formalin
- Plain sterile tube for culture (if required)

Patient preparation and positioning

- General anaesthesia is essential for both dogs and cats
- The animal should be positioned with the area to be sampled uppermost:
    - In cases of suspected tumour, bacterial osteomyelitis or mycosis, the centre of the lesion should be sampled, as sampling the periphery will often yield only samples of the reactive bone surrounding the primary lesion. The centre of the lesion is identified by radiography or another diagnostic imaging modality
    - When collecting a bone marrow core biopsy sample, the anatomical site for needle insertion is the same as for **bone marrow aspiration**. However, if following **bone marrow aspiration**, insertion at a slightly different point (on the same limb) or on the contralateral limb is preferable
    - In cases of bone tumour, the biopsy tract may need to be excised during definitive treatment; careful consideration should therefore be given to its location
- **Aseptic preparation – (a) non-surgical procedures** is performed at the site on an area approximately 10 cm × 10 cm centred on the point of needle insertion

Technique

1 Make a small skin incision with a scalpel blade over the site of needle insertion.
2 Two options are described: Jamshidi needle and the Arrow® OnControl® Powered Bone Access System.

If using a Jamshidi needle:

a With the stylet of the Jamshidi needle in place, advance the needle through the soft tissues until bone is reached (Figure B.23). If the lesion to be biopsied is at the periphery of the bone, remove the stylet. If the lesion is deeper within the bone or a bone marrow core biopsy is required, leave the stylet in place.

b Advance the needle using steady and very firm pressure with clockwise and anticlockwise drilling movements in one plane, with the needle remaining perpendicular to the bone.

c If the stylet is in place, remove it when the lesion to be biopsied has been reached or the cortex has been penetrated (when collecting a core biopsy sample).

d Advance the needle a sufficient distance into the bone (1–3 cm) such that the lumen of the needle is filled with a core of bone. The opposite cortex should not be penetrated.

e Section the core of bone from its source at the distal tip of the needle by rotating and moving the handle of the bone marrow needle vigorously in different directions (circular motion and side to side), and then twisting the needle within the bone clockwise a few times and then anticlockwise. These movements should be performed with reasonable force to ensure the core will not be left behind when the needle is withdrawn.

f Remove the needle from the bone. This is usually achieved by pulling back firmly on the needle whilst twisting it gently.

If using the Arrow® OnControl® Powered Bone Access System:

a With the stylet of the biopsy needle in place, advance it through the soft tissues until bone is reached. If the lesion to be biopsied is at the periphery of the bone, remove the stylet. If the lesion is deeper within the bone or a bone marrow core biopsy is required, leave the stylet in place. An assistant

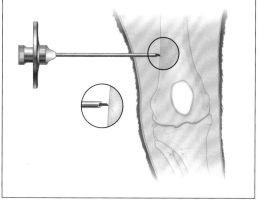

Figure B.23: The Jamshidi needle should be advanced through the soft tissues to the bone with the stylet *in situ*.

may be required to hold the needle in place. Alternatively, the needle can be attached directly into the driver without pre-placing it on to the bone.

b Open the product tray and insert the non-sterile driver into the black connector in the tray. Note: the connector contains a driver connection end (Figure B.24a) and a needle connection end (Figure B.24b).

c Using sterile gloved hands, pull the sterile sleeve over the driver. Remove the white tag on the sleeve to expose adhesive film, fold the sleeve over to adhere, and then roll the sleeve down towards the driver. Fold the blue tabs inwards to close the sleeve around the drill.

d Gently attach the driver to the biopsy needle, which can be pre-positioned on the bone; an audible click indicates attachment. Engage the driver trigger continuously and apply gentle downward pressure to penetrate the cortex.

e If the stylet is still in place, remove it when the lesion to be biopsied has been reached or (when collecting a core biopsy sample) the cortex penetrated. To do this, lift the black collar on the connector and then lift the driver and connector up and off the needle hub (Figure B.25).

f Squeeze the trigger gently to advance the biopsy needle a sufficient distance into the bone (1–3 cm) such that the lumen of the needle is filled with a core of bone. The opposite cortex should not be penetrated.

g Release the trigger when the required depth is reached.

h Remove the needle from the bone by gently squeezing the trigger on the drill whilst pulling the needle back.

i Disconnect the driver and connector from the needle by lifting the black collar on the connector and lifting the driver and connector up and off the needle hub (Figure B.25).

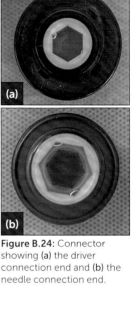

(a)

(b)

Figure B.24: Connector showing **(a)** the driver connection end and **(b)** the needle connection end.

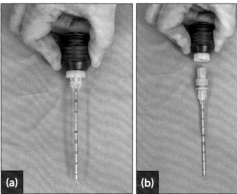

(a)

(b)

Figure B.25: (a–b) Disconnecting and removing the connector from the needle.

3   Insert the blunt probe retrograde into the tip of the needle to expel the specimen through the handle end. This is important as the needle tapers towards the free end (Figure B.26).

4   Place the specimen into an appropriate collection pot.

5   **If obtaining a sample in cases of suspected tumour, bacterial osteomyelitis or mycosis, it is very important to repeat the procedure with redirection of the needle to obtain multiple core samples (Figure B.27).**

6   The skin incision should be sutured or closed with tissue adhesive.

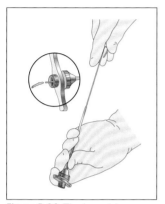

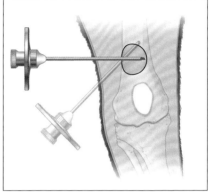

Figure B.26: The bone biopsy specimen is removed from the needle using a blunt probe.

Figure B.27: Multiple samples should be obtained from patients with suspected tumours, osteomyelitis and mycosis.

Sample handling

- The sample should be fixed in 10% neutral buffered formalin
- The sample should be sent to a histopathology laboratory. Note that the sample will have to be decalcified at the laboratory; this process may take several days
- In cases of suspected bacterial osteomyelitis or mycosis, an additional sample should be placed in a sterile plain tube and submitted to the laboratory for culture

Potential complications

- It is possible that bacterial and fungal infections may spread into the surrounding soft tissues during bone biopsy
- Lameness may be exacerbated by biopsy
- Rarely, bone can be weakened enough for a fracture to occur. This is more likely to happen if multiple samples are taken

Bone marrow aspiration

Indications/Use

To obtain a sample of bone marrow for cytology to aid diagnosis/staging in:

- Non-regenerative anaemia, neutropenia or thrombocytopenia
- Unexplained leucocytosis, polycythaemia or thrombocytosis
- Abnormal or atypical cells in circulation
- Pyrexia of unknown origin
- Hyperproteinaemia associated with a monoclonal or polyclonal gammopathy
- Unexplained hypercalcaemia

SAMPLING OPTIONS

- Two types of bone marrow sample are collected for diagnostic purposes:
  - A bone marrow aspirate provides cytological (morphological) information on individual cells
  - A bone marrow core biopsy (see **Bone biopsy – needle core**) allows evaluation of the degree of cellularity and the presence or absence of infiltration with fat or fibrous tissue
- Ideally, both should be collected, but sometimes the presence of bone marrow disease makes sample collection difficult and only one type of sample can be obtained

---

Contraindications

- Coagulopathy
- Fracture in the region to be sampled
- Significant skin or soft tissue infection over the site of collection

Equipment

- As required for **Aseptic preparation – (a) non-surgical procedures**
- Klima or Rosenthal needle with interlocking stylet (Figure B.28)
  - 14 G for dogs >5 kg
  - 16 G for dogs <5 kg and cats
- *Alternatively*, a Jamshidi bone biopsy needle can be used (see Figure B.22a):
  - 12 G for dogs >5 kg
  - 14 G for dogs <5 kg and cats
- *Alternatively*, the Arrow® OnControl® Powered Bone Access System can be used (see Figure B.22b). This comprises:
  - Power Driver
  - Bone marrow biopsy tray containing connector and sterile sleeve
  - Aspiration needle:
    - 15 G, 25 mm
    - 15 G, 68 mm
- 20 ml syringe
- Approximately 1 ml of acid citrate dextrose (ACD) removed from a blood transfusion collection bag

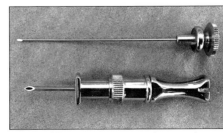

Figure B.28: A bone marrow aspirate can be obtained using a Klima needle.

B

- Local anaesthetic
- Scalpel and No.10 scalpel blade
- 10–12 clean microscope slides laid out
- Hairdryer
- EDTA collection tube
- Container of 10% neutral buffered formalin (for submission of a small core biopsy sample, if obtained)
- Tissue glue or suture materials for skin closure

> **PRACTICAL TIP**
>
> To prevent the bone marrow clotting, anticoagulant can be drawn up into the 20 ml syringe to coat the entire barrel, and then removed from the syringe while flushing the bone marrow needle with the stylet removed. The stylet should then be replaced in the bone marrow needle.

Sites used for bone marrow aspiration

- Dogs:
  - Iliac crest
  - Greater tubercle of humerus
  - Trochanteric fossa of the femur
- Cats:
  - Greater tubercle of humerus
  - Trochanteric fossa of the femur

Patient preparation and positioning

- In dogs, heavy sedation and local anaesthesia are usually sufficient, although the more inexperienced clinician may prefer general anaesthesia
- In cats, general anaesthesia should be used
- At least one assistant is necessary, to aid with positioning the animal for needle insertion and also to help with making smears of the bone marrow
- **Aseptic preparation – (a) non-surgical procedures** should be performed on an area approximately 10 cm x 10 cm, centred on the point of needle insertion
- Patient positioning varies with site of sampling:
  - Iliac crest: sternal recumbency with both hindlimbs pushed tightly under the body (Figure B.29)
  - Humerus: lateral recumbency
  - Femur: lateral recumbency
- Local anaesthetic should be infiltrated into the skin, subcutis and periosteum. The use of a long-acting local anaesthetic to provide analgesia following the procedure should be considered

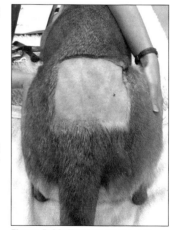

Figure B.29: The animal should be placed in sternal recumbency for obtaining bone marrow aspirates from the iliac crest.

Technique

1 Make a small stab incision in the skin over the required site (Iliac crest; greater tubercle of humerus; or trochanteric fossa of the femur).

2 Introduce the bone biopsy needle with the stylet in place through the skin and subcutis and on to the bone. If using the Arrow® OnControl® Powered Bone Access System, insert the aspiration needle associated with this, with the stylet in place. Alternatively, the needle can be attached directly into the driver without pre-placing it on to the bone.

   a **Iliac crest:** Insert the needle into the widest and most dorsal aspect of the iliac crest (Figure B.30). The needle should be aimed down the centre of the iliac crest, which can be found by placing a finger on either side of the bone or by gently redirecting the needle off either side of the bone. The needle should be directed slightly caudally and remain approximately perpendicular to the skin during insertion.

   b **Humerus:** Insert the needle into the greater tubercle of the proximal humerus and align it with the long axis (shaft) of the humerus (Figure B.31).

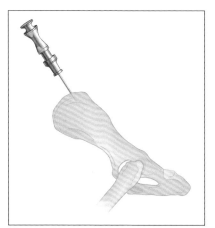

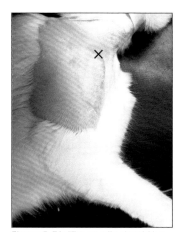

Figure B.30: The needle should be inserted into the widest and most dorsal aspect of the iliac crest.

Figure B.31: The needle should be inserted into the greater tubercle of the proximal humerus (black X).

Alternatively, in medium to large dogs, insert the needle on the craniolateral flattened aspect of the proximal humerus, perpendicular to the long axis of the bone (Figure B.32). The needle insertion point is made more accessible if an assistant rotates the elbow medially; this limb position should be maintained at all times.

   c **Femur:** Palpate the greater trochanter and insert the needle medial to this and into the trochanteric fossa. Once the needle is in the trochanteric fossa, advance it parallel to the long axis (shaft) of the femur (Figure B.33). The needle insertion point is made more accessible if an assistant stabilizes the femur by grasping the stifle and applies slight internal (medial) rotation.

A
B
C
D
E
F
G
H
I
J
K
L
M
N
O
P
Q
R
S
T
U
V
W
X
Y
Z

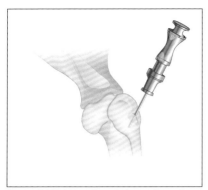

Figure B.32: In medium to large dogs, the needle can be inserted on the craniolateral flattened aspect of the proximal humerus.

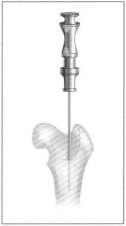

Figure B.33: The needle should be inserted into the trochanteric fossa.

WARNING

- It is important to remember that the sciatic nerve is located caudal to the femur and can be damaged if the needle slips caudal to the femur. Sciatic nerve damage can be avoided by walking the needle off the medial edge of the greater trochanter.

---

3 Enter the medullary cavity:

   a **If using a Klima, Rosenthal or Jamshidi bone biopsy needle:**

      i. Gradually advance the needle using steady and very firm pressure with a drilling action (clockwise and anticlockwise movements in one plane, with the needle perpendicular) until the needle enters the medullary cavity

      ii. Entry into the medullary cavity is detected as a decrease in resistance to needle insertion into the bone or increased stability of the needle within the bone. When the needle is properly seated within the medullary cavity, movement of the needle will result in the same movement of the bone.

   b **If using the Arrow® OnControl® Powered Bone Access System:**

      i. Open the product tray and insert the non-sterile driver into the black connector in the tray. Note the connector contains a driver connection end and a needle connection end (see Figure B.24)

      ii. Using sterile gloved hands, pull up the sterile sleeve over the driver. Remove the white tag on the sleeve to expose adhesive film, fold the sleeve over to adhere, and then roll the sleeve down towards the driver. Fold the blue tabs inwards to close the sleeve around the drill

      iii. Gently attach the driver to the biopsy needle, which is recommended to be pre-positioned on the bone; an audible click indicates attachment. Engage the driver trigger continuously and apply gentle downward pressure to penetrate the cortex

iv. Entry into the medullary cavity may be detected as a decrease in resistance to needle insertion into the bone or increased stability of the needle within the bone. Alternatively, the needle should be inserted approximately 1 cm, which is usually enough to enter the medullary cavity. When the needle is properly seated within the medullary cavity, movement of the needle will result in the same movement of the bone

v. Release the trigger when the required depth is reached

vi. Disconnect the driver and connector from the needle by lifting the black collar on the connector and lifting the driver and connector up and off the needle hub (see Figure B.25).

4 Collect the bone marrow sample:

a Remove the stylet and attach a 20 ml syringe to the needle (Figure B.34)

b Aspirate with several quite forceful withdrawals of the plunger (to around the 10 ml mark on the syringe)

c Release the plunger as soon as any blood-coloured material appears in the hub of the syringe. Bone marrow aspirate samples usually comprise <0.5 ml

d Remove the syringe, leaving the needle in place

e Immediately process the bone marrow sample (as detailed below)

f If no bone marrow is obtained, this may be due to poor needle placement or to marrow fibrosis. Replace the stylet and advance the needle a further 1.0 cm manually (or mechanically if using the Arrow® OnControl® Powered Bone Access System); remove the stylet and reapply suction. If this is still not successful, withdraw the needle, replace the stylet and redirect the needle. When two or three attempts have been unsuccessful, an alternative site should be found

g *Optional:* After obtaining a bone marrow sample, the needle may be left in place without the syringe. It can then be used to obtain a small core biopsy sample, by advancing it a further 10–20 mm into the marrow cavity, without the stylet in place. Rotate the needle vigorously in one direction and then remove it. The core sample is removed from the needle using a blunt probe or, if this is not available, the stylet. However, **bone biopsy – needle core** is the preferred method for obtaining a core sample.

5 Close the skin deficit with tissue glue or a single suture.

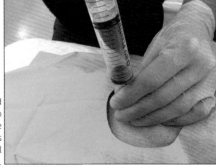

Figure B.34: A syringe should be attached to the needle to collect the sample. The plunger is released as soon as any blood-coloured material appears in the hub.

Sample handling

- Prior to aspiration, 10–20 clean microscope slides should be placed at a near-vertical angle
- A drop of marrow should be placed at the top end of each slide. Excessive blood present in the marrow sample runs down to the bottom of the slide, whilst the marrow spicules should remain at the top of the slide (Figure B.35)
- Smears of the marrow spicules should be made using the squash preparation technique (see **Fine-needle aspiration**). Smears should be made quickly, as the marrow clots rapidly (usually within 10–20 seconds). The smears should be dried by waving them in the air or by using a hairdryer
- Unstained smears should be submitted to a laboratory for analysis
- Excess marrow can be placed in an EDTA tube for cytological evaluation, although morphology will be adversely affected over time
- If a core biopsy sample is obtained, this should be placed in 10% neutral buffered formalin

Potential complications

- Significant haemorrhage is unlikely. However, in a severely thrombocytopenic patient, prolonged digital pressure should be applied to the biopsy site
- Puncture or laceration of muscles and nerves

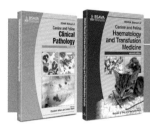

Figure B.35: A bone marrow sample should be placed at the top of the slide. Due to the near-vertical angle, any excess blood will run down to the bottom of the slide leaving the bone marrow spicules at the top.

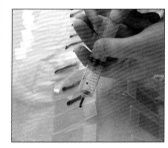

FURTHER INFORMATION

Details of the cytological evaluation of bone marrow are given in the *BSAVA Manual of Canine and Feline Clinical Pathology* and in the *BSAVA Manual of Canine and Feline Haematology and Transfusion Medicine*.

Bronchoalveolar lavage

Indications/Use

- To investigate coughing and suspected bronchial or alveolar disease
- To obtain a sample for cytology and bacteriology from the lower airways of dogs and cats

---

OPTIONS

- Bronchoalveolar lavage (BAL) is used to sample smaller airways (lower bronchioles and alveoli) and can be performed using an endoscope or 'blind'
- The upper airways of medium and large-sized dogs may also be sampled by **transtracheal wash**
- The upper airways of small dogs and cats may be sampled by **endotracheal wash**
- The advantage of BAL compared with a transtracheal wash or an endotracheal wash is that it allows more complete and accurate sampling by targeting the site of disease and is more likely to obtain a true alveolar sample. The limitation is that it requires bronchoscopic guidance and so is restricted to those practices with the appropriate facilities.

Contraindications

- Patient not stable enough to undergo anaesthesia (e.g. severe hypoxaemia, cardiac arrhythmia/dysfunction)
- Coagulopathy
- Partial tracheal obstruction
- Unstable asthma
- Pulmonary hypertension

Equipment

- As required for **Bronchoscopy** (if performed using a bronchoscope)
- A sterile bronchoalveolar lavage catheter (6 Fr, 124 cm long, with an end rather than a side hole) (Figure B.36a) or a soft urinary catheter (6–8 Fr, 30–60 cm long, with an end hole)
- 500 ml warm 0.9% sterile saline
- 5–20 ml syringes
- Sample trap (Figure B.36b)
- Suction pump and connecting tubing
- Hypodermic needles: 21 G
- Microscope slides
- EDTA and sterile plain collection tubes

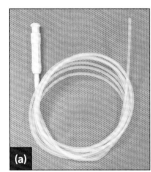

(a)

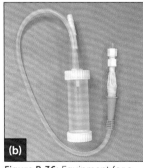

(b)

Figure B.36: Equipment for a bronchoalveolar lavage includes **(a)** a lavage catheter and **(b)** a sample trap.

Patient preparation and positioning

- Inhalation anaesthesia is generally recommended, although intravenous anaesthesia may be used. An elbow port connector can be used to provide constant gas anaesthesia when performing BAL
- Pre-oxygenation is very helpful, especially when there is compromised oxygenation. This can be provided through nasal oxygen delivery or a face mask. Supplementary oxygen can also be delivered through the channel of the endoscope or via a urinary catheter placed alongside the endoscope. Flow volumes of 1–3 litres per minute can be safely used
- The patient should be positioned in sternal recumbency with the head elevated and neck extended
- A mouth gag is essential to keep the mouth open
- A sandbag positioned under the chin can help to raise the head to a more neutral position

---

WARNING

- Care should be taken when endoscopes are placed in the airway without oxygen being delivered as significant hypoxaemia can occur. Therefore, careful monitoring of pulse oximetry is required. In addition, endoscopes can interfere with ventilation and result in hypercapnia and overventilation of the lungs, trauma and bronchospasm.

SPECIAL CONSIDERATIONS FOR CATS

Extra care should be taken when performing bronchoscopy in cats, as the airways are particularly prone to bronchospasm.

- The procedure should be performed as quickly as possible with the minimum of trauma
- As cats are prone to laryngospasm, the larynx should be sprayed with lidocaine prior to intubation. The clinician should wait 30–60 seconds for the lidocaine to desensitize the larynx before gently inserting the tube; the tube should only be inserted when the larynx is open, using a rotating motion
- If a commercially available topical lidocaine spray is being used, the clinician should be aware of the dose delivered with each depression of the pump, as toxicity may result from repeated applications. A dose of 1 mg/kg of 2% lidocaine is appropriate for use in cats (i.e. approximately 0.2 ml for a 4 kg cat)
- To reduce the risk of bronchospasm, terbutaline can be given approximately 30 minutes prior to bronchoscopy (0.015 mg/kg s.c. or i.m). The onset of action is 15–30 minutes and is usually notable by an increase in heart rate
- Terbutaline should also be available for administration during the procedure if bronchospasm still occurs. If this does not stabilize the patient, administration of a short-acting steroid (e.g. dexamethasone sodium phosphate 0.1 mg/kg i.v. once) should be considered
- A suction unit (or 10–20 ml syringe attached to a sterile urinary catheter) should be kept nearby and can be used for clearing any secretions from the oropharynx. The cat should be maintained in sternal recumbency, if possible, for this procedure. If the cat resents suctioning of the oropharynx, re-induction of anaesthesia may be required to clear the upper airway effectively

---

Technique

1 If using a bronchoscope, perform **bronchoscopy**.

2 Once the lung lobes to be sampled have been selected, pass the bronchoscope into successively smaller airways until it sits snugly (Figure B.37).

3 Pre-draw sterile saline into several syringes.

4 Instil warmed sterile saline via the biopsy channel of the endoscope:

a A bolus of 5 ml is used in cats and dogs <10 kg

b A bolus of 10–20 ml is used in dogs >10 kg.

5 Perform gentle coupage.

6 Withdraw the bronchoscope a short distance to allow you to see the sample being collected.

7 Immediately aspirate the saline from the biopsy channel using a syringe. Negative pressure during aspiration indicates the need to decrease suction to avoid airway collapse. If necessary, the bronchoscope can be repositioned slightly, taking care not to dislodge the tip of the bronchoscope from the airway in which it is wedged.

8 If air fills the syringe, eliminate it, and make additional aspiration attempts.

9 Repeat Steps 4 to 6 a maximum of three times until an adequate sample has been obtained.

10 Ideally, sample at least two lung lobes.

Alternatively, the procedure can be performed using a lavage catheter passed through the biopsy channel of an endoscope (Figure B.38). Attach either a syringe to the end of the lavage catheter for aspiration or, preferably, a sample trap connected to a suction pump.

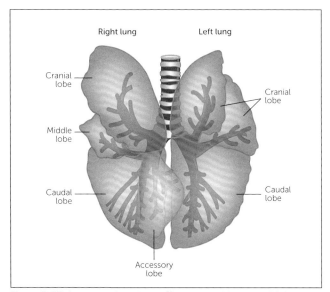

Right lung　　　Left lung

Cranial lobe

Cranial lobe

Middle lobe

Caudal lobe

Caudal lobe

Accessory lobe

Figure B.37: Anatomy of the lungs. (Reproduced from the *BSAVA Manual of Canine and Feline Endoscopy and Endosurgery*)

Alternatively, although less advisable, the procedure can be performed 'blind' using a lavage catheter or soft urinary catheter passed without endoscopic assistance. Gently introduce the catheter aseptically into the endotracheal (ET) tube just until resistance is felt; at this point the catheter should be lodged within a distal airway (Figure B.39). Sterile saline is then instilled and re-aspirated as described above.

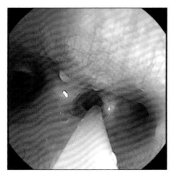

Figure B.38: A lavage catheter should be passed through the biopsy channel of an endoscope and enter a distal airway in order to perform a bronchoalveolar lavage.

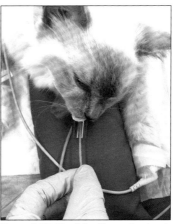

Figure B.39: The 'blind' bronchoalveolar lavage technique involves inserting a lavage catheter into a distal airway without the use of an endoscope.

11   Following BAL, continue administration of 100% oxygen and volatile agent for 5 minutes, to allow time to detect any immediate complications (e.g. bronchospasm). Continue oxygen supplementation via the ET tube until extubation. Utilize pulse oximetry to measure the patient's oxygenation throughout the recovery from anaesthesia, and during the postoperative period.

NOTE

- A total recovery of 40–90% of the instilled volume of saline represents good sample recovery. Recovered fluid is typically slightly turbid, with a foamy layer at the top (representative of surfactant) (Figure B.40)

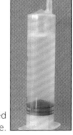

Figure B.40: Fluid sample recovered following bronchoalveolar lavage.

Sample handling

- A portion of the sample should be submitted in a sterile plain tube for culture
- An aliquot should be placed in an EDTA tube for cytology
- The cells collected are fragile, so samples should be processed as soon as

possible. If samples are to be sent to an external laboratory, fresh air-dried unstained smears of any flocculent/mucoid material should also be made (see **Fine-needle aspiration**). Direct smears of the fluid can be made, but most samples contain few cells

Potential complications

- Catheter breakage and aspiration of the catheter into the airway
- Bronchospasm
- Laryngospasm and coughing
- Haemorrhage
- Iatrogenic infection
- Pneumothorax

Bronchoscopy

Indications/Use

- Evaluation of tracheal and lower airway disorders
- Acquisition of samples (see also **Bronchoalveolar lavage**)
- Foreign body removal

Contraindications

- Patient not stable enough to undergo anaesthesia
- Significant coagulopathy
- Partial tracheal obstruction
- Unstable asthma
- Pulmonary hypertension

Equipment

- Flexible endoscope: diameter 2.5–6 mm, length 50–80 cm
- Endoscopic viewing equipment
- Topical local anaesthetic spray
- Mouth gag

BRONCHOSCOPES

The preferred bronchoscope is a 3.5–6.0 mm diameter fibreoptic endoscope with a working length of at least 55 cm. These are the typical dimensions for human bronchoscopes and an endoscope of 5 mm diameter will be adequate for most sizes of dog. For endoscopy of cats a narrower bronchoscope is needed. Endoscopes with a working length of 55 cm can be too short to adequately inspect the lobar bronchi of large breeds of dogs. Longer veterinary endoscopes are available to overcome this problem, but an alternative approach is to use a gastroduodenoscope. While such endoscopes are up to 8 mm in diameter, occlusion of the airway is relative as the dog is also larger. One problem with using an endoscope longer than 55 cm and <6 mm in diameter, or an endoscope of even narrower dimensions, is that the image tends to be less clear because there are fewer fibres to transmit light. The latest advance is the development of videobronchoscopes.

- Elbow port (Figure B.41): this connects the endotracheal (ET) tube to the breathing circuit and allows simultaneous insertion of the endoscope whilst oxygen and the volatile agent are delivered
- Pulse oximeter
- For foreign body retrieval: forceps including basket, rat-toothed, alligator, net and polyp snare-type

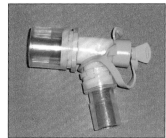

Figure B.41: An Elbow port is used to connect the endotracheal tube to the breathing circuit.

Patient preparation and positioning

- Inhalation anaesthesia is recommended; however, intubation should only be performed if the endoscope can fit easily through the ET tube, allowing for the movement of air and the endoscope at the same time. An elbow port connector can be used to provide constant gas anaesthesia whilst the endoscope is passed through the ET tube
- If it is not possible to pass the endoscope through the ET tube, intravenous anaesthesia must be used. To reduce the risk of hypoxaemia, an additional oxygen supply can be delivered via a urinary or other type of flexible narrow-gauge catheter passed adjacent to the bronchoscope. Flow volumes of 1–3 litres per minute can be used safely
- Pre-oxygenation is very helpful, especially when there is compromised oxygenation. This can be provided through nasal oxygen delivery or a face mask
- The patient should be placed in sternal recumbency with the head elevated and neck extended (Figure B.42). However, some operators prefer the patient to be in lateral recumbency as handling, introducing and operating the endoscope can be easier

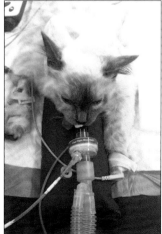

Figure B.42: Patient positioned in sternal recumbency for bronchoscopy. Unless a very narrow diameter endoscope is used, the patient will need to be extubated and the endoscope passed directly into the trachea.

- A mouth gag is essential to keep the mouth open and prevent the patient biting down on to the endoscope in the event of contact with the pharynx stimulating the gag reflex

---

WARNING

- Care should be taken when endoscopes are placed in the airway without oxygen being delivered as significant hypoxaemia can occur. Therefore, careful monitoring of pulse oximetry is required. In addition, endoscopes can interfere with ventilation and result in hypercapnia and overventilation of the lungs, trauma and bronchospasm.

SPECIAL CONSIDERATIONS FOR CATS

Extra care should be taken when performing bronchoscopy in cats, as their airways are particularly prone to bronchospasm.

- The procedure should be performed as quickly as possible with the minimum of trauma
- As cats are prone to laryngospasm, the larynx should be sprayed with lidocaine prior to intubation. The clinician should wait 30–60 seconds for the lidocaine to desensitize the larynx before gently inserting the tube; the tube should only be inserted when the larynx is open, using a rotating motion
- If a commercially available topical lidocaine spray is being used, the clinician should be aware of the dose delivered with each depression of the pump, as toxicity may result from repeated applications. A dose of 1 mg/kg of 2% lidocaine is appropriate for use in cats (i.e. approximately 0.2 ml for a 4 kg cat)
- To reduce the risk of bronchospasm, terbutaline can be given approximately 30 minutes prior to bronchoscopy (0.015 mg/kg s.c. or i.m). The onset of action is 15–30 minutes and is usually notable by an increase in heart rate
- Terbutaline should also be available for administration during the procedure if bronchospasm still occurs. If this does not stabilize the patient, administration of a short-acting steroid (e.g. dexamethasone sodium phosphate 0.1 mg/kg i.v. once) should be considered
- A suction unit (or 10–20 ml syringe attached to a sterile urinary catheter) should be kept nearby and can be used for clearing any secretions from the oropharynx. The cat should be maintained in sternal recumbency, if possible, for this procedure. If the cat resents suctioning of the oropharynx, re-induction of anaesthesia may be required to clear the upper airway effectively

Technique

1 In cats, spray the larynx with topical local anaesthetic and wait 30–60 seconds.
2 Advance the endoscope into the larynx and examine this region (Figure B.43).
3 If the patient is to be intubated, evaluate the proximal trachea prior to intubation. Intubation can be performed after evaluation of the length of the trachea that would otherwise be covered by the ET tube.

A

B

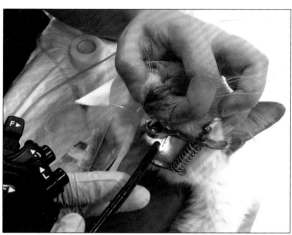

Figure B.43: Examination of the larynx with an endoscope prior to intubation.

4 Centre the endoscope as it is advanced; take care not to irritate the surface of the trachea with the endoscope.

5 As the endoscope is advanced, the carina or bifurcation is seen. The patient's right side is on the operator's left side; therefore, the right mainstem bronchus will be seen on the left side of the image. The left and right mainstem bronchi branch off crisply with sharp edges (see Figure B.37).

6 The right mainstem bronchus is in line with the trachea and should be examined first.

7 Then pass the endoscope into the left mainstem bronchus.

8 Evaluate segmental and subsegmental airways on the left and right sides as thoroughly and systematically as possible.

9 Take samples as required (see **Bronchoalveolar lavage**).

10 Following bronchoscopy, continue administration of 100% oxygen and volatile agent for 5 minutes, to allow time to detect any immediate complications (e.g. bronchospasm). The animal's respiratory rate and pattern, and ideally pulse oximetry, should be monitored continuously during the procedure and in the recovery period to observe for complications such as dyspnoea and hypoxaemia.

11 Oxygen supplementation may need to be continued following extubation until the animal is able to maintain sternal recumbency and pulse oximetry shows adequate levels of oxygen saturation (S_pO_2 >95%). Monitor respiratory pattern and rate over the following 12 hours, ideally in the hospital.

12 If complications occur in the recovery period and rapid reversal of hypoxaemia and dyspnoea cannot be achieved medically, re-induction of anaesthesia for intubation and ventilation may be required to increase oxygenation and enable investigations to determine the cause of dyspnoea.

Foreign body removal

1 Position the endoscope several centimetres proximal to the foreign body.

2 Pass the retrieval forceps, in the closed position, down the biopsy channel (if there is sufficient room) or adjacent to the endoscope.

3 Open the forceps, grasp the foreign body and close the forceps.

4 Remove the endoscope and forceps at the same time.

WARNING

- Care must be taken to provide adequate ventilation during the retrieval procedure.
- Foreign body removal can be very challenging. The veterinary surgeon should be prepared to stop and refer the animal for surgery if the procedure becomes prolonged.
- There is a risk of airway damage or rupture and the development of a pneumothorax. The equipment for thoracocentesis or thoracostomy tube placement should therefore be available.

Potential complications

- Hypoxaemia
- Bronchospasm
- Laryngospasm and coughing
- Haemorrhage
- Pneumothorax

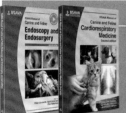

FURTHER INFORMATION

Further information on endoscope equipment and techniques can be found in the *BSAVA Manual of Canine and Feline Endoscopy and Endosurgery*. Further information on bronchoscopy and its interpretation can be found in the in the *BSAVA Manual of Canine and Feline Cardiorespiratory Medicine*.

Buccal mucosal bleeding time

Indications/Use
- Suspected primary coagulopathy

Contraindications
- Thrombocytopenia
- Known other primary haemostatic abnormality

Equipment
- Spring-loaded cutting device (e.g. Surgicutt Vet H or Simplate II)
- 2 cm wide gauze bandage
- Tissue paper/filter paper
- Stopwatch or timer

Patient preparation and positioning
- If possible, the procedure should be performed with the animal conscious
- Light sedation may be required in fractious dogs and in cats
- The patient is restrained in lateral or sternal recumbency, either on a table or on the floor

Technique
1. Fold back the patient's upper lip and hold it in place, either via an assistant or with a gauze bandage. This will impede the venous return from the lip and cause congestion.
2. Position the cutting device on the buccal mucosa, avoiding any obvious superficial vessels. Hold firmly but avoid excessive pressure.
3. Depress the trigger on the device to create a small incision in the buccal mucosa and simultaneously start the timer. Remove the cutting device approximately 1 second after triggering.
4. At 15 seconds, blot the flow of blood with filter paper placed a few millimetres below the incision, *without dislodging the clot* (Figure B.44).
5. Blot in a similar manner every 15 seconds until blood no longer stains the filter paper.

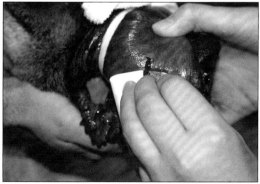

Figure B.44: Filter paper should be used to blot the blood flow every 15 seconds until the bleeding ceases.

6 Stop the timer when bleeding has ceased.

7 Record the time from making the incision to cessation of bleeding.

Results

- In healthy dogs, the buccal mucosal bleeding time (BMBT) is 1.7–3.3 minutes; this can be mildly prolonged (to 4.2 minutes) in anaesthetized or sedated dogs. The BMBT of healthy anaesthetized cats is 1.0–2.4 minutes. However, these values may differ depending on operator technique.
- A prolonged BMBT may indicate moderate to marked thrombocytopenia, thrombopathies, vasculitis or von Willebrand's disease

Potential complications

- Prolonged bleeding can occur (uncommon) but should cease with continued pressure over the incision site. If it does not, the administration of fresh frozen plasma may be required

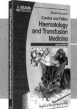

FURTHER INFORMATION

Further details on coagulation tests and abnormalities can be found in the *BSAVA Manual of Canine and Feline Haematology and Transfusion Medicine.*

Cardiopulmonary resuscitation

Indications/Use

- Confirmed cardiopulmonary arrest (CPA) or in any unresponsive apnoeic cat or dog until CPA is ruled out

---

WARNING

- Requires recognition of unresponsive apnoeic patient only, as basic cardiopulmonary resuscitation (CPR) must not be delayed.
- *Rapid* assessment of Airway, Breathing and Circulation required.

Equipment

- Organized and regularly audited crash trolley (Figure C.1), containing:
    - Cuffed endotracheal (ET) tubes: full range of sizes with stylets and dog urinary catheters for difficult intubation
    - Laryngoscope with different size blades
    - Syringe to inflate ET tube cuff
    - Open weave bandage (to secure ET tube)
    - Ambu bag (self-re-inflating bag)
    - Intravenous catheters: range of sizes
    - Intraosseous catheters
    - Dog urinary catheters for intratracheal drug administration
    - Relevant drugs (Figure C.2)
    - Needles and syringes to match drug doses required
    - Electrical defibrillator and paste/gel
    - Clippers
    - Bags of sterile fluids for intravenous administration: 0.9% sterile saline, lactated Ringer's (Hartmann's) solution and hypertonic saline or mannitol
    - Intravenous fluid administration sets
    - 0.9% sterile saline to flush intravenous/intraosseous catheters

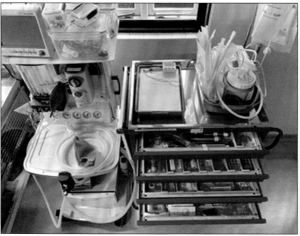

Figure C.1: Crash trolley. The drawers of the trolley are labelled to indicate the contents and the trolley should be regularly checked to ensure it is well stocked and the expiry dates of drugs have not been exceeded. An oxygen supply, breathing system and monitoring equipment should also be available.

- Monitor, pads and gel for electrocardiography
- End-tidal CO_2 (ETCO$_2$) monitor
- Oxygen saturation (S_pO_2) monitor
- Stethoscope
- Blood pressure monitor
- Equipment as required for **Thoracocentesis – needle**
- Thermometer
- Blood sample pots/tubes
- Suction machine (set up, ready to use)
- Charts (clear; in CPR area)
  - Local CPR protocol
  - Drug dosages – preferably in mg/kg and in ml for weights 5–50 kg
- Plastic trough positioning aids: range of sizes
- Oxygen supply with necessary tubing/breathing circuit
- Pen, paper and stopwatch

Patient preparation and positioning

- The patient should be placed in lateral recumbency
- Cats and small dogs may be positioned on a table; the table should be lowered for medium-, large- and giant-breed dogs or a foot stool may be required. Alternatively, larger patients can be positioned on the floor
- The operator delivering chest compressions should stand on the dorsal side of the patient

Technique

- **Priority is to begin basic life support (BLS)**
- **Advanced life support (ALS) should be started and monitored simultaneously if possible**

TIPS FOR A SUCCESSFUL OUTCOME

- Well trained team with team leader
- Regular rehearsals
- The team leader must give clear orders, which are repeated back by the team member carrying out the task, to ensure the task is completed correctly
- A nominated scribe should keep a record of the time and type of interventions performed whilst CPR is being carried out

---

Basic life support

Figure C.3 shows the CPR algorithm for BLS.

NOTES

- Each BLS cycle lasts 2 minutes
- Begin the first cycle as soon as possible and complete it uninterrupted
- Chest compressions and ventilation are carried out simultaneously
- Change person performing chest compressions between cycles to avoid fatigue

---

Indication	Drug and concentration	Dose
Cardiac arrest	Adrenaline (1:1000; 1 mg/ml) – Low dose	0.01 mg/kg
	Adrenaline (1:1000; 1 mg/ml) – High dose	0.1 mg/kg
	Vasopressin (20 IU/ml)	0.8 IU/kg
	Atropine (0.6 mg/ml)	0.04 mg/kg
Ventricular tachycardia	Lidocaine (20 mg/ml)	2 mg/kg
Ventricular fibrillation and/ or ventricular tachycardia	Amiodarone (150 mg/100 ml or 360 mg/200 ml bag sizes) Only use preparations without polysorbate 80 and benzyl alcohol solvents, which can cause anaphylactic reactions	2 mg/kg bolus over 10 minutes; can be followed by a CRI at 0.8 mg/kg/h for 6 hours, then 0.5 mg/kg/h
Drug reversal	Naloxone (0.4 mg/ml)	0.04 mg/kg
	Flumazenil (0.1 mg/ml)	0.01 mg/kg
	Atipamezole (5 mg/ml)	100 µg/kg

Figure C.2: Relevant drugs for cardiopulmonary resuscitation in cats and dogs.

Chest compressions

1 **Perform 100–120 compressions per minute.**

2 Compress the thorax by a third to a half of its resting width and allow full chest recoil between compressions.

  a **Medium and large dogs:** Place the palm of one hand over the back of the other hand with your fingers interdigitated. Apply the palms of the hands to the thorax of the animal. Keep your elbows locked in extension and push downwards through the palms of your hands. Your shoulders should be positioned vertically over your hands. For most dogs, place hands centrally over the thorax such that compressive force acts on the widest part (Figure C.4). Place hands directly over the heart for dogs with deep narrow chests. For flat-chested dogs (e.g. Bulldogs), sternal compressions can be delivered with the patient positioned in dorsal recumbency.

  b **Cats and small dogs:** Wrap a single hand around the sternum at the level of the heart and compress the thorax between your thumb and fingers (Figure C.5); or use the technique for deep narrow-chested dogs.

Ventilation

1 Carry out **endotracheal intubation** of the animal in lateral recumbency.

2 Secure the ET tube to the animal's muzzle or mandible.

3 Inflate the cuff of the ET tube.

4 Attach an Ambu bag to the ET tube or connect it to a breathing system, anaesthetic machine and oxygen source.

5 **Ventilate at 10 breaths/min with a tidal volume of 10 ml/kg and inspiratory time of 1 second.**

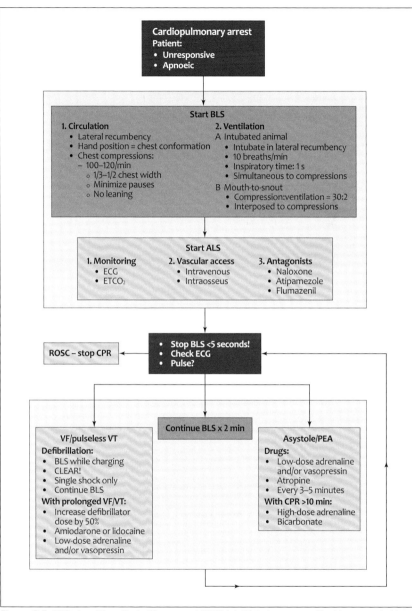

Figure C.3: CPR algorithm. Basic life support (BLS) is initiated once a patient is suspected to be in cardiopulmonary arrest (CPA) and is continued until return of spontaneous circulation (ROSC) is confirmed. Advanced life support (ALS) measures are instituted as soon as possible alongside BLS, which is only interrupted for short patient evaluations (electrocardiogram (ECG) and pulse). $ETCO_2$ = end-tidal carbon dioxide; PEA = pulseless electrical activity; VF = ventricular fibrillation; VT = ventricular tachycardia. (Reproduced from the *BSAVA Manual of Canine and Feline Emergency and Critical Care*)

C

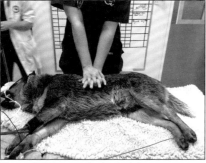

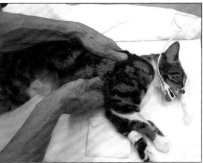

Figure C.4: In round-chested dogs, compressions should be delivered over the widest part of the chest. (Reproduced from the *BSAVA Manual of Canine and Feline Emergency and Critical Care*)

Figure C.5: Chest compression technique for basic life support in a cat or small dog.

NOTE

- If the patient is under anaesthesia when CPA occurs, immediately cease delivery of the anaesthetic agent. If using inhalational anaesthetic agents, temporarily disconnect the ET tube from the breathing system and flush the breathing system with oxygen before reconnecting to the patient and commencing ventilation

---

Advanced life support

Monitoring

- **Electrocardiography** should be carried out to identify arrhythmias
- ETCO$_2$: an indicator of correct placement of the ET tube in the trachea, adequacy of ventilation and circulation status. ETCO$_2$ of >15 mmHg (dog) or >20 mmHg (cat) should be aimed for
- Pulse: palpation should be carried out between BLS cycles; useful for the detection of return of spontaneous circulation
- Electrolytes and arterial blood gas: not mandatory but useful where electrolyte disturbance may be involved in causing CPA

Vascular access

- **Intravenous catheter placement** (preferable)
- **Intraosseous cannula placement**

NOTE

- Whilst intravenous drug administration is preferred, intratracheal drug dosing can be considered for adrenaline (0.02–0.1 mg/kg) and atropine (0.15–0.2 mg/kg); however, it may be ineffective. Insert a dog urinary catheter via the ET tube to the level of the carina. Dilute drug with saline or sterile water

---

Drug administration and defibrillation

1 If implicated in CPA, administer reversal agents for opioids (naloxone), alpha-2 agonists (atipamezole) or benzodiazepines (flumazenil) (see Figure C.2 for doses).

2 Give low-dose adrenaline (0.01 mg/kg i.v.) during every other cycle of BLS. If CPA for >10 min, consider single high-dose adrenaline injection (0.1 mg/kg i.v.). Vasopressin can be given as an alternative to, or in combination with, adrenaline during every other cycle of CPR (0.8 IU/kg).

3 If asystole or pulseless electrical activity, give atropine (0.04 mg/kg iv) during every other cycle of BLS.

4 If ventricular fibrillation (VF) or pulseless ventricular tachycardia (VT), perform electrical defibrillation.

   a If VF or pulseless VT is detected within 4 minutes of CPA, perform defibrillation immediately.

   b If VF or pulseless VT is detected after 4 minutes of CPA, perform 1 cycle of BLS before defibrillation.

     i To avoid the risk of fire, make sure there is no alcohol on the fur of the thorax.

     ii Set the electrical dose (Figure C.6).

Biphasic defibrillation	
Electrical dose	2–4 J/kg

Figure C.6: Electrical dose for biphasic defibrillation.

     iii Apply defibrillator gel or paste to the paddles.

     iv Press the paddles firmly against opposite sides of the thorax, over the heart, at the level of the costochondral junctions.

     v If two hand paddles are used, the animal will need to be placed in dorsal recumbency; a plastic trough positioning aid will help (Figure C.7a).

     vi If a posterior paddle is available, the animal can remain in lateral recumbency. The posterior paddle is positioned between the table and the animal, and the hand paddle is placed on the opposite side of the thorax (Figure C.7b).

     vii Charge the defibrillator.

     viii Operator calls 'Clear!' and ensures that no-one (including themselves) is touching the patient or the table.

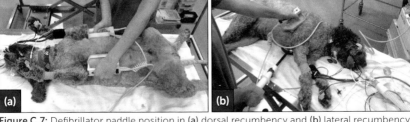

Figure C.7: Defibrillator paddle position in **(a)** dorsal recumbency and **(b)** lateral recumbency when a posterior paddle is available. (Reproduced from the *BSAVA Manual of Canine and Feline Emergency and Critical Care*)

ix Apply current to the thorax.

x Perform 1 cycle of BLS immediately.

xi Reassess electrocardiogram (ECG).

xii If VF or pulseless VT, repeat electrical defibrillation with a 50% increased dose. If VF is unresponsive to three or more attempts at defibrillation, administer amiodarone (see Figure C.2 for doses).

NOTE

- Medical conversion of VF is ineffective – electrical defibrillation is required. Lidocaine or amiodarone can be administered for VT

---

5 Supplement inspired oxygen:

  a If arterial blood gas data are available, titrate to a partial pressure of oxygen in arterial blood (P_aO_2) of 80–105 mmHg

  b If arterial blood gas data are unavailable, giving 100% of fraction of inspired oxygen (F_iO_2) is reasonable.

6 Consider intravenous fluid therapy:

  a In euvolaemic or hypervolaemic patients, do not give fluids

  b In hypovolaemic patients, give intravenous fluids to restore blood volume, but cautiously (1–2 ml/kg/h).

7 Open-chest CPR – external CPR may be ineffective in certain situations (e.g. pneumothorax, diaphragmatic hernia). *Only consider this if a specialist veterinary team and a dedicated intensive care unit are available.*

Post-CPR care

- Referral to a specialist centre should be considered
- Monitoring should be continued: ECG; $ETCO_2$; S_pO_2; arterial blood gases; blood pressure; blood electrolyte, lactate and glucose concentrations; and body temperature
- The patient should be assessed for return of spontaneous respiration. Normal respiratory function is associated with:
  - $ETCO_2$ 27–38 mmHg (dog) or 21–31 mmHg (cat)
  - P_aCO_2 32–43 mmHg (dog) or 26–36 mmHg
  - S_pO_2 94–98%
  - P_aO_2 80–100 mmHg
- The amount of supplemental oxygen should be changed appropriately in cases of hypoxaemia or hyperoxaemia
- Intermittent positive pressure ventilation (IPPV) will be required if the P_aCO_2 is abnormal, or the animal is hypoxaemic despite an F_iO_2 of 60%
- Haemodynamic status should be assessed. A normal haemodynamic status is associated with:
  - Mean arterial pressure 80–120 mmHg
  - Systolic arterial pressure 100–200 mmHg
- If hypertensive, any vasopressor treatment should be decreased, pain should be treated and antihypertensives should be considered
- If hypotensive, fluid therapy if hypovolaemic, vasopressors if vasodilated, inotropes if decreased heart contractility and blood transfusion if anaemic should be considered

- If normotensive but lactate >2.5 mmol/l, treatment for poor perfusion should be considered and the guidelines above for hypotension followed
- Temperature should be assessed:
  - Mild hypothermia (32–34°C) may be advantageous during CPA
  - Hypothermic animals should be rewarmed slowly – by 0.25–0.5°C per hour
- Neurological status should be assessed:
  - Assess for signs of cerebral oedema: coma, cranial nerve deficits, decerebrate postures and abnormal mentation. If cerebral oedema suspected, treatment with mannitol or hypertonic saline should be considered
  - Assess for signs of seizures, although seizure activity may be undetectable. Overt seizures should be treated. Prophylaxis with phenobarbital loading may be considered in an apparently normal patient

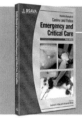

FURTHER INFORMATION

Further information on CPR is available in the *BSAVA Manual of Canine and Feline Emergency and Critical Care*. See also Fletcher *et al.* (2012) RECOVER evidence and knowledge gap analysis on veterinary CPR. Part 7: Clinical guidelines. *Journal of Veterinary Emergency and Critical Care* **22**(S1), 102–131.

Cast application

Indications/Use

- Additional external support to supplement internal fixation for:
  - Arthrodesis of the carpus/tarsus
  - Fractures of the distal limb
- Primary coaptation of selected long bone fractures that meet the following criteria:
  - Fractures distal to the elbow and stifle
  - Relatively stable fracture configuration (e.g. greenstick fractures, interdigitating transverse fractures, or fracture of one member of a pair of bones)
- Minimally displaced fractures with at least 50% overlap of the fracture ends in orthogonal radiographic views
  - Non-articular fractures
  - A predicted fracture union time of 4–6 weeks, as assessed by radiography; juvenile animals are better candidates than adults

Contraindications

- Soft tissue swelling
- Primary coaptation of fractures that do not fit the above criteria, including unstable spiral and oblique fractures, all comminuted fractures and all articular fractures

- Primary coaptation of fractures of the distal radius and ulna in small-breed dogs
- Athletic or working animals

NOTES

- Effective cast application is challenging in obese animals and chondrodystrophoid breeds
- Sighthounds have a higher incidence of cast complications

Equipment

- Non-adhesive dressing for any wounds
- Adhesive tape for stirrups (2.5 cm wide)
- Tongue depressor
- Stockinette (not absolutely essential)
- 2 to 3 rolls of cast padding (5–7.5 cm wide)
- 2 to 3 rolls of conforming gauze bandage (5–7.5 cm wide)
- 2 to 3 rolls of resin-impregnated fibreglass cast materials
- Outer protective bandage material (e.g. self-adhesive non-adherent bandage or adhesive bandage (optional))
- Oscillating saw

Patient preparation and positioning

- The animal should be sedated heavily or anaesthetized
- The haircoat should be clipped if it is likely to interfere with cast application, and the limb should be clean and dry
- The animal should be placed in lateral recumbency with the affected limb uppermost and supported in a weight-bearing position by an assistant

Technique

1 Place two strips of adhesive tape (stirrups) on the distal limb on *either* the dorsal and palmar/plantar surfaces, or the medial and lateral surfaces. These stirrups should extend beyond the tip of the toes and should be stuck to each other or to a tongue depressor. The assistant can now maintain the limb elevated away from the body by holding the stirrups.
2 Roll the stockinette up the limb and apply tension to eliminate creases (optional).
3 Insert padding between the toes.
4 Beginning distally, apply cast padding in a spiral fashion up the limb, overlapping by 50% on each turn. Two layers are generally indicated. Take particular care to ensure even padding over pressure points. Excessive padding around pressure points should be avoided, and consideration should be given to increasing the padding in adjacent depressed regions to create a bandage of even diameter.
5 Apply conforming gauze to compact the cast padding, again overlapping turns by 50%.
6 Follow the manufacturers' recommendations regarding wetting and handling of the cast material.

7 Apply the cast material over the bandage, again with a 50% overlap on each turn. Two (for cats and most dogs) or three (for large- or giant-breed dogs) layers of cast material should be applied. Leave a 1–2 cm margin of cast padding exposed proximal to the cast. Increase tension as the cast is applied proximal to the elbow or stifle, to give a snug fit about the muscle masses and to prevent loosening. Do not make indentations in the cast material with fingers.

8 Once the cast has hardened, use an oscillating saw to trim excess casting material proximally and distally to prevent rubbing and to permit weight bearing, respectively.

9 Split the cast into halves along either the sagittal or frontal planes using an oscillating saw: the plane chosen should result in the least compromise to the supportive function of the cast, as determined by fracture configuration and forces acting on the cast. Hold the cast together with adhesive tape. Splitting the cast in half simplifies and facilitates cast changes, encouraging regular checking of the limb for healing and complications.

10 Roll the stockinette and padding over the proximal edge of the cast and secure them to the cast with adhesive tape.

11 Peel apart the stirrups, twist them through 180 degrees and stick them to the distal cast. The pads and nails of the axial digits should remain exposed.

Cast maintenance and monitoring

- Written instructions should always be given out at discharge and owners must understand their role in cast maintenance
- Casts should be checked every 4 hours for the first 24 hours and then weekly by a veterinary surgeon; rapidly growing dogs and other high-risk patients may require more frequent assessment
- Animals with a cast should have restricted exercise levels
- The cast must be kept clean and dry. A plastic bag may be placed over the foot while the dog is walking outside. The plastic bag should be removed when the dog is indoors

---

CHECKING PROCEDURE

- Splitting the cast in half simplifies and facilitates cast changes, encouraging regular checking of the limb for healing and complications.
  1. Remove the adhesive tape securing the two halves of the cast and remove the cast.
  2. Remove conforming gauze and cast padding.
  3. Remove dressing if present.
  4. Examine any wounds and the limb for cast complications.
  5. Reapply dressing as required.
  6. Reapply cast padding and gauze padding, taking care to use the same amount as before to prevent undue pressure or looseness.
  7. Reapply both halves of the cast and secure with adhesive tape.
- Points to monitor for are:
  - Swelling of the toes or proximal limb
  - Toe discoloration and coolness
  - Skin abrasion about the toes or proximal cast
  - Cast loosening *continues* ▶

C

> **CHECKING PROCEDURE continued**
>
> ▪ Points to monitor for are:
> - Angular deformity
> - Cast damage or breakage
> - Discharge or foul odour
> - Chewing at the cast
> - Deterioration in weight-bearing function
> - Signs of general ill health (e.g. inappetence, dullness)
> - These signs should prompt cast removal, assessment and replacement only if appropriate

Potential complications

- Venous stasis
- Limb oedema
- Moist dermatitis
- Skin maceration under a wet bandage
- Infection
- Pressure sores/skin necrosis
- Cast loosening
- Deterioration in fracture apposition
- Fracture non-union, malunion or delayed union
- Joint stiffness or laxity

Cast removal and aftercare

- The timing of cast removal should be aided by radiography. In most instances, radiographic evidence of bridging callus formation across fracture sites or arthrodesis sites is desired prior to cast removal
- After cast removal, it is important that a regimen of progressively increasing controlled exercise is enforced. The goal is stimulation of callus remodelling without jeopardizing fracture/arthrodesis repair

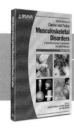

> **FURTHER INFORMATION**
>
> For more information on cast application, see the *BSAVA Manual of Canine and Feline Musculoskeletal Disorders.*

Cerebrospinal fluid sampling – (a) cerebellomedullary cistern

C

SITE SELECTION

- Cerebrospinal fluid (CSF) is more commonly collected from the **cerebellomedullary cistern** as it is technically easier, usually results in a larger sample volume and is typically associated with less iatrogenic blood contamination than collection from the lumbar cistern
- In cases of focal central nervous system (CNS) disease, samples are more likely to be abnormal when they are collected caudal to the lesion. Therefore, in animals with lesions involving the spinal cord or canal, **lumbar cistern** samples are more consistently abnormal than samples collected from the cerebellomedullary cistern
- Collection from both sites can be considered in cases of diffuse pathology or when one of the samples is contaminated, and has been shown to have higher sensitivity for steroid-responsive meningitis–arteritis (SRMA) than collection from a single site

Indications

- Suspected meningitis
- Infectious or inflammatory CNS disease
- Pyrexia of unknown origin
- Suspected CNS lymphoma
- CNS disease where other diagnostic tests prove inconclusive

Contraindications

- Signs suggestive of raised intracranial pressure (e.g. progressive obtundation; initial miosis then later fixed mydriasis; extensor rigidity; opisthotonos; irregular respiration)
- Evidence of a large intracranial space-occupying mass on computed tomography (CT)/magnetic resonance imaging (MRI)
- Evidence of severe hydrocephalus or severe cerebral oedema on CT/MRI
- Evidence of brain herniation on CT/MRI
- Suspected active intracranial haemorrhage or haemorrhagic diathesis
- Atlantoaxial luxation or other causes of cervical vertebral instability
- Infection of the soft tissues overlying the puncture site
- Patient with a high risk of anaesthetic complications

WARNING

- Caution should be employed with Cavalier King Charles Spaniels. Chiari-like malformations are more common in this breed, and sampling from the cerebellomedullary cistern may lead to needle penetration of the cerebellum and brainstem. It is therefore advisable to obtain a **lumbar cistern** sample unless there is MRI evidence to show that the cerebellum is not caudally displaced.

Equipment

- As required for **Aseptic preparation – (a) non-surgical procedures**
- Spinal needle:
  - 20 G (large dogs) to 22 G (cats and most dogs)
  - 1.5 inches (cats and most dogs) to 3.0 inches (some large- or giant-breed dogs)
- EDTA and sterile plain collection tubes
- Microscope slide
- Sedimentation chamber (optional)

Patient preparation and positioning

- General anaesthesia is essential
- The animal is placed in lateral recumbency with the dorsum near the edge of the table
- The head is flexed to at least 90 degrees and an assistant should hold it in place (Figure C.8)

> ### WARNING
>
> - Flexing the neck may compromise respiration. The animal's respiratory rate and character should be monitored at all times. Ideally, an armoured endotracheal (ET) tube should be placed (see **Endotracheal intubation**). If not, then silicone tubes are preferable to rubber ones as the latter may kink and obstruct the airways.

- The muzzle is raised until its sagittal plane is parallel with the table top
- **Aseptic preparation – (a) non-surgical procedures** is performed on a wide area at the base of the skull, from the occipital protuberance to the crest of the axis, including the wings of the atlas
- Sterile gloves should be worn to reduce the likelihood of introducing infection during the procedure

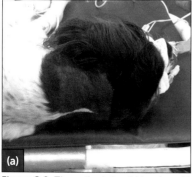 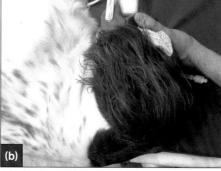

Figure C.8: The patient should be placed in **(a)** lateral recumbency with **(b)** an assistant holding the head in position to obtain a cerebrospinal fluid sample from the cerebellomedullary cistern.

Technique

1   Palpate a triangle of landmarks formed by the occipital protuberance and the most rostral points of the lateral wings of the atlas. The location for needle insertion is on the dorsal midline in the centre of the triangle formed by these landmarks (Figure C.9).

2   Insert the spinal needle parallel to the table surface in the direction of the mandible, with the bevel facing caudally. This usually results in the needle being inserted approximately perpendicular to the skin surface (Figure C.10a). *Alternatively*, the occipital protuberance can be used to identify the midline and the needle inserted just rostral to the most rostral aspect of the wings of the atlas and angled slightly caudally.

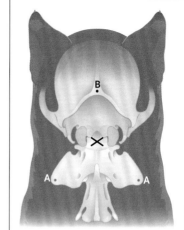

Figure C.9: Needle insertion site (**X**). **A** = atlas; **B** = occipital protuberance.

3   Once the skin is penetrated, remove the stylet.

4   Advance the needle very slowly (1–2 mm at a time) whilst watching for CSF to appear in the hub (Figure C.10b). If the needle hits bone while being advanced, it may be redirected cranially or caudally, moving the needle off the bone until the subarachnoid space is penetrated. If this is not successful after a few redirections, remove the needle and try again.

5   A characteristic 'pop' might be felt when the needle passes through the atlanto-occipital membrane. When the subarachnoid space has been entered, CSF will appear in the needle hub. If blood is seen in the needle hub, entry into a local blood vessel is likely and the sample will be less useful for cytological evaluation. Remove the needle and make a fresh attempt with a new needle.

6   Collect CSF by allowing it to drip passively from the hub into collecting tubes (Figure C.10cd). Suction with a syringe should *not* be applied.

7   When a minimum of 0.5 ml of CSF has been collected, withdraw the needle in a single motion.

Sample handling

▪   CSF is hypotonic compared with serum; the cells within CSF swell rapidly and burst due to osmotic lysis soon after collection. Ideally, CSF should be either analysed or preserved for analysis within 30–60 minutes of collection

▪   Most CSF samples contain relatively few cells; therefore, the sample can be concentrated by some means prior to microscopic examination. Cells can be concentrated using a homemade sedimentation chamber. The flanged end of a 2 ml syringe barrel (the end where the plunger would be inserted) is clamped to a clean microscope slide using bulldog clips after smearing Vaseline® or another occlusive lubricant around the base to form an airtight seal. A 0.25–0.5 ml sample of CSF is put into the chamber and left for 30 minutes; the supernatant is then removed using a pipette. The slide with adherent cells is then air-dried and submitted to the laboratory unstained. Other tests can be performed on the supernatant

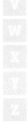

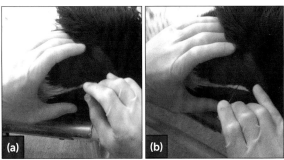

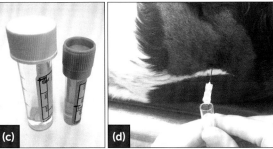

Figure C.10: (a) The needle should be inserted parallel to the table surface and perpendicular to the skin. **(b)** The needle should be advanced slowly into the subarachnoid space. **(c)** Collection tubes for samples. **(d)** Cerebrospinal fluid should be allowed to drip passively from the needle hub into a collection tube.

- *Alternatively*, a simple modification of the sedimentation chamber technique involves placing the needle used for CSF sampling directly on to a microscope slide hub down and leaving to stand for a minimum of 1 hour (the upright needle must be protected to avoid accidental injury). The needle is then removed and the slide carefully blotted before air drying and staining. This provides a rapid and sensitive qualitative analysis useful for the detection of inflammatory disease
- *Alternatively*, rather than concentrating the cells, they can be preserved by the addition of 30–50% by volume of the animal's own serum (i.e. 0.3–0.5 ml serum to 1.0 ml CSF). This will preserve the CSF cells for up to 48 hours after collection. **If this is done, it is important also to submit a CSF sample in a plain tube without the addition of serum to enable total protein measurement and any other analyses**
- CSF in an EDTA tube is submitted for cytological examination, total protein and total nucleated cell count
- CSF in an EDTA tube can also be submitted for the detection of infectious diseases by polymerase chain reaction (PCR)
- CSF in a sterile plain tube can be submitted for serology, bacteriological or fungal culture if required

Potential complications

- Cerebral and/or cerebellar herniation due to changes in intracranial pressure, resulting in brainstem signs, respiratory arrest and death
- Brainstem trauma due to needle puncture
- CNS haemorrhage
- Loss of airway patency due to patient positioning and use of an unarmoured ET tube
- Iatrogenic infection

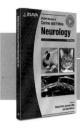

FURTHER INFORMATION

For more information on cerebrospinal fluid sampling, see the *BSAVA Manual of Canine and Feline Neurology.*

Cerebrospinal fluid sampling – (b) lumbar cistern

SITE SELECTION

- Cerebrospinal fluid (CSF) is more commonly collected from the **cerebellomedullary cistern** as it is technically easier, usually results in a larger sample volume and is typically associated with less iatrogenic blood contamination than collection from the lumbar cistern
- In cases of focal central nervous system (CNS) disease, samples are more likely to be abnormal when they are collected caudal to the lesion. Therefore, in animals with lesions involving the spinal cord or canal, **lumbar cistern** samples are more consistently abnormal than samples collected from the cerebellomedullary cistern
- Collection from both sites can be considered in cases of diffuse pathology or when one of the samples is contaminated, and has been shown to have higher sensitivity for steroid-responsive meningitis–arteritis (SRMA) than collection from a single site

Indications

- Suspected meningitis
- Infectious or inflammatory CNS disease
- Pyrexia of unknown origin
- Suspected CNS lymphoma
- CNS disease where other diagnostic tests prove inconclusive

Contraindications

- Signs suggestive of raised intracranial pressure (e.g. progressive obtundation; initial miosis then later fixed mydriasis; extensor rigidity; opisthotonos; irregular respiration)
- Evidence of brain herniation on computed tomography (CT)/magnetic resonance imaging (MRI)
- Suspected active intracranial haemorrhage or haemorrhagic diathesis
- Luxation or vertebral instability of the caudal lumbar vertebrae
- Empyema or spinal epidural abscess
- Infection of the soft tissues overlying the puncture site
- Patient with a high risk of anaesthetic complications

Equipment

- As required for **Cerebrospinal fluid sampling – (a) cerebellomedullary cistern**
- Spinal needle:
  - 20 G (large- or giant-breed dogs) to 22 G (cats and most dogs)
  - 1.5 inches to 3 inches

Patient preparation and positioning

- General anaesthesia is essential
- The animal is placed in lateral recumbency with its dorsum near the edge of the table
- The lumbar spine is flexed by moving the hindlimbs cranially and an assistant should hold the animal in this position (Figure C.11)
- The appropriate intervertebral space should be located:
  - Cats: L6–L7
  - Dogs: L5–L6 or occasionally L6–L7
- This is done by palpating the iliac crests and lumbar dorsal spinous processes: the small, difficult-to-palpate vertebral spinous process found between the iliac crests is L7; the much more prominent vertebral spinous process immediately cranial to the iliac crests is that of L6
- **Aseptic preparation – (a) non-surgical procedures** is performed over an area at least 5 cm wide

Technique

1 Insert the needle perpendicular to the skin, in the midline, on to the most prominent point (the top) of the appropriate (caudal) vertebral dorsal spinous process (i.e. on to the spinous process of L6 to reach the L5–L6 space, or on to the L7 process to reach the L6–L7 space), with the bevel facing cranially (Figure C.12a).

2 Once the needle is on the dorsal spine, walk it cranially staying on the midline, and then remove the stylet and advance the needle towards the dorsal interarcuate ligament.

3 'Walking' the needle over the dorsal lamina is often required to arrive at the resistant interarcuate ligament. Pass the needle through the interarcuate ligament (some force is occasionally required) and continue to advance, feeling

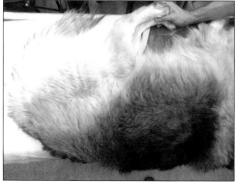

Figure C.11: The patient should be placed in lateral recumbency with the hindlimbs held cranially to flex the lumbar spine to obtain a cerebrospinal fluid sample from the lumbar cistern.

for a distinct 'pop' as the needle enters the dorsal subarachnoid space. Note: if the needle passes through the cauda equina/caudal spinal cord, this often elicits a tail or leg twitch and means that the dorsal space has been missed.

4 The needle may then be either retracted into the dorsal subarachnoid space, or advanced to the ventral floor of the vertebral canal before being retracted slightly into the ventral subarachnoid space. It is easier if the stylet has been removed by this point in order to look for CSF flow, which can be very slow.

5 When the subarachnoid space has been entered, CSF will appear in the needle hub. If no CSF appears, retract the needle slightly or turn the hub gently. If blood emerges from the needle hub, entry into a local blood vessel is likely and the sample will be less useful for cytological evaluation. Remove the needle and make a fresh attempt with a new needle.

6 Collect CSF by allowing it to drip passively from the hub into collecting tubes (Figure C.12b). Suction with a syringe should *not* be applied.

7 When a minimum of 0.5 ml CSF has been collected, withdraw the needle in a single motion.

8 Fluoroscopic/radiographic needle guidance might be helpful in some cases.

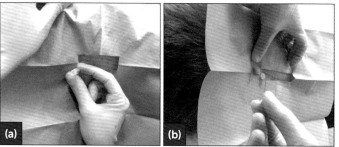

Figure C.12: (a) The needle should be inserted perpendicular to the skin in the midline. (b) Cerebrospinal fluid should be allowed to drip passively from the needle hub into a collection tube.

Sample handling

As for **Cerebrospinal fluid sampling – (a) cerebellomedullary cistern**.

Potential complications

- Cerebral and/or cerebellar herniation due to changes in intracranial pressure resulting in brainstem signs, respiratory arrest and death
- Spinal cord trauma due to needle puncture
- CNS haemorrhage
- Iatrogenic infection

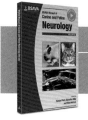

FURTHER INFORMATION

For more information on cerebrospinal fluid sampling, see the *BSAVA Manual of Canine and Feline Neurology.*

Cystocentesis

Indications/Use

- Collection of urine directly from the bladder without contamination from the urethra or genital tract. This method should be used for bacterial culture of urine
- Decompression of a severely overdistended bladder pending urethral catheterization or, in exceptional circumstances, when urethral catheterization is not possible

Contraindications

- Severely diseased bladder (rupture possible)
- Inadequate bladder volume or excessive body fat such that the bladder cannot be palpated or immobilized manually
- Potential pyometra or prostatic abscess that could be inadvertently ruptured by this technique
- Bladder tumour that could potentially be seeded

Equipment

- As required for **Aseptic preparation – (a) non-surgical procedures**
- Hypodermic needles:
  - Dogs: 21–23 G, 1–2 inches
  - Cats: 23 G, 1–2 inches
- 10 ml syringe
- Two sterile plain collection tubes capable of holding at least 5 ml each

---

BACTERIOLOGY

- If bacteriology is to be performed at an external laboratory, urine should be placed in a sterile plain collection tube and analysed within 24 hours of collection
- Note that the use of a tube containing boric acid preservative (red top universal tube) is no longer recommended

---

Patient preparation and positioning

- Cystocentesis can usually be performed with the patient under physical restraint or light sedation
- It can be performed with the animal in either dorsal or lateral recumbency, or with the animal standing
- *Alternatively*, cystocentesis can be performed under ultrasound guidance
- **Aseptic preparation – (a) non-surgical procedures** is performed over the appropriate area

Technique

1. Entering the bladder:
   a. If the animal is in *dorsal or lateral recumbency,* with one hand palpate and stabilize the bladder by pushing it in a caudal direction against the pelvic

brim. Then, with the other hand, attach the needle to the syringe and insert it through the abdominal wall, in the midline, just in front of the pelvic brim (Figure C.13a)

b   If the animal is *standing*, urine should ideally be obtained from the right side (to avoid penetrating the descending colon), while gently pushing the bladder from the left side towards the right side of the caudal abdomen. Alternatively, a left-sided approach can be used, with the bladder gently pushed from the right side toward the left (Figure C.13b)

c   The ideal site of bladder penetration is a short distance (a few centimetres, but will depend on how much urine is in the bladder) cranial to the junction of the bladder and the urethra. If possible, insert the needle in a caudal direction and at a 45-degree angle to the bladder wall; the layers of the bladder wall will help to seal the puncture site

d   Apply slight negative pressure to the syringe while inserting the needle.

2   Once the bladder lumen is penetrated, urine will be seen filling the syringe (Figure C.14). Continue to stabilize the bladder until the needle is withdrawn from the abdomen.

3   Once sufficient urine has been collected to perform the required diagnostic tests (usually a minimum of 5 ml), remove the needle in one motion.

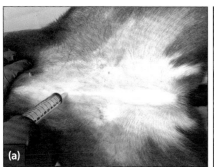
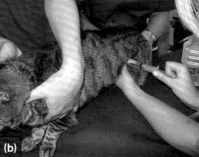

Figure C.13: Cystocentesis can be performed with the patient **(a)** in dorsal recumbency or **(b)** standing. (Courtesy of Langford Veterinary Services and reproduced from the *BSAVA Manual of Feline Practice*)

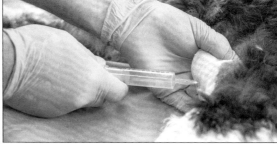

Figure C.14: Urine is seen filling the syringe following penetration of the bladder lumen.

Sample handling

- Urine should be placed into a sterile plain tube for bacterial culture and should reach the laboratory as soon as possible (within 24 hours)
- A separate sample in a plain tube can be used for **urinalysis**

Potential complications

- Very rarely, an overdistended and traumatized bladder will rupture during cystocentesis. Surgical repair is then required
- Uroperitoneum, following urine leaking from the needle site

Cystostomy tube placement

Indications/Use

- Urethral trauma
- Urethral obstruction (uroliths, neoplasia, stricture, granulomatous urethritis)
- Bladder trauma
- Bladder neoplasia, if causing obstruction of the neck
- Neurogenic bladder atony
- Detrusor–urethral dyssynergia

Equipment

- Mushroom-tipped catheter with 'regular' mushroom or Foley catheter (8–20 Fr)
  - Cats and small dogs: 8–16 Fr
  - Dogs: 16–20 Fr
  - Low profile, silicone, human gastrostomy tube may be preferred if long-term use is anticipated

---

NOTE

- Foley catheters can be placed as cystostomy tubes for short-term use. However, the Foley balloon may deflate with time, meaning an increased risk of tube dislodgement compared with mushroom-tipped catheters

---

- Sterile intravenous fluid administration set and empty fluid bag, or commercial closed urine collection system with appropriate adapters for connection to the catheter. Alternatively, an adapter and bung can be used for intermittent bladder drainage
- As required for **Aseptic preparation – (b) surgical procedures**
- Suture materials
- Soft tissue surgical instrument set

Patient positioning and preparation

- General anaesthesia is required
- Patient should be placed in dorsal recumbency
- **Aseptic preparation – (b) surgical procedures** is required

---

Technique

1. Approach the bladder via a ventral midline caudal coeliotomy. Extend the incision parapreputially in male dogs.
2. Place stay sutures in the bladder to allow it to be handled during cystostomy tube placement.
3. Make a full-thickness paramedian stab incision in the right or left abdominal wall cranial to the flank fold; this incision should be located such that the bladder will be lying in an anatomically normal position when the tube is placed, allowing for changes in bladder size.
4. Pass the catheter through the stab incision so that the mushroom tip (or balloon if using a Foley catheter) is in the abdomen and the catheter tip is outside. Place an adapter and bung on the catheter tip to prevent urine leakage when the tube is inserted into the bladder.
5. Place a full-thickness purse-string suture (absorbable) in the bladder; unless pathology dictates otherwise, this should be on the ventral aspect of the bladder, between the apex and mid-body. The diameter of the purse-string suture should be large enough to allow tube placement through the centre. Hold the ends of the suture material with haemostats; do not tie at this point.
6. Make a stab incision in the middle of the purse-string suture, just large enough to push the tip of the catheter through into the bladder lumen; if using a mushroom-tip catheter, fold the tip before inserting the catheter.
7. Once the mushroom tip has opened in the lumen of the bladder (or following inflation of the Foley catheter balloon), tighten and secure the purse-string suture around the shaft of the tube, sealing the bladder wall around the tube (Figure C.15)

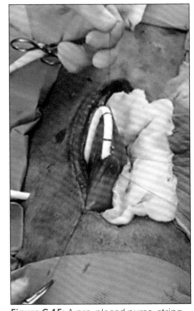

8. Place three or four interrupted (absorbable) sutures between the seromuscular layer of the bladder wall and the corresponding abdominal wall to appose the bladder to the body wall around the tube. Pre-place all sutures before tying.
9. Pull the external (catheter tip) end of the tube so that the mushroom tip or Foley balloon is positioned snugly against the bladder wall.
10. Secure the tube to the skin using a finger-trap suture.
11. Close the coeliotomy wound routinely.
12. Apply a sterile dressing around the tube stoma site.
13. Place gauze or a loose body wrap around the tube to prevent patient interference. An Elizabethan collar should also be worn whilst the tube is in place.

Figure C.15: A pre-placed purse-string suture is tightened around the cystostomy tube after the mushroom tip has been inserted into the bladder. The catheter tip is exiting the abdomen via a paramedian incision. Note the use of stay sutures to help exteriorize and manipulate the bladder during tube placement. (Courtesy of Laura Owen)

C

MINIMALLY INVASIVE APPROACH

As an alternative to coeliotomy, cystostomy tubes can be placed through a minimally invasive inguinal approach. The patient is positioned in lateral recumbency with the upper pelvic limb retracted caudally. The bladder is exposed by separating the abdominal wall musculature via a 2–3 cm skin incision in the inguinal region. Once located, the tube should be placed through a separate abdominal wall incision into the bladder (as per the coeliotomy technique; Figure C.16). It is recommended that the clinician becomes familiar with cystostomy placement via coeliotomy before attempting this technique, which is described in full by Bray *et al.* (2009).

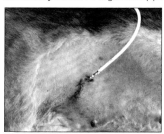

Figure C.16: Cystostomy tubes can be placed via a minimally invasive inguinal approach. (Courtesy of Laura Owen)

LOW PROFILE TUBES

If long-term urinary diversion is required, a low profile, balloon tip gastrostomy tube is preferred. Unlike conventional mushroom-tip or Foley catheters, these tubes sit flush with the skin so there is a lower risk of tube breakage or removal by patient interference. An extension set is connected for urine drainage. Low profile tubes are usually placed once a mature stoma has been established via the technique(s) described above (Figure C.17).

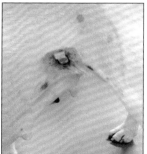

Figure C.17: A low profile gastrostomy tube can be placed for long-term urinary diversion. (Courtesy of Laura Owen)

Tube maintenance and removal

- The stoma site should be inspected and cleaned daily and the sterile dressing replaced as required
- The collection system should be kept in a clean environment and aseptic technique should be followed when emptying the urine bag or directly emptying the tube
- The urine bag should be emptied and the volume of urine retrieved recorded as clinically indicated (usually 4 times per day)
- If tube obstruction is suspected, the collection system should be disconnected and the catheter flushed with sterile saline using aseptic technique
- The cystostomy tube should remain in place for at least 7–10 days before it is removed, to allow time for adhesion formation between the bladder and abdominal wall

- To remove the tube:
  - If using a Foley catheter, the balloon should be deflated and the catheter pulled out
  - If using a mushroom-tip catheter, a sterile, blunt-ended stylet should be inserted into the catheter to extend the tip as it is removed. With the non-dominant hand, counter-traction should be applied to the flank whilst the dominant hand applies traction to remove the tube. In dogs, this procedure can usually be performed without sedation; however, sedation is often required in cats
  - The catheter tip should be inspected to ensure it has been removed in its entirety
- Urine leakage via the stoma is expected for 3–5 days after tube removal. During this time the stoma should be kept clean and petroleum jelly can be applied to the peristomal skin to protect against urine scald

Potential complications

- Urinary tract infection
- Haematuria
- Tube dislodgement or premature removal
- Tube obstruction
- Leakage of urine around the tube site
- Fistula formation and persistent urine leakage after tube removal
- Breakage of tube caused by patient interference
- Breakage of the mushroom tip during tube removal

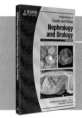

FURTHER INFORMATION

For further information, see Bray *et al.* (2009) Minimally invasive inguinal approach for tube cystostomy. *Veterinary Surgery* **38(3)**, 411–416 and the *BSAVA Manual of Canine and Feline Nephrology and Urology.*

Ehmer sling

Indications/Use

- To support the hip joint following closed reduction of craniodorsal hip joint luxation (to permit stabilization and healing of the periarticular tissues)
- The Ehmer sling holds the pelvic limb in flexion, while internally rotating and mildly abducting the hip joint

Contraindications

- Hip instability following closed reduction of hip luxation, such that the Ehmer sling would not hold the hip in the reduced position; if the hip re-luxates immediately after reduction or within 4 weeks, internal reduction and stabilization should be considered
- Ventral hip luxation
- Patient's temperament will not tolerate prolonged immobilization of limb
- Patient's conformation (e.g. chondrodystrophoid, well-muscled) does not permit effective sling application
- Concurrent hip fractures or pre-existing disease (e.g. hip dysplasia)
- Concurrent injuries such as fractures or open wounds
- Poorly tolerated in cats

Equipment

- Padded bandage material or cast padding
- Conforming gauze bandage
- Adhesive outer protective bandage material (e.g. Elastoplast)

Patient preparation and positioning

- General anaesthesia is required for closed reduction of hip luxation and is preferred for Ehmer sling application
- The patient should be positioned in lateral recumbency with the affected limb uppermost
- At the beginning of the procedure, the pelvic limb should be held in a gently flexed position

Technique

1 Confirm successful hip joint reduction by radiography and check range of motion and stability of the hip joint. Confirm that conservative management of hip luxation is appropriate (see **Hip luxation – closed reduction**).

2 Apply padded bandage material around the metatarsal region to lightly pad this area.

3 Secure the padded bandage material around the metatarsal region with conforming gauze bandage (Figure E.1a). It is important to pass the conforming gauze bandage from lateral to medial around the *dorsal* aspect of the metatarsus and from medial to lateral around the plantar aspect of the metatarsus.

4 Completely flex the whole limb.

5 Pass the conforming gauze bandage from the *lateral* aspect of the metatarsus across the *cranial* aspect of the mid-tibia, to the *medial* aspects of the mid-tibia and mid-femur (Figure E.1b).

6 Pass the bandage over the *cranial* aspect of the mid-femur to the *lateral* aspect of the mid-femur (Figure E.1c).

7 Pass the bandage *caudal* to the stifle to the *medial* aspects of the distal tibia and proximal metatarsal region, before returning to the plantar aspect of the metatarsus.

8 The result should be a figure-of-eight bandage, which passes medial to the crus in both directions.

9 Apply a few more layers of conforming gauze bandage to secure the pelvic limb in the flexed position (Figure E.1d)

10 Apply an adhesive protective bandage material over the conforming bandage to overhang the edge of the conforming gauze to secure the bandage to the skin/fur.

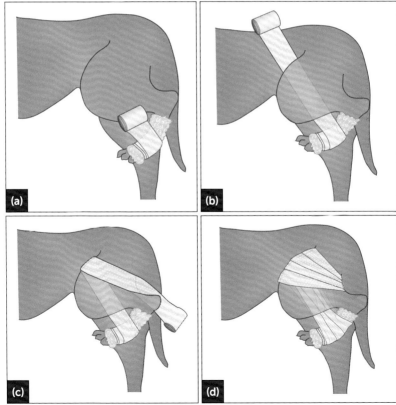

Figure E.1: (a–d) Technique for applying an Ehmer sling.

Alternative techniques

- Ehmer slings are prone to slipping, especially over the cranial aspect of the stifle. These slings can be made using an elastic adhesive bandage alone, with some metatarsal padding. This decreases slipping but the sling is more difficult to remove, and skin irritation is more likely
- The sling can also be secured around the abdomen by extending the bandage from the *plantarolateral* aspect of the metatarsus, *lateral* to the flexed pelvic limb and over the dorsal aspect of the body, before wrapping it around the abdomen
- In long-haired dog breeds, shaving the fur of the limb before applying an Ehmer sling may reduce the risk of slippage

Sling maintenance

- Recommendations for the duration of time for which Ehmer slings need to be maintained to prevent hip re-luxation vary: 7 to 10 days is frequently quoted
- Ehmer slings must be checked several times daily for complications, ideally every 4 hours
- Exercise restriction must be enforced

Potential complications

- If applied too tightly, potential complications include:
  - Paw swelling due to venous stasis
  - Irritation of the skin, especially over the medial thigh
  - Sloughing of the metatarsal pad
  - Pressure necrosis of the soft tissues
- If the sling becomes wet, moist dermatitis and soft tissue maceration may occur
- Ehmer sling loosening and slipping over the stifle are frequent problems
- Hip re-luxation can also occur due to inappropriate case selection or incorrect technique

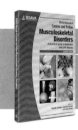

FURTHER INFORMATION

For more information on hip luxation and Ehmer sling application, see the *BSAVA Manual of Canine and Feline Musculoskeletal Disorders.*

Electrocardiography

Indications/Use
- Detection of an arrhythmia during clinical examination
- As part of the investigation of heart disease
- Investigation of collapse, weakness or exercise intolerance
- Suspected electrolyte abnormality, particularly hyperkalaemia
- Monitoring during pericardiocentesis
- Monitoring during anaesthesia or in a critical care setting

Equipment
- Electrocardiograph
- Limb leads x4
- Non-traumatic alligator or other clips (with teeth filed down) or disposable pre-gelled self-adhesive electrodes
- Adhesive tape
- Electrocardiography gel
- 70% surgical spirit

Patient preparation and positioning
- The animal should be calm and relaxed, before being placed on a surface that is electrically insulated, such as a rubber mat or thick blanket
- Dogs should ideally be placed in right lateral recumbency, with the fore- and hindlimbs as perpendicular to the long axis of the body as possible (Figure E.2)
- To decrease stress in cats, electrocardiography can be performed in sternal recumbency, sitting or standing. These positions are also acceptable for dyspnoeic or uncooperative patients. Complex amplitude and morphology are more variable in these non-standard positions; however, improved patient compliance (especially in cats) may produce a better quality trace with fewer artefacts
- Chemical restraint may cause changes in rhythm, but can be used as a last resort if the alternative is an uninterpretable trace. Drugs known to have a minimal effect on the cardiovascular system should be used
- When using non-traumatic alligator or other clips, it is not necessary to remove hair before attaching them
- Disposable pre-gelled self-adhesive electrodes are applied directly to the pads without previous preparation (Figure E.3)

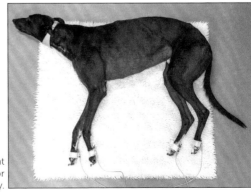

Figure E.2: Patient positioning for electrocardiography.

E

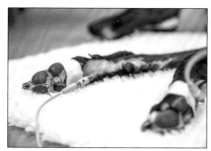

Figure F.3: Self-adhesive electrodes should be applied directly to the footpads.

Technique

Electrocardiography leads

- The electrodes may be colour-coded and marked for use on human patients. They are attached to the limbs as described in Figure E.4
- When using non-traumatic alligator or other clips, it is not necessary to remove hair before attaching them. The clips are generally placed on skin overlying bony protuberances, to minimize the effect of muscle interference. They are then sprayed with surgical spirit or covered in electrocardiography gel to achieve good electrical conductivity
- Limb electrodes are usually positioned fairly near to the body to reduce movement artefact, using the relatively hairless areas of skin just behind both elbows and in front of the left stifle. Hindlimb electrodes may also be attached to the skin overlying the gastrocnemius tendon
- The neutral electrode may be placed anywhere, but is usually placed in front of the right stifle

Machine controls

- Sensitivity control: allows the operator to vary the number of centimetres on the paper that are equivalent to 1 mV. Most traces are recorded at 1 cm/mV, but if the complexes are so tall that they cannot be accommodated, decreasing the sensitivity will give a readable trace. Or, if complexes are too small (commonly seen in cats), the sensitivity can be increased
- Paper speed control: allows the operator to choose how quickly the trace is run, usually either 25 or 50 mm/s
    - 50 mm/s is generally preferred as it helps with the measurement of intervals and waves/complexes
    - Slow running may be useful to save paper in a long recording if looking for intermittent arrhythmias; alternatively, the trace could be run at a fast paper speed for an animal with a fast heart rate or tachyarrhythmia

Lead	Attachment site	Colour
RA ('right arm')	Right elbow	Red
LA ('left arm')	Left elbow	Yellow
F or LL ('left leg')	Left stifle	Green
N or RL ('right leg', earth lead)	Right stifle	Black

Figure E.4: Electrocardiography lead colours and attachment sites.

- Filter: allows artefacts to be suppressed, evening out the trace. Its use might cause a marked decrease in the height of the QRS complexes and this should be taken into account when the trace is interpreted
- Lead selector: manual lead selection is preferred and the operator should select the six frontal plane leads (lead I, II, III, aVR, aVL and aVF) in turn

Recording

1 Once the patient is positioned and the leads attached, switch on the unit and check the sensitivity and paper speed.
2 Ensure that the sensitivity (vertical axis scale) is set to optimize complex size to a height that is clearly seen, without overlapping of leads, and fits the paper.
3 Ensure that the filter is turned off.
4 Normally at least five good quality complexes should be recorded in all four leads at 50 mm/s.
5 For rhythm analysis, record a longer (20–30 seconds) lead II strip at 50 mm/s (Figure E.5).
6 If intermittent arrhythmias are suspected, it may be necessary to record for several minutes with lead II at 25 mm/s.

Reference ranges

Reference ranges for electrocardiography are given in Figure E.6.

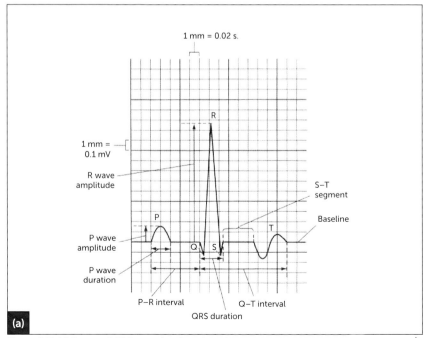

Figure E.5: (a) A normal ECG complex. (continues) ▶

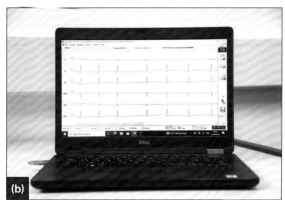

Figure E.5: (continued) **(b)** A computer-based six lead ECG recording.

(b)

Parameter	Unit	Dogs	Cats
Heart rate	beats per minute	70–160 for adult dogs 60–140 for giant breeds up to 180 for toy breeds up to 220 for puppies	120–240
P wave duration	seconds	<0.04 (<0.05 in giant breeds)	<0.04
P wave amplitude	mV	<0.4	<0.2
P–R interval	seconds	0.06–0.13	0.05–0.09
QRS duration	seconds	<0.06	<0.04
R wave amplitude	mV	<2.5–3.0	<0.9
Q–T interval	seconds	0.15–0.25	0.12–0.18
Mean electrical axis (MEA)	degrees	+40 to +100	0 to +160

Figure E.6: Reference ranges used in electrocardiography. (Data from Tilley LP (1992) *Essentials of Canine and Feline Electrocardiography: Interpretation and Management,* 3rd edition. Lea & Febiger, Philadelphia)

Endoscopy of the gastrointestinal tract – (a) upper tract

Indications/Use

- Investigation of clinical signs of oesophageal, gastric and small intestinal (primarily duodenal) disease
- Investigation of radiographic or ultrasonographic abnormalities of the upper gastrointestinal (GI) tract
- Collecting samples from the upper GI tract
- Removal of selected foreign bodies

Contraindications

- Care should be taken with insufflation and lavage if oesophageal and/or gastric perforation is suspected
- Inadequate investigation prior to endoscopy
- Poorly prepared patient (food not withheld so stomach full)
- Uncorrected bleeding disorder

Equipment

- Flexible endoscope: diameter 7–9 mm; insertion tube at least 1 m long (1.5 m in giant breeds of dog); 4-way tip deflection; minimum 2.2 mm biopsy channel; ability to insufflate with air; ability to remotely wash lens
- Endoscopic viewing equipment
- Facilities for suction
- Flexible endoscopic biopsy forceps
- Mouth gag
- Sterile aqueous lubricant (e.g. K-Y jelly)
- Container of 10% neutral buffered formalin
- Hypodermic needle: 21 G
- Tissue cassette with foam insert (e.g. CellSafe+ biopsy capsule)

Patient preparation and positioning

> **NOTE**
>
> - **Do not** perform barium studies in the 24-hour period prior to upper GI endoscopy

- Food must be withheld from at least 12 (ideally 24) hours prior to the procedure
- Water should be withheld from 4 hours prior to the procedure
- If delayed gastric emptying is suspected, a plain lateral radiograph should be obtained prior to anaesthesia to ensure the stomach and small intestines are empty. If preparation is inadequate, withhold food for a further 12–24 hours
- General anaesthesia is essential. The endotracheal (ET) tube should be tied to the *mandible*, not the maxilla (see **Endotracheal intubation**). Avoid atropine if possible, as it affects both motility and secretions of the gastrointestinal tract
- A mouth gag must always be placed to avoid damage to the endoscope
- The patient should be positioned in left lateral recumbency (air fills the antrum, making pyloric intubation possible), with the head and neck extended (Figure E.7)

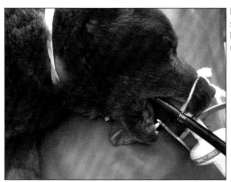

Figure E.7: The patient should be positioned in left lateral recumbency for upper GI endoscopy.

Technique

1 Lubricate the tip of the endoscope with K-Y jelly, avoiding the lens.

2 Pass the endoscope along the midline of the hard palate into the pharynx, reaching the upper oesophageal sphincter.

3 Apply gentle pressure to pass the sphincter.

4 Advance the endoscope in short segments down the oesophagus whilst insufflating with air. Try to keep the entire mucosal circumference in view at all times. A better view of the oesophagus will be obtained at the end of the procedure while the endoscope is withdrawn.

5 Pass the endoscope until the gastro-oesophageal junction is visualized, usually seen as a star- or slit-like opening.

6 Align the tip of the endoscope with the lower oesophageal sphincter and gently advance, overcoming slight resistance.

7 If the lower oesophageal sphincter is closed, slightly angle the tip (30 degrees), with continued insufflation, to pass into the stomach.

8 Once inside the stomach, inflate with moderate amounts of air to allow orientation. The initial view on entering the stomach is of the junction of the fundus and the body on the greater curvature.

9 If duodenoscopy is to be performed, the stomach should be examined in detail *after* examination of the duodenum. Delay in intubating the pylorus can make pyloric intubation more difficult. Perform a quick inspection to locate the antrum and pylorus, and identify any lesions to be examined more closely later in the procedure. Initial examination of the stomach will detect foreign material, food, fluid, bile and blood.

10 Follow the rugal folds toward the antrum. Once in the antrum there are few rugal folds, the mucosa is paler in colour and the lumen tapers toward the pylorus (see Figures E.10 and E.11). A ring of contraction passing toward the pylorus is also often present.

11 Once the tip is engaged with the pylorus and centred in the lumen, advance the endoscope forward while continually readjusting the tip to keep it in the centre of the pyloric canal.

12 Maintain gentle pressure on the pylorus until the next antral contraction and the endoscope may be 'accepted' into the pylorus.

NOTE

- In order to navigate around the stomach, it is helpful to have a mental image of the gastric anatomy (Figure E.8). On entering the stomach, once any red-out has been corrected, the initial view is of the greater curvature at the junction of the fundus and body (Figure E.9). If there is red-out, slight withdrawal of the tip and insufflation will enable a view of the lumen. Slight deviation of the tip will then give a panoramic view of the body of the stomach towards the antrum; rugal folds, which tend to run parallel to the long axis of the stomach, will be seen

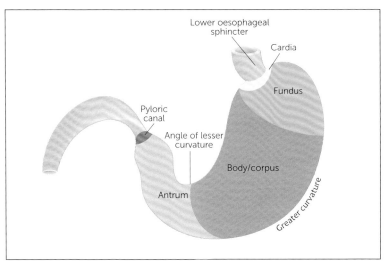

Figure E.8: Ventrodorsal diagrammatic representation of the regions of the stomach. (Reproduced from the *BSAVA Manual of Canine and Feline Endoscopy and Endosurgery*)

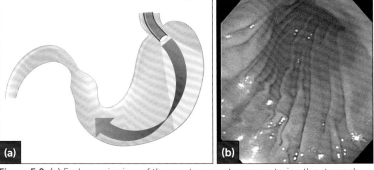

Figure E.9: (a) Endoscopic view of the greater curvature on entering the stomach and (b) parallel rugal folds running along the greater curvature. (Reproduced from the *BSAVA Manual of Canine and Feline Endoscopy and Endosurgery*)

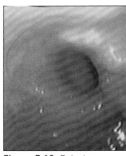

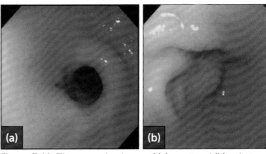

Figure E.10: Pyloric sphincter viewed from the antrum.

Figure E.11: The normal pylorus of **(a)** a cat and **(b)** a dog. (Reproduced from the *BSAVA Manual of Canine and Feline Endoscopy and Endosurgery*)

PARADOXICAL MOVEMENT

- In some patients, as the endoscope approaches the antrum, there is a tendency either for the tip to get stuck in the greater curvature or, as the endoscope is advanced, the tip may appear to move backwards (i.e. away from the pylorus). In these situations, it is difficult to enter the antrum and virtually impossible to reach the pylorus or intubate the duodenum.
- This so-called *paradoxical movement* (Figure E.12) happens particularly when the stomach is overinflated. It can be prevented by **deflating the stomach as much as possible**, or by turning the tip slightly into the greater curvature so that it advances into the antrum, or by rotating the endoscope slightly as it is advanced. Finally, if all else fails, external compression on the right body wall flattens the flexure and may assist entry into the antrum.

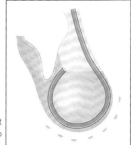

Figure E.12: Paradoxical movement may occur and prevent access into the antrum and pylorus.

MANOEUVRES TO AID PYLORIC INTUBATION

- Deflate the stomach as much as possible
- Intermittent puffs of air may assist the passage of the tip, but continual insufflation will probably cause overinflation
- Gently rotate the endoscope around its long axis, but be careful as too much torque can be damaging
- Position the patient in dorsal or right lateral recumbency. This is best done with the endoscope already positioned in the antrum, as orientation can be more difficult once the animal is repositioned
- Pass biopsy forceps 'blindly' through the pylorus and then pass the endoscope along this temporary 'guidewire'. However, there is a risk of GI perforation with this technique and so it should be performed with great care

13 Red-out occurs as the endoscope passes into the pyloric canal. The colour will change from 'red-out' to 'yellow-out', indicating the presence of bile in the duodenum.

14 As the endoscope is passed into the duodenum, angle the tip downwards and to the right.

15 Once in the duodenum, stop advancing the endoscope and inflate with small amounts of air.

16 Advance the endoscope along the duodenum examining the lumen.

17 Once the duodenum has been examined, return the endoscope to the stomach.

18 Inflate the stomach to allow a complete examination.

19 At some point during the examination, briefly overinflate the stomach to almost completely flatten the rugal folds and check that no lesions remain hidden between the folds.

20 Retroflex and partially withdraw the endoscope (the so-called 'J manoeuvre') to allow visualization of the cardia, which lies in the 'blind spot' on entry to the stomach (Figure E.13).

21 Deflate the stomach at the end of the procedure and withdraw the endoscope slowly, whilst examining the oesophagus.

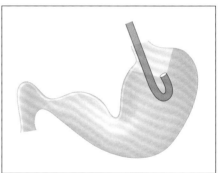

Figure E.13: A 'J manoeuvre' is required to examine the cardia.

Biopsy and sample handling

- Where gross lesions are detected during gastroscopy, multiple biopsy samples should be collected from the lesion and the surrounding (apparently normal) tissue
- If no macroscopic lesions are observed, samples should be collected from:
  - The gastric fundus (take at least 2)
  - The body of the stomach (take at least 4)
  - The antral canal (take at least 2)
  - The periphery of any ulcer
  - Different areas of the duodenum (take 8–10)
- **Samples should always be taken, even if no lesions are apparent**

Technique

1 Position the endoscope in the region to be sampled.

2 Pass the biopsy forceps down the biopsy channel of the endoscope with the cup firmly closed.

3 Pass the forceps out of the end of the endoscope, open the cup, position on to the mucosa, and close the cup.

4 Withdraw the biopsy forceps through the biopsy channel of the endoscope with the cup firmly closed.

PRACTICAL TIPS

- Position the biopsy forceps perpendicular to the mucosa whenever possible (see Figure E.17). This will maximize sample collection
- Avoid overinflation as this stretches the mucosa and smaller samples will be obtained
- Advance the forceps until the mucosa 'tents' and then close them

---

5 To remove samples from the biopsy forceps, immerse in 10% neutral buffered formalin. Then rinse the forceps well in saline before reinserting them into the endoscope. *Alternatively*, carefully remove samples from the biopsy forceps with a needle and place directly into formalin or lay on the foam insert of a tissue cassette (e.g. CellSafe+ biopsy capsule).

Potential complications

- Gastrointestinal perforation is rare, but can result from forceful insertion of the endoscope, especially when attempting duodenal intubation. Excessive insufflation can also rupture ulcerated areas
- Significant haemorrhage is rare. Minor and clinically insignificant haemorrhage is very common
- To avoid gastric dilatation, air should be removed from the stomach after gastroscopy
- Overdistension of the stomach causes compression of the caudal vena cava and a drop in venous return. Compression of the diaphragm may also result in decreased tidal volume
- Acute bradycardia most commonly occurs when the duodenum is entered, especially in toy breeds or in patients with severe gastrointestinal disease

Endoscopy of the gastrointestinal tract – (b) lower tract

Indications/Use

- Investigation of clinical signs of lower gastrointestinal (GI) tract disease including constipation
- Investigation of radiographic or ultrasonographic abnormalities of the lower GI tract
- Collecting samples from the lower GI tract

Contraindications

- Inadequate investigation prior to endoscopy
- Poorly prepared patient (food not withheld and enemas not administered so the colon contains ingesta)
- Uncorrected bleeding disorder

Equipment

- As required for **Endoscopy of the gastrointestinal tract – (a) upper tract** (mouth gag not required). A flexible endoscope the same size as required for examination of the upper GI tract can be used. *Alternatively*, a rigid endoscope or proctoscope can be used, as this allows excellent visualization of the mucosa, though only of the distal colon and rectum
- Bowel cleansing solution (e.g. Klean Prep, Golytely, Nulytely, Moviprep, Dulcobalance)
- Equipment for giving an enema (e.g. soft enema tube, Higginson's pump)

Patient preparation and positioning

A variety of protocols for colonic preparation in advance on colonoscopy can be employed and may largely be dictated by the experience and preference of the operator.

> **WARNING**
>
> - Careful preparation of the large intestine is essential if the entire mucosal surface is to be thoroughly examined. The presence of faeces severely restricts the ability to carry out this examination.

- Food must be withdrawn from at least 24 hours prior to the procedure
- Ideally, a bowel cleansing solution should be administered:
  - Dogs: 2–4 doses of 30 ml/kg of an oral solution at least 2 hours apart, with the final dose being administered approximately 12 hours before the endoscopic procedure. Some dogs will voluntarily ingest the solution, especially when mixed with chicken flavoured water. For those that do not, it is difficult to administer adequate volumes via an oral drench, and therefore an orogastric tube is required for administration
  - Cats: 20 ml/kg of an oral solution should be given slowly via a **naso-oesophageal tube** 12–24 hours prior to the procedure
- Water should be withheld from 4 hours prior to the procedure
- Two warm water enemas should be given on the morning of the procedure, with the last one approximately 1–2 hours before the procedure. A well lubricated soft enema tube should be inserted per rectum to the level of the last rib and approximately 15 ml/kg of warm water instilled under gravity, whilst the tube is gently agitated back and forth. Alternatively, a Higginson's pump or equivalent can be used to administer the water. A rectal examination must first be performed, to make sure it is safe to insert the enema tubing
- If inadequate preparation is suspected, a plain lateral radiograph should be obtained prior to anaesthesia. If preparation is inadequate, the steps above should be repeated
- General anaesthesia is essential. Atropine should be avoided if possible, as it affects both motility and secretions of the gastrointestinal tract
- The patient should be positioned in left lateral recumbency

Technique

1. Lightly lubricate the distal 20 cm of the endoscope, taking care to avoid the lens.
2. Insert the endoscope gently through the anus and into the rectum (Figure E.14).

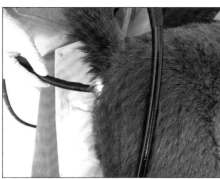

Figure E.14: The endoscope should be inserted gently through the anus and into the rectum.

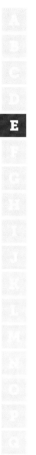

3 Once in the rectum, inflate with air to enable the mucosa to be visualized. Pinching the anus will prevent air from escaping.

4 Pass the endoscope along the descending colon, while insufflating with air.

5 At the cranial end of the descending colon, the junction between the descending and transverse colon (splenic flexure) will be encountered as an obvious 'bend' (Figure E.15). Move the tip of the endoscope in the direction of the bend and advance slowly. Some resistance may be felt, but excessive pressure should not be needed, and could result in rupture of the colon. It is not uncommon to induce red-out whilst doing this.

6 Once in the transverse colon, the lumen should be inflated with air to re-establish a clear image.

7 The next 'bend' marks the junction of the transverse and ascending colon; manoeuvre the endoscope in the direction of the bend and advance slowly, as before. Gently moving the endoscope backwards and forwards, while inflating with air, can aid its passage.

8 The ascending colon is short and ends at the ileocolic junction. This is recognized by the adjacent blind-ending sac, the caecum (Figure E.16). Carefully examine the caecum.

9 Direct the tip of the endoscope towards the ileocolic sphincter while advancing slowly. The ability to advance the endoscope into the ileum will depend on the size of the patient and the diameter of the endoscope insertion tube. If it is not possible to intubate the ileum for visual examination, it is permissible to advance the biopsy forceps 'blindly' into the ileum to collect biopsy samples. This must be done with care.

10 Withdraw the endoscope slowly and take biopsy samples. It is often easier to examine and sample the colon while the endoscope is being withdrawn.

Biopsy and sample handling

- Samples should be collected from any lesions found
- If no lesions are observed, samples should be collected from:
  - The ascending and transverse colon (take 2 or 3 from each)
  - The descending colon (take 4 or 5)
- **Samples should always be taken, even if no lesions are apparent**

Technique

1 Position the endoscope in the region to be sampled.

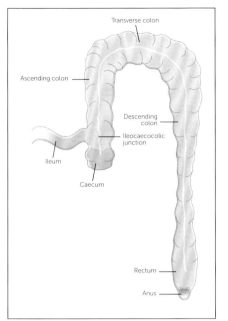

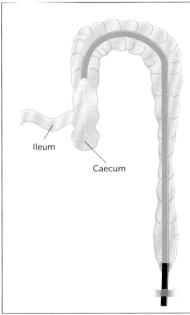

Figure E.15: Anatomical structure of the large intestine. (Reproduced from the *BSAVA Manual of Canine and Feline Endoscopy and Endosurgery*)

Figure E.16: The caecum is visible as a blind-ending sac adjacent to the ileocolic junction.

2 Pass the biopsy forceps down the biopsy channel of the endoscope with the cup firmly closed.

3 Pass the forceps out of the end of the endoscope, open the cup, position on to the mucosa, and close the cup.

4 Withdraw the biopsy forceps through the biopsy channel of the endoscope with the cup firmly closed.

PRACTICAL TIPS

- Position the biopsy forceps perpendicular to the mucosa whenever possible (Figure E.17). This will maximize sample collection
- Avoid overinflation, as this stretches the mucosa and smaller samples will be obtained
- Advance the forceps until the mucosa 'tents' and then close them

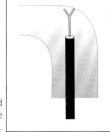

Figure E.17: The biopsy forceps should be positioned perpendicular to the mucosal wall to obtain a sample.

5 To remove the samples from the biopsy forceps, immerse in 10% neutral buffered formalin. Then rinse the forceps well in saline before reinserting them into the endoscope. Alternatively, carefully remove samples from the biopsy forceps with a needle and place directly into formalin or lay on the foam insert of a tissue cassette (e.g. CellSafe+ biopsy capsule).

Potential complications

- Gastrointestinal perforation is rare, but can result from forceful insertion of the endoscope. Excessive insufflation can also rupture ulcerated areas. Exploratory surgery is required if either of these occur
- Significant haemorrhage is rare. Minor and clinically insignificant haemorrhage is very common

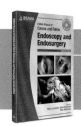

FURTHER INFORMATION

Further information on endoscopy of the GI tract can be found in the *BSAVA Manual of Canine and Feline Endoscopy and Endosurgery.*

Endotracheal intubation

Indications/Use

- Delivery of oxygen alone, or oxygen and inhalational agents, during general anaesthesia
- Severe upper respiratory tract obstruction (e.g. brachycephalic obstructive airway syndrome, laryngeal paralysis, laryngeal oedema, upper airway neoplasia)
- Delivery of oxygen and for manual ventilation during **cardiopulmonary resuscitation**

Equipment

- Endotracheal (ET) tubes (red rubber, PVC or silicone) of various sizes and lengths (Figure E.18)

NOTE

- Red rubber ET tubes are more likely to deteriorate over time and their opacity means that intraluminal obstructions may be overlooked. Consequently, PVC or silicone tubes are preferred

- Sterile, water-soluble lubricant
- Stylet, particularly if using silicone tubes
- Laryngoscope with appropriate length(s) of blade

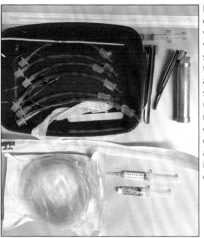

Figure E.18: Equipment prepared for intubation of a canine patient, including: ET tubes of various widths and lengths; laryngoscope with various blade lengths; open weave bandage for securing the tube to the patient; syringe for ET tube cuff inflation; induction agent drawn up in a syringe and 0.9% saline intravenous flush syringe; a dog urinary catheter and a rigid stylet (most commonly used with silicone ET tubes, not shown) which may be useful if a challenging intubation is anticipated; a tongue depressor which allows a thorough upper airway examination to be conducted prior to induction; suction tubing and a flexible suction catheter in case of regurgitation.

- Open weave bandage
- Syringe for cuff inflation
- Topical lidocaine spray for larynx (routinely used in cats only)

NOTE

- If using a commercially available topical lidocaine spray, the clinician should be aware of the dose delivered with each depression of the pump, as toxicity may result from repeated applications. A dose of 1 mg/kg of 2% lidocaine is appropriate for use in cats (i.e. approximately 0.2 ml for a 4 kg cat)

- An assistant
- Additional induction agent if intubating for anaesthesia
- An oxygen supply and breathing system (or Ambu bag) if intubating to establish a patent airway or for cardiopulmonary resuscitation
- If challenging intubation is anticipated:
  - Additional assistant to pass equipment or provide flow-by oxygen
  - Additional lighting (e.g. head torch)
  - Dog urinary catheters or feeding tubes to use as stylets; with appropriate connectors, oxygen can be delivered into the airway via a dog urinary catheter
  - Suction machine and tubing

Patient preparation and positioning

- The patient should be positioned in sternal recumbency; lateral or dorsal recumbency is also possible according to patient pathology or preference of the clinician
- Cats and small- and medium-breed dogs are usually placed on an appropriate trolley or table prior to intubation; large- and giant-breed dogs are more safely restrained on the floor for intubation
- Unless the pathology dictates otherwise, or when performed for cardiopulmonary resuscitation, patients should be premedicated and an adequate plane of anaesthesia induced prior to intubation

E

ET TUBE CHECKS

Before use, the following checks are advised:

- Is the ET tube clean and the lumen clear of any possible obstruction?
- Is there an appropriate connector to allow attachment to a breathing system?
- Ensure that the cuff does not leak – it should be inflated and left for 10 minutes or tested under water
- Premeasure the tube against the patient – it should reach from the incisors to the thoracic inlet when the neck is flexed. In cats and small dogs, the length of excess ET tube outside the patient's mouth should be minimized to reduce dead space
- Ensure that when water-soluble lubricant is applied to the tube it does not occlude the bevel or Murphy eye (vent hole)

Technique

1 An assistant holds the patient's upper jaw in one hand using a bandage tie placed behind the canine teeth. The patient's head and neck should be extended towards you at an approximately 45-degree angle.

2 Grasp the lower jaw, draw out the tongue gently and open the mouth wide; this can be facilitated by the assistant (Figure E.19).

3 Hold the laryngoscope and the tongue in your non-dominant hand and place the tip of the laryngoscope on the base of the tongue, just rostral to the epiglottis. It should not be placed on the epiglottis itself.

4 If the soft palate is obscuring the view of the larynx, use the ET tube or a stylet to gently lift it out of the way. If the patient has respiratory signs, assess the structure and function of the larynx at this point. Flow-by oxygen should also be provided.

5 As cats are prone to laryngospasm, spray the larynx with lidocaine prior to intubation. Wait 30–60 seconds for the lidocaine to desensitize the larynx before continuing and gently insert the tube only when the larynx is open using a rotating motion.

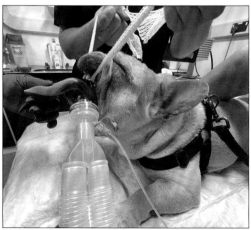

Figure E.19: An assistant holds the patient's upper jaw using a bandage tie behind the canine teeth and extends the head and neck towards the operator who grasps the lower jaw and draws out the tongue. Flow-by oxygen is provided by an additional assistant.

6 Advance the ET tube over the epiglottis. Direct the tube ventrally to pass through the arytenoid cartilages and vocal folds, into the trachea.

7 Confirm correct positioning of the ET tube in the trachea following intubation (e.g. via capnography but note that a trace may be absent prior to cuff inflation, observing movement of a small piece of cotton wool held over the end of the ET tube, or visualizing synchronous movement of the patient's thorax and the reservoir bag on the breathing system). If the patient is apnoeic, a breath can be given and synchronous chest excursion should be seen.

8 Secure the ET tube in place by tying the open-weave bandage around the tube or connector and then tying the ends around the upper or lower jaw or behind the ears. Once secured, the connector should sit external to the incisors.

9 Connect the ET tube to a breathing system and turn the oxygen supply on.

10 Inflate the cuff and check for gas leakage.

ET TUBE CUFFS

Red rubber and silicone ET tubes have high-pressure, low-volume cuffs, which better protect the airway from aspiration but increase the risk of tracheal mucosal injury. PVC ET tubes can have high-volume, low-pressure cuffs, which reduce the risk of tracheal mucosal injury but may be less protective against aspiration. Cuff inflation should be to a maximum pressure of 25 mmHg. Cuffs may deflate (or inflate if using nitrous oxide) during anaesthesia and therefore they should be checked regularly, particularly after a change in recumbency.

---

11 Always disconnect and reconnect the breathing system from the ET tube when turning the patient to reduce the risk of tracheal injury.

Potential complications

- Laryngospasm in cats
- Oesophageal intubation (this may promote regurgitation under anaesthesia and lead to hypoxaemia)
- Endobronchial intubation (premeasuring the tube against the patient helps reduce the risk of this complication)
- Kinking or obstruction of the ET tube whilst *in situ*
- Extubation during patient transport or change in recumbency
- Tracheal mucosal injury due to overinflation of the ET tube cuff, especially in cats. This may lead to tracheal stricture
- Tracheal rupture due to twisting of the ET tube whilst *in situ*
- Whilst rare, it is possible for ET tubes to be bitten and inhaled

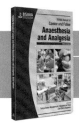

FURTHER INFORMATION

For more information on intubation, see the *BSAVA Manual of Canine and Feline Anaesthesia and Analgesia.*

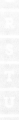

Endotracheal wash

Indications/Use

- To obtain a sample from the airways for cytology and bacteriology. Blind sampling via an endotracheal (ET) tube can be reasonably effective, especially in cats, and is a valuable technique if bronchoscopy is not available
- Generally yields samples representative of the trachea and primary or (at best) secondary bronchi, although some material from the lower bronchioles and alveoli may be collected

---

OPTIONS

- The upper airway of medium- and large-breed dogs may also be sampled by **transtracheal wash**
- The lower airways of dogs and cats may be sampled using **bronchoalveolar lavage**

Contraindications

- Compromised respiratory function
- Patients with pulmonary parenchymal disease, rather than tracheal or bronchial disease

Equipment

- Sterile ET tube
- Male dog urinary catheter (4–6 Fr). The tip of the catheter can be cut off to remove the side holes, but care must be taken to ensure that the tip is not sharp. Alternatively, a lavage catheter (e.g. one designed for a bronchoscope biopsy channel) can be used
- Topical lidocaine spray for larynx (routinely used in cats only)
- Warmed 0.9% sterile saline
- 10 ml and 20 ml syringes
- 3-way tap
- Sterile plain and EDTA collection tubes
- Microscope slides

Patient preparation and positioning

- The patient should be preoxygenated using a face mask prior to induction of general anaesthesia
- General anaesthesia is essential
- The patient is placed in either lateral or sternal recumbency

---

SPECIAL CONSIDERATIONS FOR CATS

- Extra care should be taken when performing bronchoscopy in cats, as the airways are particularly prone to bronchospasm.
- The procedure should be performed as quickly as possible with the minimum of trauma
  continues ▶

> ### SPECIAL CONSIDERATION FOR CATS continued
>
> - As cats are prone to laryngospasm, the larynx should be sprayed with lidocaine prior to intubation. The clinician should wait 30–60 seconds for the lidocaine to desensitize the larynx before gently inserting the tube; the tube should only be inserted when the larynx is open, using a rotating motion
> - If a commercially available topical lidocaine spray is being used, the clinician should be aware of the dose delivered with each depression of the pump, as toxicity may result from repeated applications. A dose of 1 mg/kg of 2% lidocaine is appropriate for use in cats (i.e. approximately 0.2 ml for a 4 kg cat)
> - To reduce the risk of bronchospasm, terbutaline can be given approximately 30 minutes prior to bronchoscopy (0.015 mg/kg s.c. or i.m). The onset of action is 15–30 minutes and is usually notable by an increase in heart rate
> - Terbutaline should also be available for administration during the procedure if bronchospasm still occurs. If this does not stabilize the patient, administration of a short-acting steroid (e.g. dexamethasone sodium phosphate 0.1 mg/kg i.v. once) should be considered
> - A suction unit (or 10–20 ml syringe attached to a sterile urinary catheter) should be kept nearby and can be used for clearing any secretions from the oropharynx. The cat should be maintained in sternal recumbency, if possible, for this procedure. If the cat resents suctioning of the oropharynx, re-induction of anaesthesia may be required to clear the upper airway effectively

Technique

1. Premeasure the length of the catheter needed to reach the tracheal bifurcation (approximately the 4th intercostal space) and mark this on the packaging.
2. If intubating a cat, apply topical local anaesthetic spray to the larynx. Topical lidocaine spray for larynx (routinely used in cats only).
3. Insert a sterile ET tube into the trachea, avoiding oral contamination (see **Endotracheal intubation**).

> ### NOTE
>
> - Take care to minimize contact between the tip of the ET tube and the oropharynx during intubation, to avoid oropharyngeal contamination

4. Pass the sterile catheter down the ET tube to the pre-marked length. To avoid contamination, the catheter should be inserted by feeding it *through the sterile packaging (if present)*.
5. Attach a 3-way tap to the catheter.
6. Inject warmed sterile saline (0.5 ml/kg) into the catheter via the 3-way tap.
7. Immediately aspirate back the saline.

8 Repeat the injection of saline and the aspiration two or three times as required. A total recovery of 1–3 ml of a slightly turbid fluid with a foamy layer at the top (representative of surfactant) represents good sample recovery. Coupage and turning the patient may improve cell yield.

9 Following completion of an endotracheal wash, continue administration of 100% oxygen and volatile agent for 5 minutes, to allow time to detect any immediate complications from the procedure (e.g. bronchospasm). Continue oxygen supplementation via the ET tube until extubation. Pulse oximetry should be utilized to measure the patient's oxygenation throughout recovery from anaesthesia and during the postoperative period.

Sample handling

- A portion of the sample should be placed in a sterile plain tube and submitted for culture
- A portion of the sample should be placed in an EDTA tube and submitted for cytology
- The cells collected are fragile, so samples should be processed as soon as possible. If samples are to be sent to an external laboratory, fresh air-dried unstained smears of any flocculent/mucoid material should also be made (see **Fine-needle aspiration**). Direct smears of the fluid can be made, but most samples are poorly cellular

Potential complications

- Bronchospasm
- Laryngospasm and coughing
- Haemorrhage
- Iatrogenic infection
- Placement of catheters with excessive force can damage the lungs and airways and, in the worst case scenario, result in pneumothorax

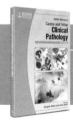

FURTHER INFORMATION

Details on cytology of upper respiratory tract samples can be found in the *BSAVA Manual of Canine and Feline Clinical Pathology*

Fine-needle aspiration

Indications/Use

- To obtain a sample for cytology. Some tissues or masses give much better cell yields and/or greater chance of a definitive diagnosis than others

Contraindications

- Aspiration of internal organs of patients with severe thrombocytopenia or a coagulopathy
- Aspiration of highly vascular masses (particularly if internal)
- Cases in which the results would not affect decision making (e.g. a lesion that clearly requires surgical management)

WARNING

- Clotting times (activated partial thromboplastin time (APTT) and one-stage prothrombin time (OSPT)) should ideally be checked before aspirating masses associated with the liver, spleen, kidney or other well vascularized organs.

Equipment

- As required for **Aseptic preparation – (a) non-surgical procedures**
- Hypodermic needles: 21–23 G for cutaneous/subcutaneous masses and lymph nodes; 23 G for internal organs; 16–25 mm (depending on depth of tissue to be sampled)
- 5 ml syringe
- Microscope slides
- Hairdryer
- Ultrasound equipment (where required)

Patient preparation and positioning

- Fine-needle aspiration of superficial masses can usually be performed with the patient under physical restraint or light sedation
- Fine-needle aspiration of abdominal viscera or masses may require heavy sedation or general anaesthesia
- The animal is positioned with the area to be sampled uppermost
- **Aseptic preparation – (a) non-surgical procedures** is performed on the skin over the site to be aspirated, or the skin overlying the needle insertion site (for abdominal viscera/mass aspiration)

Technique

1. For superficial masses, immobilize the mass with one hand and insert the needle into it using the other hand. For deep masses, or masses or viscera within the abdomen or thorax, immobilization is usually not possible.
2. Aspiration may be performed using the 'needle-only' method or by using continuous suction.
   a. **Needle-only method:** this method is useful for aspirating soft masses and

lymph nodes. It has the advantages that fragile cells are not damaged by suction and haemodilution is minimized.

i   Insert the needle into the mass without a syringe attached.

ii Gently redirect the needle several times within the mass to gather a core of cells in the barrel of the needle (Figure F.1). The needle should not exit the mass during redirection.

iii Remove the needle from the mass.

b **Continuous suction method:** this method is useful for aspirating firm masses such as soft tissue sarcomas, which tend not to exfoliate cells well. It can, however, cause more damage to fragile cells and may increase blood contamination.

i   Insert the needle into the mass with a 5 ml syringe attached.

ii With the needle in the mass, withdraw the plunger to one-half to three-quarters of the volume of the syringe (to apply 2–3 ml suction).

iii Maintain suction and move the needle to and fro, redirecting the needle several times within the mass (Figure F.2).

iv Release the suction and remove the needle from the mass.

v   Disconnect the needle from the syringe.

3 Attach an air-filled syringe to the needle.

4 Expel the contents of the needle containing the sample on to one or more clean microscope slides (Figure F.3) and prepare smears using one of the techniques described below.

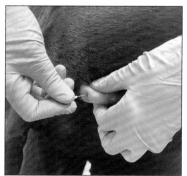

Figure F.1: The needle-only aspiration method can be used to collect samples from soft masses or lymph nodes.

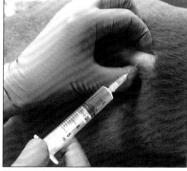

Figure F.2: The continuous suction aspiration method can be used to collect samples from firm masses.

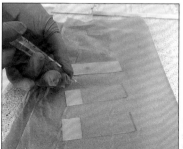

Figure F.3: The contents of the needle should be expelled on to microscope slides and prepared for examination.

Ultrasound guidance

- Fine-needle aspiration of internal organs and of intra-thoracic or intra-abdominal masses is best performed under ultrasound guidance
- Care should be taken to remove excess ultrasound gel from the area of skin through which the needle is to be inserted, as gel can obscure cellular detail and alter the staining characteristics of the sample
- The needle should be introduced close to the ultrasound probe, to make visualization and tracking of the needle point easier
- Although a one-handed active aspiration technique with a syringe attached is possible, in many cases introducing the needle alone and redirecting its path within the area of interest is not only adequate but easier if single-handed

Sample handling

Squash preparation

With experience, this technique produces excellent smears. However, in inexperienced hands cells may be damaged/ruptured, resulting in an unreadable smear.

1 Expel the aspirate on to the centre of a microscope slide (Figure F.4a).
2 Place a second 'spreader' slide horizontally and at right angles to spread the sample, taking care not to exert downward pressure that could rupture the cells.
3 Using only the surface tension between the two slides, draw the 'spreader' slide quickly and smoothly across the bottom slide (Figure F.4b).
4 Rapidly dry the smear by waving it in the air or under a hairdryer. **Note that it is the smear produced on the _underside of the 'spreader' slide_ that will be examined.**

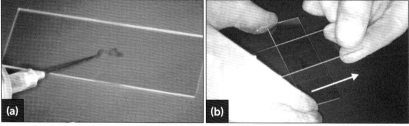

Figure F.4: Squash preparation. **(a)** The aspirate should be expelled on to a microscope slide. **(b)** A 'spreader' slide is then drawn across the bottom slide to create the smear.

Blood film technique

This technique has less potential for causing cell rupture and is useful for lymph node aspirates since lymphocytes are fragile. It is not suitable for samples of low cellularity, e.g. fluid aspirates. A 'spreader' slide with one corner missing is used to prepare the smear in order to avoid spreading the cells over the edges of the slide.

1 Expel the aspirate near to one end of a microscope slide in the centre line.
2 Hold the 'spreader' between the thumb and middle finger, placing the index finger on top of the 'spreader'.

3 Place the 'spreader' in front of the aspirate, at an angle of about 30 degrees, and draw it backwards until it comes into contact with the sample, allowing the sample to spread out rapidly along the edge of the 'spreader'.

4 Advance the 'spreader' forwards smoothly and quickly.

5 After the 'spreader' has been advanced two-thirds of the way along the bottom slide, lift it abruptly upwards in order to concentrate cells at the end of the smear.

6 Rapidly dry the smear by waving it in the air or under a hairdryer.

Potential complications

- Haemorrhage. Any haemorrhage should be controlled by firm pressure over the site for several minutes. Continued haemorrhage from an internal organ is an indication for exploratory surgery
- Tissue inflammation (e.g. mast cell tumour degranulation)
- Introduction of infectious material into a previously sterile space following aspiration of an abscess
- Seeding from tumours, especially urothelial cell (transitional cell) carcinoma or from the urinary tract, as well as carcinomas of the lung, liver and kidney

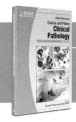

FURTHER INFORMATION

For information on fine-needle aspiration and cytological interpretation, see the *BSAVA Manual of Canine and Feline Clinical Pathology.*

Gallbladder aspiration

Indications/Use
- Investigation of biliary tract disease
- To obtain samples for cytology and bacteriology

Contraindications
- Biliary tract obstruction, as this may result in leakage or rupture
- Severe disease of the gallbladder wall, as this may result in leakage or rupture

Equipment
- As required for **Aseptic preparation – (a) non-surgical procedures**
- Ultrasound machine (for ultrasound-guided aspiration)
- 10–20 ml syringe
- Hypodermic or spinal needles: 21–23 G; 1.5 to 3 inches (depending on depth of the gallbladder)
- EDTA and sterile plain collection tubes

Patient preparation and positioning

APPROACH

Gallbladder aspiration is performed under ultrasound guidance or at the time of an exploratory laparotomy. When performed under ultrasound guidance, a transhepatic approach may be used to minimize leakage of bile. Gallbladder aspiration should never be performed 'blind'.

ASSESSMENT OF COAGULATION

It may be best practice to perform a coagulation panel (prothrombin and activated partial thromboplastin times) prior to gallbladder aspiration, especially in patients with suspected chronic liver disease. If coagulation abnormalities are found, vitamin K at 0.5–1.5 mg/kg s.c. q12h should be given; re-evaluate coagulation times after 24–48 hours to confirm normalization prior to aspiration. If vitamin K has no effect, a transfusion of fresh frozen plasma should be administered and coagulation testing repeated before aspiration is carried out. Provided no coagulation abnormalities are detected, aspiration should be performed as soon as possible after a plasma transfusion.

- If performed under ultrasound guidance, general anaesthesia or heavy sedation is essential
- The patient is placed in dorsal or lateral recumbency, depending on which position allows optimal visualization of the liver and gallbladder
- Using ultrasonography, the optimal site for gallbladder aspiration is identified. This is often on the left side of the patient as this is more likely to allow the needle to be inserted through adjacent liver tissue prior to entry into the gallbladder. In large dogs, an intercostal approach may be required
- **Aseptic preparation – (a) non-surgical procedures** is performed on the skin over a wide area around the site of needle entry

Technique

1   If using ultrasonography, the site previously identified is used. If performed during surgery, identify a site in the body of the gallbladder and away from its neck; there is no need to use a transhepatic approach, as the site of needle insertion can be monitored for leakage.

2   Insert the needle with the syringe attached into the gallbladder, ideally at an angle of approximately 45 degrees to the body wall. This will help to minimize leakage of bile following withdrawal of the needle.

3   Aspirate bile into the syringe, removing as much as possible in order to minimize leakage after needle removal.

4   Monitor for bile leakage for approximately 5–10 minutes after aspiration, either visually at the time of surgery or with ultrasonography.

5   If there is evidence of significant bile leakage, an exploratory laparotomy is required.

> **WARNING**
>
> - It should be remembered that there is still a risk of haemorrhage even if coagulation parameters are normal, and it is therefore essential to have the option of prompt surgical intervention in case of complications. The animal also needs to be kept under close observation after the procedure and monitored for evidence of haemorrhage (e.g. tachycardia, pallor, weakness, reduced pulse quality).

Sample handling

- A portion of the sample should be submitted in a sterile plain tube for culture and sensitivity testing
- An aliquot should be placed in an EDTA tube for cytology

Potential complications

- Leakage of bile, leading to bile peritonitis
- Gallbladder rupture
- Haemorrhage

Gastric decompression – (a) orogastric intubation

Indications/Use

- Stabilization of dogs with gastric dilatation and volvulus (GDV) prior to surgery
- Orogastric intubation is superior to percutaneous needle decompression (see below)

> **WARNING**
>
> - Fluid therapy for the treatment of hypovolaemic shock must be initiated prior to gastric decompression.

Equipment

- Wide-bore stomach tube
- 7.5 cm wide roll of adhesive bandage with a hollow plastic core
- Funnel
- Bucket
- Warmed 0.9% sterile saline, lactated Ringer's (Hartmann's) solution or tap water

Patient preparation and positioning

- Sedation may be required to reduce anxiety, but the patient should be monitored for hypotension
- A right lateral abdominal radiograph should be obtained to confirm the diagnosis of GDV if there is any doubt
- The patient should be placed on a table or trolley to allow gravity to aid in gastric emptying
- A 'sitting' position or sternal recumbency is often best, but gastric decompression may be achieved in right lateral recumbency

Technique

1. Mark the distance from the dog's nose to its 11th rib on the stomach tube. The tube should not be passed beyond this length, to minimize the risk of rupture of a potentially compromised gastric wall.
2. Insert the bandage roll longitudinally into the dog's mouth. The mouth is held closed around the bandage roll by an assistant or by applying tape around the dog's muzzle (Figure G.1ab).
3. Apply a small amount of lubricant on to the end of the tube. Insert the stomach tube through the core of the bandage roll and gently down into the dog's stomach. Rotating the stomach tube gently about its long axis may aid passage through the gastro-oesophageal junction.
4. Gaseous decompression is achieved spontaneously.
5. Further emptying of the stomach can be achieved by lavage with copious volumes of warm saline, lactated Ringer's (Hartmann's) solution or tap water.
   a. Pour the solution from a height into the stomach, using a funnel attached to the end of the stomach tube.
   b. Allow the contents to flow out of the stomach by lowering the tube below the level of the dog.

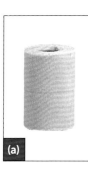
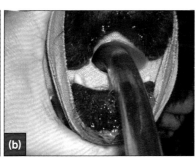

Figure G.1: (a) A 7.5 cm adhesive bandage roll with plastic core. (b) The roll placed 'end-on' orally with similar tape wrapped around the dog's muzzle to facilitate passage of a stomach tube. (© John Williams)

(a)

(b)

Potential complications

- Trauma to the gastro-oesophageal junction
- Passage of the stomach tube through a compromised gastric wall

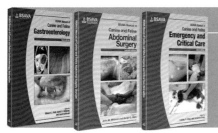

FURTHER INFORMATION

For more detail on gastric dilatation and volvulus, see the *BSAVA Manual of Canine and Feline Abdominal Surgery*, the *BSAVA Manual of Emergency and Critical Care* and the *BSAVA Manual of Canine and Feline Gastroenterology*.

Gastric decompression – (b) percutaneous needle

Indications/Use

- May facilitate orogastric intubation
- Should be performed when orogastric intubation is not possible

> **WARNING**
>
> - Fluid therapy for the treatment of hypovolaemic shock must be initiated prior to gastric decompression.

Equipment

- As for **Aseptic preparation – (a) non-surgical procedures**
- 16 or 18 G over-the-needle intravenous catheter

Patient preparation and positioning

- Sedation may be required to reduce anxiety, but the patient should be monitored for hypotension
- A right lateral abdominal radiograph should be obtained to confirm the diagnosis of GDV if there is any doubt
- The patient is placed in left lateral or sternal recumbency
- **Aseptic preparation – (a) non-surgical procedures** is performed on an area of skin over the most distended part of the right abdominal wall

Technique

1 Percuss the right abdominal wall and define the site of greatest tympany, where the distended stomach is likely to be directly abutting the abdominal wall.

2 Insert the catheter percutaneously directly into the stomach.

3 Remove the stylet of the catheter to allow air to escape freely from the stomach.

Potential complications

- Entry of the catheter into another abdominal organ

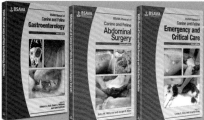

FURTHER INFORMATION

For more detail on gastric dilatation and volvulus, see the *BSAVA Manual of Canine and Feline Abdominal Surgery*, the *BSAVA Manual of Emergency and Critical Care* and the *BSAVA Manual of Canine and Feline Gastroenterology*.

Gastric decontamination

Indications/Use

- In most cases of acute toxin ingestion. However, decontamination can only be performed within a narrow window of time for most substances; it is therefore important to obtain a thorough history and time since exposure

---

METHOD SELECTION

- Gastric decontamination is performed either by induction of **emesis** or by **gastric lavage**. Gastric lavage is not as effective as emesis, so if emesis can be safely induced this is preferred
- Activated charcoal should be administered following emesis/gastric lavage; it acts as an adsorbent for many toxins and further reduces gastrointestinal absorption
- When a toxin cannot be identified but there is a high suspicion of poisoning, it is reasonable to give a single dose of activated charcoal
- However, it should not be given where the toxin does not reliably bind to activated charcoal (e.g. heavy metals, xylitol, ethylene glycol, alcohol) or when it is contraindicated (e.g. salt toxicosis, corrosives, hydrocarbons)
- In addition, symptomatic patients who are at risk of aspiration pneumonia (e.g. have a decreased gag reflex) should not receive oral activated charcoal
- Other contraindications for activated charcoal administration include patients requiring endoscopy (due to decreased visualization), when there is risk of a pharmacobezoar (functional ileus) or in patients with mechanical ileus

---

Emesis

- Induction of emesis should be attempted when ingestion is recent (e.g. 1–2 hours) in asymptomatic patients
- Delayed induction of emesis (up to 4–6 hours post-ingestion) is only recommended if the patient remains asymptomatic and the toxin is known to stay in the stomach for long periods of time (e.g. chocolate, grapes, large wads of chewing gum containing xylitol, massive ingestions of toxins)

Contraindications

- Emesis induction should not be performed:
  - If the ingested substance is caustic or corrosive, due to the risk of further damage to the oesophagus
  - If the ingesta contains paraffin, petroleum products or other oily or volatile organic compounds, due to the risk of inhalation
  - If the patient is unconscious, fitting, in respiratory distress or unable to stand

Equipment

- An emetic agent such as apomorphine, an alpha-2 agonist (e.g. xylazine or medetomidine) or sodium carbonate (washing soda) (see below for doses in different species)

Patient preparation and positioning

- Patients should be conscious and standing

Technique

There are different options for the induction of emesis in different species.

Dogs

- Apomorphine at 0.1 mg/kg s.c. (licenced dose)
- Sodium carbonate (washing soda) crystals. The dose is empirical but usually a large crystal in a medium- to large-breed dog and a small crystal in a small dog. **DO NOT confuse with caustic soda (sodium hydroxide)**

Cats

- Alpha-2 agonists such as xylazine at 0.6 mg/kg i.m. or 1.0 mg/kg s.c. once (effective in >75% of cats), i.m. or dexmedetomidine at 7 µg (micrograms)/kg i.m. *Note that these drugs may also result in the unwanted effect of sedation*
- Sodium carbonate (washing soda) crystals. The dose is empirical but usually a small crystal is appropriate for a cat. **DO NOT confuse with caustic soda (sodium hydroxide)**

WARNING

- Other options such as syrup of ipecacuanha, household remedies (table salt, mustard) and hydrogen peroxide are not recommended and can be dangerous.

Gastric lavage

Equipment

- As required for **Gastric decompression – (a) orogastric intubation** (adhesive bandage not required)

Patient preparation and positioning

- The patient should be anaesthetized and the trachea intubated with a cuffed endotracheal tube (see **Endotracheal intubation**)
- The patient should be placed in lateral or sternal recumbency, ideally with the head at a level below that of the body

Technique

1 Mark the distance from the animal's nose to its 11th rib on the stomach tube. The tube should not be passed beyond this length, to minimize the risk of rupture of a potentially compromised gastric wall.

2 Insert a lubricated stomach tube into the animal's mouth, down the oesophagus and into the stomach using gentle twisting motions. Simultaneous inflation (e.g. blowing into the tube) will assist with passage of the tube into the stomach.

3 Confirm appropriate orogastric tube placement. This can be achieved by:
   a Palpating the neck for two tube-like structures (i.e. the trachea and the orogastric tube within the oesophagus)
   b Palpating the body wall for the orogastric tube within the abdomen
   c Obtaining gastric contents or gas upon orogastric tube placement
   d Insufflating the orogastric tube while simultaneously auscultating for gurgling sounds within the stomach.

4 Instil approximately 10 ml/kg tepid or warm water via the bilge/stomach pump or via gravity through a funnel.

5 During the procedure, frequently palpate the stomach to prevent overdistension. Aggressive agitation of the stomach during lavage can enhance recovery.

6 Allow the fluid to drain out of the stomach tube, by lowering the tube and the animal's head.

7 Perform multiple lavage cycles. The procedure should be repeated until the fluid returned is relatively clear (commonly 10–20 times).

8 The orogastric tube must be 'kinked off' prior to removal in order to prevent fluid from being accidentally aspirated.

Activated charcoal

- Activated charcoal is usually given via a stomach tube after gastric lavage, but can also be administered orally after the induction of emesis
- Slurries of activated charcoal are more effective than tablets or capsules
- Recommended dose is 0.5–4.0 g/kg orally and can be repeated every 4–6 hours for the first 24–48 hours, or until charcoal is seen in the faeces
- Repeat dose administration of activated charcoal is particularly important when the agent is enterohepatically recirculated (e.g. salicylates, barbiturates, theobromine, methylxanthines)
- Activated charcoal can slow gastrointestinal transit time, thus co-administration of a cathartic (e.g. sorbitol or magnesium sulphate) can be considered, although this is not recommended in dehydrated patients or patients where there is a suspicion of ileus

> **WARNING**
> - Activated charcoal reduces the absorption of, and therefore the efficacy of, orally administered drugs.

Potential complications

- Damage to the oesophagus from caustic or corrosive ingesta or the stomach tube
- Inhalation of stomach contents
- Passage of the stomach tube through a damaged gastric wall

Gastrostomy tube placement – (a) endoscopic

Indications/Use

- Long-term (months to years) nutritional support
- Where naso-oesophageal or oesophagostomy tube feeding is not possible (e.g. vomiting, severe oesophageal disease or following oesophageal surgery, head/neck trauma)

Contraindications

- Gastric outflow obstruction
- Severe oesophageal strictures (may impede endoscope passage)
- Likely temporary anorexia, especially when an alternative feeding method could be used (e.g. **naso-oesophageal tube placement**, **oesophagostomy tube placement**)
- Comatose, recumbent or dysphoric animals that are at risk of aspiration
- Surgical placement of a gastrostomy tube may be preferable in obese patients or those with ascites where close apposition of the stomach to the abdominal wall may be difficult to achieve with an endoscopic approach

Equipment

- A commercial percutaneous endoscopic gastrostomy (PEG) kit (Figure G.2) containing a radiopaque polyurethane 60–80 cm gastrostomy tube, introducer needle, guidewire, fixation device and Y-adaptor:
  - Cats and small dogs: 16 Fr
  - Medium and large dogs: 20–22 Fr
- Endoscope: 7–10 mm diameter; 1 m long
- Endoscopic grasping or biopsy forceps
- As required for **Aseptic preparation – (a) non-surgical procedures**
- Scalpel and No. 10 scalpel blade
- Sterile dressing to cover the tube site
- Tube gauze or loose body wrap

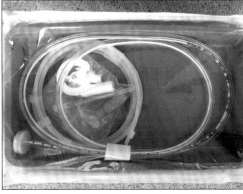

Figure G.2: Commercial PEG kit.

Patient preparation and positioning

- General anaesthesia is required
- The patient is positioned in right lateral recumbency
- **Aseptic preparation – (a) non-surgical procedures** is performed on an area on the left flank (approximately 15 cm x 15 cm in a medium-sized dog), extending caudally from the costal arch and dorsoventrally from the transverse processes of the lumbar vertebrae to the level of the ventral end of the 13th rib

Technique

1 Insert the endoscope down the oesophagus and into the stomach. Insufflate the stomach so it is moderately distended.
2 An assistant applies pressure on the stomach with a finger just behind the last rib, and the endoscopist visualizes the indented mucosa. This allows identification of the site into which the tube will be inserted. *Alternatively,* the light of the endoscope may be seen shining through the body wall and used to locate the site of catheter insertion. Ideally, the tube should enter the stomach at the junction of the body and the antrum; if it is too near the pylorus it may cause an obstruction.
3 Make a 5–10 mm skin incision over the site identified for tube insertion.
4 Withdraw the endoscope back into the cardia.
5 Insert the introducer needle percutaneously into the inflated stomach via the skin incision (Figure G.3).
6 Pass endoscopic grasping or biopsy forceps down the biopsy channel and out the end of the endoscope. Open the forceps and position them by the tip of the introducer needle ready to grab the guidewire.
7 Pass the guidewire through the introducer catheter and thread it into the stomach.
8 Grasp the guidewire with the endoscopic grasping or biopsy forceps (Figure G.4). Without withdrawing the forceps into the biopsy channel, hold the forceps and endoscope as one unit and slowly pull this out of the stomach, up the oesophagus and out of the mouth. **Keep the forceps closed at all times**.

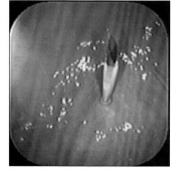

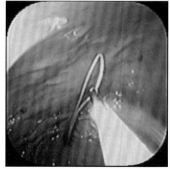

Figure G.3: The introducer needle is inserted percutaneously into the inflated stomach ideally at the junction of the body and the antrum.

Figure G.4: The guidewire should be grasped with the forceps.

9 Once the tip of the endoscope, forceps and guidewire come out of the animal's mouth, release the guidewire from the forceps.
10 Attach the guidewire to the end of the gastrostomy tube (Figure G.5).

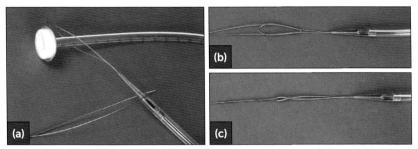

Figure G.5: (a) The mushroom tip of the PEG tube is looped through the swaged-on wire loop to join it to the wire loop passing out of the mouth. (b) The wire loops are interlocked. (c) The wires are pulled tight to produce a knotless connection.

11 Pull the other end of the guidewire, from where it exits the animal's flank, to draw the feeding tube into the mouth, down the oesophagus, into the stomach, and out through the stomach wall (Figure G.6). Firm traction is needed to pull the feeding tube through the stomach and body wall layers and out through the skin incision.
12 Once the gastrostomy tube has exited the body wall, pull it so that the bumper on the end of the tube that is to remain in the stomach lies snugly against the stomach wall (Figure G.7).

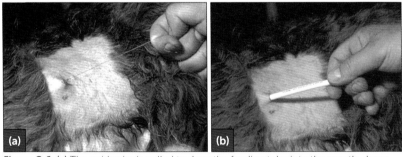

Figure G.6: (a) The guidewire is pulled to draw the feeding tube into the mouth, down the oesophagus, into the stomach and (b) out through the stomach wall.

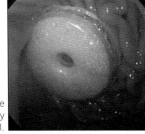

Figure G.7: The bumper on the end of the tube should fit snugly against the stomach wall.

13 Pass the endoscope back into the stomach to check that the tube is positioned in the correct area and that the bumper is flat against the stomach wall.

14 Secure the tube with the fixation device contained within the kit. Note that the tube should not be pulled and fixed excessively tightly, as this could result in skin and stomach wall necrosis.

15 In case of future migration, note the correct position of the tube relative to the body wall, based on the centimetre graduations on the side of the tube.

16 If the kit allows, cut the tube to the desired length. Attach the adaptor contained within the kit on to the end of the tube (Figure G.8).

17 Apply a sterile dressing to the skin stoma site.

18 Place tube gauze or a loose body wrap to protect the remaining tube and prevent it from being removed (Figure G.9).

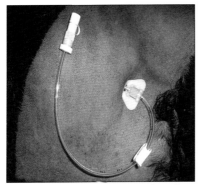

Figure G.8: Once the tube is in place, it should be cut to the desired length and an adapter attached to the end of the tube.

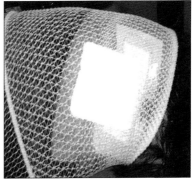

Figure G.9: The tube should be protected by gauze to prevent it from being removed by the patient.

Feeding technique

NOTE

- Do not use the tube for the first 24 hours, to allow a primary seal to form between the stomach and body wall

1 Instil sterile saline initially, in case the tube has migrated. If there is any doubt as to its position, take abdominal radiographs with or without sterile **iodinated contrast medium**.

2 Before feeding each time, flush the tube with small amounts (5–10 ml) of lukewarm tap water.

3 Aspirate the contents of the stomach with an empty syringe prior to feeding. If gastric emptying is delayed and there is more than half the previous meal in the stomach, skip the feed and consider motility modifiers such as metoclopramide.

4 Food should be warmed to body temperature and injected into the tube over approximately 5 minutes.

a Feed only one-third of the resting energy requirement (RER) on the first day.

b On the second day, feed two-thirds of the RER, increasing to the entire RER on the third day.

c Divide the daily requirement into multiple (5 or 6) feeds per 24 hours.

5 Flush the tube *after every feed* with 5–10 ml of lukewarm tap water.

RESTING ENERGY REQUIREMENT

The resting energy requirement is now used as the 'baseline' energy recommendation for hospitalized dogs and cats, regardless of the disease or surgery.

The following equation can be used to calculate the RER in kcal/day for cats or dogs:

RER = 70 × bodyweight (kg)$^{0.75}$

Alternatively, for animals >2 kg the following equation can be used:

RER = 30 × bodyweight (kg) + 70

Note: to convert kcal to kilojoules (kJ) multiply by 4.185

Tube maintenance and removal

- The stoma site should be inspected and cleaned daily, and antibiotic cream applied if necessary
- If the tube becomes blocked, 3 ml of a carbonated drink (e.g. cola or soda water) can be instilled and left for 5–10 minutes to help dislodge blockages
- The gastrostomy tube should remain in place for at least 7–10 days before removal. This period of time allows a permanent adhesion to form between the stomach and the body wall, and to prevent leakage of gastric contents into the peritoneal cavity
- If a gastrostomy tube is accidentally removed before intended, it can be re-placed through the same stoma site if the procedure is performed rapidly (e.g. within 24 hours of the tube removal)
- Some commercial PEG tubes have a collapsible soft bumper. To remove these tubes, the gauze dressing at the skin stoma site and the loose body wrap are removed, and the fixation device undone. Using firm pressure, the tube is pulled out of the stomach through the skin. Other types of tubes may require endoscopic removal (see the manufacturer's instructions)

Potential complications

- Major complications of gastrostomy tube placement in dogs and cats are uncommon and can usually be avoided with proper technique and careful client counselling
- The most common complications are:
  - Tube blockage
  - Leakage around the tube site
  - If the tube is not capped, leakage of gastric acid can cause acid burns on the skin
  - Infection at the tube site

- Tube dislodgement or removal
- Vomiting following feeding
■ Other complications include:
  - Diarrhoea due to overfeeding
  - Delayed gastric emptying due to effects of the tube on gastric motility
  - Splenic laceration
  - Necrosis of the gastric wall if the tube is too tight

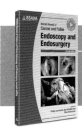

FURTHER INFORMATION

Further information on endoscopic placement of gastrostomy tubes can be found in the *BSAVA Manual of Canine and Feline Endoscopy and Endosurgery.*

Gastrostomy tube placement – (b) surgical

Indications/Use

■ As for **Gastrostomy tube placement – (a) endoscopic**, but surgical placement is usually selected when a patient is undergoing abdominal surgery or if endoscopic equipment is not available. A surgical approach permits suture placement between the stomach and abdominal wall (gastropexy), which results in a more secure seal around the tube. This may be preferable in obese patients or those with ascites.

Contraindications

■ Gastric outflow obstruction
■ Likely temporary anorexia, especially when an alternative feeding method could be used (e.g. naso-oesophageal tube placement, oesophagostomy tube placement)
■ Comatose, recumbent or dysphoric animals that are at risk of aspiration

Equipment

■ Mushroom-tipped catheter with large ('XL') mushroom
  - Cats and small dogs: 16 Fr
  - Medium and large dogs: 20–24 Fr
■ Gastrostomy tube connector and bung
■ As required for **Aseptic preparation – (b) surgical procedures**
■ Suture materials
■ Soft tissue surgical instrument set

Patient positioning and preparation

- General anaesthesia is required
- The animal should be placed in right lateral recumbency or in dorsal recumbency
- **Aseptic preparation – (b) surgical procedures** is required

Technique

1 The stomach is approached via a left paracostal coeliotomy or a ventral midline coeliotomy.
2 Make a full-thickness stab incision in the left abdominal wall just caudal to the costal arch at the level of the fundus of the stomach.
3 Pass the feeding tube through the incision so that the mushroom tip is within the abdomen and the external (catheter tip) end is outside.
4 Place a full-thickness purse-string suture (absorbable) in the fundus, midway between the lesser and greater curvatures. The diameter of the purse-string suture should be large enough to facilitate passage of the feeding tube through the centre. Do not tie the ends of the suture, but hold them with haemostats.
5 Make a stab incision in the centre of the purse-string suture, just large enough to push the folded mushroom tip of the catheter through.
6 Tighten the purse-string suture and secure it around the shaft of the gastrostomy tube; this seals the stomach wall around the tube.
7 Place four horizontal mattress sutures (absorbable) around the feeding tube between the stomach wall and the transversus abdominis muscle in a square configuration, to appose the stomach to the left abdominal wall. Place all the sutures before any is tied.
8 Omentum can be wrapped around the gastropexy site to promote healing.
9 Pull the external (catheter tip) end of the tube so that the mushroom tip is positioned snugly against the stomach wall.
10 Secure the tube to the skin using a finger-trap suture (non-absorbable).
11 Close the coeliotomy wound routinely.

Feeding technique; Tube maintenance and removal; Potential complications

As for **Gastrostomy tube placement – (a) endoscopic**.

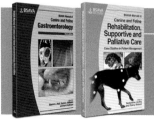

FURTHER INFORMATION

Further details on placement and use of gastrostomy tubes can be found in the *BSAVA Manual of Canine and Feline Gastroenterology* and the *BSAVA Manual of Canine and Feline Rehabilitation, Supportive and Palliative Care*.

Haemagglutination (in-saline agglutination) test

Indications/Use

- Confirmation of suspected immune-mediated haemolytic anaemia (IMHA)

> **NOTES**
>
> - A negative haemagglutination (in-saline agglutination) test result does not rule out IMHA. The direct antiglobulin or Coombs' test, which detects antibodies associated with the surface or red blood cells, should be performed if IMHA is suspected and autoagglutination cannot be demonstrated
> - A positive haemagglutination test is regarded as being diagnostic for IMHA and precludes the need to perform the Coombs' test

Equipment

- 1 ml of venous blood, freshly collected in an EDTA tube (see **Blood sampling – (b) venous**)
- Microhaematocrit tube
- Microscope slide and coverslip
- 0.9% saline
- 2 ml syringe and needle
- Microscope

Technique

1 Using a microhaematocrit tube, place 2–4 drops of blood on a microscope slide.
2 Using a syringe and needle, withdraw saline from a bag and add an equal volume to the blood on the slide.
3 Rock the slide gently for 30 seconds.
4 Examine the slide grossly for agglutination (i.e. clumping of red cells; Figure H.1).
5 Add a coverslip and examine the slide microscopically under high power.
6 A positive result is confirmed by the *microscopic* visualization of clumps of randomly oriented red blood cells (Figure H.2).

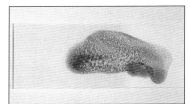

Figure H.1: Gross appearance of cell agglutination.

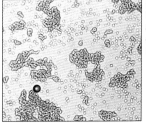

Figure H.2: Microscopic appearance of clumps of red blood cells.

ROULEAUX

It is very important to examine the slide using a microscope, as rouleaux formation appears identical to true agglutination on gross examination (Figure H.3). If rouleaux formation persists, additional saline should be added in an attempt to disperse this natural phenomenon.

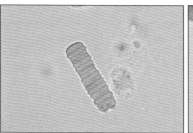
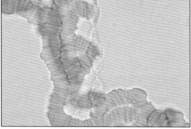

Figure H.3: Microscopic appearance of rouleaux formations.

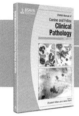

FURTHER INFORMATION

Further details of the test and its interpretation can be found in the *BSAVA Manual of Canine and Feline Clinical Pathology.*

Hip luxation – closed reduction

Indications/Use
- Recent traumatic hip luxation

Contraindications
- If luxation has been present for longer than 7–10 days, closed reduction is unlikely to be successful
- Fractures of the femoral head
- If there is pre-existing hip dysplasia, the risk of re-luxation following closed reduction is high

Equipment
- Soft cotton rope or towel sling
- Sandbag
- As required for **Ehmer sling**

Patient preparation and positioning

- General anaesthesia is required
- Ventrodorsal and lateral radiographs of the pelvis should be obtained to confirm hip luxation and to evaluate the direction of the luxation. Radiography is also required to detect avulsion fractures of the teres ligament, chip fractures of the dorsal acetabular rim, other pelvic fractures and the presence of pre-existing coxofemoral osteoarthritis, which may complicate management of hip luxation
- The patient should be positioned in lateral recumbency, with the affected limb uppermost
- For large dogs it may be beneficial to secure their hindquarters to the table, using a soft cotton rope placed within the inguinal region of the affected limb and secured caudodorsally to the table. Alternatively, the affected pelvic limb may be supported using a towel sling: the towel is passed through the inguinal region and both ends are held by an assistant standing on the dorsal side of the patient

Technique

Craniodorsal luxation (the majority of cases)

1 Manipulate the femoral head to loosen any adhesions.
2 Externally rotate the limb and apply caudodistal traction to lift the femoral head over the dorsal rim of the acetabulum. Internal rotation of the limb will then engage the femoral head in the acetabulum. The greater trochanter may be guided caudally and distally with the non-dominant hand.
3 A palpable/audible click may be noted at reduction. Apply pressure to the trochanter and rotate the joint to express any haematoma from the joint space.
4 Manipulate the hip and check it for range of motion and stability.
5 Confirm reduction radiographically.
6 If appropriate, apply an **Ehmer sling** for 7–10 days.

Cranioventral luxation

1 Manipulate the femoral head to the craniodorsal position and reduce as described above. Alternatively, it may be possible to manipulate the femoral head directly back into the acetabulum by palpation.
2 Confirm reduction radiographically.

Caudoventral luxation

1 If the femoral head is within the obturator foramen, first release it from this position. Apply traction to the affected limb by grasping it proximal to the stifle, whilst applying counter-traction to the tuber ischium.
2 Lift the femoral head laterally and cranially into the acetabulum. This may be aided by placing a sandbag between the thighs: the sandbag then acts as a fulcrum to lever the femoral head back into the acetabulum.
3 Confirm reduction radiographically.
4 Further support following closed reduction is not required in the majority of cases.
   a **An Ehmer sling is contraindicated.**
   b Stifle hobbles may be used:

i.   Create a loop out of strong adhesive tape folded on to itself, with adhesive sides together. The width of the folded adhesive tape should be sufficient for strength and comfort. The length of the loop should be sufficient to encircle the pelvic limbs at the level of the stifles with the animal in a normal standing position
ii. Place the loop of adhesive tape around the stifles and secure in position by wrapping further adhesive tape around the loop between the stifles
iii. The hobble can be further secured in position with a length of tape which passes from the lateral aspect of the hobble on one side, over the dorsum of the animal, to the lateral aspect of the hobble on the other side.

Aftercare

- Exercise should be restricted for 4–6 weeks following closed reduction of hip luxation, to allow for healing of the periarticular tissues
- Appropriate analgesia should be provided

Potential complications

- Re-luxation of the hip
- Hip osteoarthritis
- Iatrogenic damage to the cartilage of the femoral head

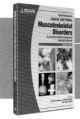

FURTHER INFORMATION

Further information on hip problems and their treatment can be found in the *BSAVA Manual of Canine and Feline Musculoskeletal Disorders*.

Intraosseous cannula placement

Indications/Use
- Fluid administration:
  - Where direct intravenous access is not possible (e.g. hypovolaemic puppies/kittens, severe vascular collapse), fluids normally administered intravenously can be administered via an intraosseous cannula
  - To provide *initial* fluid resuscitation and medication until intravenous access is possible

---

> **WARNING**
>
> - Most substances that can be given intravenously can be given into the medullary space of bone and absorption into the vasculature is extremely rapid. However, hypertonic and alkaline fluids may cause pain and lameness.

Contraindications
- Sites with high risk of bacterial contamination/infection (e.g. due to local tissue damage, local skin infection, diarrhoea, urinary incontinence)
- Where intravenous access is possible

Equipment
- As required for **Aseptic preparation – (a) non-surgical procedures**
- Intraosseous cannulas:
  - Ideally, intraosseous cannulas should have a central stylet to prevent a core of bone from obstructing the cannula
  - Cannula size should be appropriate for the estimated diameter of the bone marrow canal, size of the point of access into the bone and proposed fluid administration rates
  - Cannulas that may be suitable for intraosseous use include:
    - Commercially available intraosseous cannulas
    - Spinal needle
    - Bone marrow aspiration needle
    - Hypodermic needle (may be able to penetrate the soft cortex of young puppies and kittens)
- Scalpel and No.11 scalpel blade
- Local anaesthetic
- T-connector or extension set containing heparinized saline (1 IU of heparin per ml of 0.9% saline)
- Sterile non-adherent dressing or swab
- Adhesive tape or suture material
- Soft padded bandage and outer protective bandage

Patient preparation and positioning
- The animal's limb must be held still; this can usually be achieved by manual restraint but sedation may be required

- **Aseptic preparation – (a) non-surgical procedures** should be carried out on a large area of skin surrounding the proposed site of cannula entry
- Possible sites:
    - The medial aspect of the trochanteric fossa of the femur (see **Bone marrow aspiration**)
    - The flat medial surface of the proximal tibia, 1–2 cm distal to the tibial tuberosity
    - The cranial aspect of the greater tubercle of the humerus (see **Bone marrow aspiration**)
    - The wing of the ilium (see **Bone marrow aspiration**)
    - The preferred sites are those in the femur and tibia (Figure I.1)

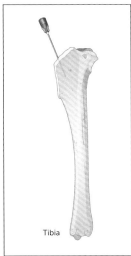

Figure I.1: An intraosseous cannula can be placed in the medial surface of the proximal tibia.

Tibia

Technique

1. Infiltrate local anaesthetic down to the level of the periosteum.
2. Make a stab incision in the skin over the proposed entry point into the bone.
3. Insert the cannula through the skin and directly down on to the bone.
4. Insert the cannula or needle into the bone, using a firm twisting motion until it has passed through the cortex and a small way into the medullary cavity. Entry into the medullary cavity is detected as a decrease in resistance to insertion into the bone, or increased stability of the cannula within the bone. When the cannula is properly seated within the medullary cavity, movement of the cannula will result in the same movement of the bone.
5. Remove the stylet, if present.
6. Flush the cannula with heparinized saline and attach a T-connector or infusion set.
7. Secure the cannula to the surrounding skin with sutures or tape.
8. Cover the entry site through the skin with a sterile swab or sterile non-adherent dressing.
9. Apply a bandage to the limb to protect the cannula.

Cannula maintenance and removal

- Intraosseous cannulas are most often a short-term solution
- Catheter patency should be maintained by any fluid running through it. If the catheter is not being used continuously, intermittent flushing with saline or heparinized saline should be performed several times a day (up to every 4 hours), as well as before and after use. If a catheter becomes blocked it should be removed
- The bandage should be replaced and the cannula examined at least twice a day, using aseptic technique
- The site of insertion should be monitored for signs of heat, erythema, swelling, pain or subcutaneous leakage of fluid. If these signs are noted the cannula should be removed
- The cannula should be removed as soon as it is no longer required

Potential complications

- Sciatic nerve damage; this can be avoided during placement of a femoral cannula by walking the needle off the medial edge of the greater trochanter
- Growth plate damage in young animals
- Cannula displacement
- Subcutaneous leakage of fluids or medications
- Infection

Intravenous catheter placement – (a) peripheral veins

Indications/Use

- Intravenous fluid administration
- Intravenous drug administration
- Repeat intravenous blood sampling, although a central line is preferable for this indication

Contraindications

- Sites with a high risk of bacterial contamination/infection (e.g. due to local tissue damage, local skin infection, diarrhoea, urinary incontinence)

Equipment

The equipment required for intravenous catheter placement is shown in Figure I.2.

- Over-the-needle intravenous catheter (Figure I.3), comprising a needle (or stylet) with a closely associated catheter fitted over the needle. Fluid flow rate is related to catheter length and radius. For rapid fluid administration, the shortest catheter with the largest radius that can pass into the vein should be selected:
  - Dogs: usually 22 G (blue), 20 G (pink) or 18 G (green)
  - Cats: usually 22 G (blue)
  - Puppies/kittens or patients with collapsed veins may require 24 G (yellow)
- Scalpel and No.11 scalpel blade

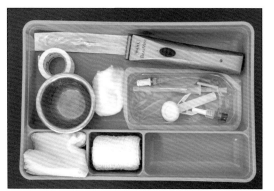

Figure I.2: Equipment required for intravenous catheter placement in a peripheral vein. The tray contains a 22 G over-the-needle intravenous catheter, T-connector, adhesive tape, conforming bandage, clippers and materials for skin preparation (cotton wool, swabs, 4% chlorohexidine gluconate and ChloraPrep [sterile applicator containing 2% chlorhexidine gluconate and 70% isopropyl alcohol]).

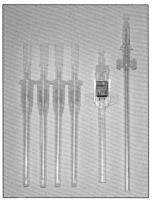

Figure I.3: Over-the-needle catheters can be used for intravenous access to a peripheral vein. (Reproduced from the BSAVA Manual of Canine and Feline Emergency and Critical Care)

- T-connector or extension set containing heparinized saline (1 IU of heparin per ml of 0.9% saline) or injection cap
- Adhesive tape
- Soft padded bandage and outer protective bandage
- Appropriate skin antiseptic
- Clippers
- Cotton wool
- Swabs

NOTE

- Sterile applicators containing 2% chlorhexidine gluconate and 70% isopropyl alcohol, designed specifically for skin antisepsis are now available. They should be used according to the manufacturer's recommendations

---

Patient preparation and positioning

- An area of skin surrounding the point of vein entry should be clipped. Long hair on the caudal aspect of the limb may need to be removed if it will interfere with securing the catheter and to help prevent contamination. In some dogs a complete 360-degree clip of the limb may be necessary
- Using cotton wool or gauze swabs, the skin over the vein should be aseptically prepared (see **Aseptic preparation – (a) non-surgical procedures**)
- Possible sites:
    - Cephalic vein and accessory cephalic vein (below the carpus) in the distal forelimb (see **Blood sampling – (b) venous**)
    - Medial and lateral saphenous veins in the distal hindlimb (see **Blood sampling – (b) venous**)
    - Auricular veins in breeds with large ears (e.g. Basset Hound)

- Dorsal common digital vein (over the metatarsal bones)
- The cephalic vein is most commonly used as it is familiar and the majority of animals will tolerate gentle restraint for catheter placement while in sternal recumbency
■ The animal's limb must be held still. This can usually be achieved by manual restraint but sedation may be useful in animals whose temperament does not permit restraint (Figure I.4)

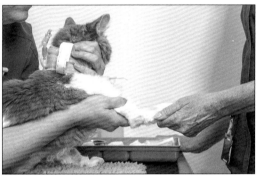

Figure I.4: Restraint for placement of a catheter in the cephalic vein.

Technique

ASEPSIS

Hands should be washed with an antiseptic solution prior to catheter placement. Sterile gloves are not necessary but the precise point of catheter insertion should not be contaminated after aseptic preparation.

1 The vein is raised by an assistant placing pressure over the vein proximal to the site of catheter placement.
2 The catheter can usually be placed directly through the skin, but in some patients a small facilitative skin nick made with a No. 11 blade may ease insertion. This is especially useful in dehydrated animals or those with very thick skin and prevents burring of the catheter tip as it passes through the subcutaneous tissues.
3 Advance the over-the-needle catheter through the skin into the vein, at an angle of 30–40 degrees, with the bevel of the stylet uppermost.
4 Once blood is visualized in the flash chamber of the catheter, flatten the stylet and catheter (i.e. reduce the angle between the catheter and the limb). Then advance the stylet/catheter unit a small distance further into the vein to ensure that the catheter lies fully within the lumen.
5 Hold the stylet in position while advancing the catheter forward off the stylet and completely into the vein.
6 Remove the stylet.
7 The assistant can now occlude the vein by applying pressure over it at the distal end of the catheter to prevent the spillage of blood.
8 Connect a T-connector or extension set containing heparinized saline or an injection cap to the catheter to close it.

9 Secure the catheter firmly in place with adhesive tape and cover with a bandage.

Peripheral venous catheter maintenance and removal

- The bandage should be replaced and the catheter examined at least twice a day
- The site of insertion should be monitored for signs of heat, erythema, swelling, pain and leakage of fluid. If signs of phlebitis are present the catheter should be removed and the tip sent for microbiological culture
- The leg and foot should be checked for swelling above the catheter site (indicating extravasation of fluid) and swelling of the toes (indicating the bandage or tape is too tight). Either of these complications necessitates catheter removal
- Catheter patency should be maintained by any fluid running through it. If the catheter is not being used continuously, intermittent flushing with heparinized saline should be performed two or three times a day as well as before and after use

> **NOTE**
>
> - In some studies, there has been no benefit associated with the use of heparinized saline as opposed to normal saline for maintaining catheter patency in dogs or humans. In low use situations, it may be more cost-effective and safer to use small bottles of normal saline because bags of heparinized saline contain no preservative and therefore have a short shelf-life

- If a catheter becomes blocked it should be removed
- When a catheter is not in use, a sterile injection cap should be used to close the catheter from the environment. Disconnection of fluid lines should be avoided and only performed when absolutely necessary to reduce contamination of the catheter

Potential complications

- Catheter displacement/extravasation of fluids or medications
- Phlebitis/thrombophlebitis
- Thrombosis/thromboembolism
- Infection
- Air embolism
- Exsanguination

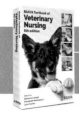

> **FURTHER INFORMATION**
>
> Further information on intravenous catheter placement can be found in the *BSAVA Textbook of Veterinary Nursing*.

Intravenous catheter placement – (b) jugular veins (modified Seldinger technique)

Indications/Use

- When administration of intravenous fluids is expected to be required over several days
- Administration of intravenous hypertonic fluids or medications
- Repeated blood sampling
- For central venous pressure measurements
- Where maintenance of a peripheral catheter may be challenging (e.g. due to patient conformation or temperament)
- When access to a peripheral vein is not possible

Contraindications

- Coagulopathy
- Local tissue damage or skin infection in the ventral cervical region
- When inpatient hospitalization and regular monitoring is not possible

Equipment

- As required for **Aseptic preparation – (a) non-surgical procedures**
- Sterile gloves
- Central venous Seldinger catheter pack: 4, 5 or 7 Fr double- or triple-lumen catheters would be appropriate, depending on vein diameter and length
- Over-the-needle catheter of appropriate diameter to receive the guidewire, if preferred to the introducer needle in the Seldinger pack
- Scalpel and No.11 scalpel blade
- Heparinized saline (1 IU of heparin per ml of 0.9% saline) in two or three 5 ml syringes
- Suture materials
- Fenestrated sterile drape
- Sterile dressing
- Bandaging material
- Electrocardiogram (ECG) monitoring equipment

Patient preparation and positioning

- Although central lines (jugular catheters) may be placed in conscious patients if they are very weak or debilitated, heavy sedation or anaesthesia is required in most animals to prevent movement during the procedure
- Anaesthetized animals should be placed in lateral recumbency, with a sandbag positioned under the neck, and the jugular vein to be catheterized uppermost (Figure I.5a)
- Either jugular vein can be used, but ideally one which has not had venepuncture previously performed should be selected
- **Aseptic preparation – (a) non-surgical procedures** is necessary, with the use of a fenestrated drape (Figure I.5b). Clipping and aseptic preparation should extend from the dorsal midline to lateral to the ventral midline and from the angle of the mandible to the thoracic inlet

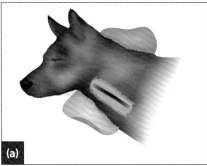
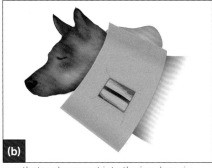

Figure I.5: (a) Patient positioning for intravenous catheter placement into the jugular vein. (b) A fenestrated drape should be placed over the site of catheter placement.

Technique

1 With their hand under the sterile drape, an assistant raises the jugular vein.

2 Make a 2–3 mm stab incision in the skin over the jugular vein (Figure I.6).

3 Insert the introducer needle or an over-the-needle catheter (pre-flushed with heparinized saline) into the vein in a rostrocaudal direction (Figure I.7). If using an over-the-needle catheter, then remove the needle. The assistant should then stop raising the jugular vein.

4 Insert the guidewire through the introducer needle or catheter into the vein.

    a The guidewire is usually held within an adapter to aid placement and may have a J-shaped tip. The J-shaped tip should be straightened by withdrawal into the adapter prior to insertion into the introducer needle or catheter (Figure I.8).

    b The ECG should be monitored for arrhythmias, as overlong wires can enter the heart.

    c Care must be taken to ensure that the guidewire is held at all times for the remainder of the procedure to prevent loss of the wire into the vein.

5 Remove the introducer needle or catheter, leaving the guidewire in place.

6 Advance the vessel dilator (contained in a Seldinger catheter pack) over the guidewire and into the vein to enlarge the subcutaneous tunnel. Twist the dilator as it passes into the vein to aid insertion (Figure I.9); then remove the dilator.

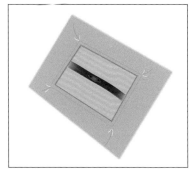
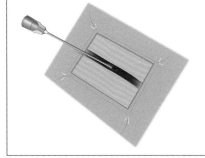

Figure I.6: An incision should be made over the jugular vein.

Figure I.7: The needle should be inserted into the jugular vein.

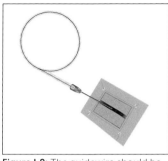

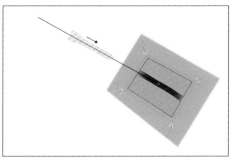

Figure I.8: The guidewire should be inserted into the jugular vein through the introducer needle.

Figure I.9: The vessel dilator should be advanced over the guidewire into the vein.

7 Advance the catheter over the wire and into the vein (Figure I.10). Note that the catheter should be premeasured to an appropriate length (i.e. to approximately the 2nd intercostal space; for the measurement of central venous pressure, the length is approximately the 4th intercostal space).

> **NOTE**
>
> - The catheter and all lumina should be prefilled with saline or heparinized saline prior to placement. However, as air will enter the catheter as it is threaded over the guidewire, this does not negate the need to check for air within the catheter after placement

8 Remove the guidewire. (Note: if the guidewire does not exit one of the ports of the catheter, too much has been placed into the patient. The wire should be pulled out by an appropriate amount and the catheter re-advanced over the wire.)

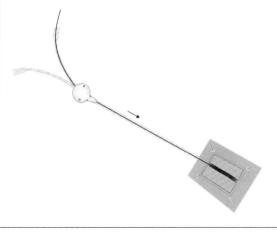

Figure I.10: The catheter should be advanced over the guidewire into the vein.

9 Place sterile injection caps, ideally incorporating on/off valves, on the end of each port of the catheter. Withdraw any air, plus some blood, from each port into a syringe part-filled with heparinized saline, to prevent air embolism and ensure intravascular placement. Then immediately flush through each port with heparinized saline.

10 Secure the catheter to the patient with sutures placed through specific suture grooves or holes in a suture wing at the base of the catheter (Figure I.11). If the catheter is too long, it can be placed a little shorter and a blue then white wing (contained in a Seldinger catheter pack) inserted over the top of the catheter to be able to suture it at the venotomy site. Ensure the wing grips the catheter properly before securing.

11 Place a sterile dressing over the entry site of the catheter and bandage the catheter carefully in place. The bandage should not be too tight; it should be possible to pass a hand under it comfortably.

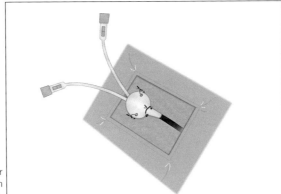

Figure I.11: The catheter should be secured in place with sutures.

Jugular catheter maintenance and removal

- The bandage should be replaced and the catheter examined at least once a day. The site of insertion should be monitored for signs of heat, erythema, swelling, pain or leakage of fluid. If signs of phlebitis are present, or the animal develops unexplained pyrexia, the catheter should be removed and the tip sent for microbiological culture
- Catheter patency should be maintained by any fluid running through it. If the catheter is not being used continuously, intermittent flushing with saline or heparinized saline (1 IU of heparin per ml of 0.9% saline) should be performed two or three times a day (up to every 4 hours) as well as before and after use

> **NOTE**
>
> - In some studies, there has been no benefit associated with the use of heparinized saline as opposed to normal saline for maintaining catheter patency in dogs or humans. In low use situations, it may be more cost-effective and safer to use small bottles of normal saline because bags of heparinized saline contain no preservative and therefore have a short shelf-life

- When a catheter is not in use, sterile injection caps should be used to close access ports; ports should never be left open to the air. Disconnection of fluid lines should be avoided and only performed when absolutely necessary to reduce catheter contamination

Potential complications

- Catheter displacement/extravasation of fluids or medications
- Phlebitis/thrombophlebitis
- Thrombosis/thromboembolism
- Infection
- Air embolism
- Exsanguination (more likely than with peripheral catheters)

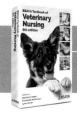

FURTHER INFORMATION

Further information on intravenous catheter placement can be found in the *BSAVA Textbook of Veterinary Nursing*.

Iodinated contrast media

Iodinated contrast media appear radiopaque on a radiograph due to iodine having a higher atomic number than soft tissues. Water-soluble iodinated contrast media are available in ionic and non-ionic forms, and a wide range is available. The more commonly used ones are detailed in Figure I.12. None is authorized for veterinary use and most are POM.

Use

- Iodinated contrast agents are used for:
  - Intravascular studies (e.g. upper urinary tract) and angiography of the cardiovascular and portal systems
  - Lower urinary tract (see **Retrograde urethrography/vaginourethrography**)
  - Joints (arthrography)
  - Salivary glands (sialography)
  - Lacrimal sac and duct
  - Investigation of peripheral sinuses and fistulae
  - Myelography
  - Lymphangiography
- Iodinated contrast media can be used to evaluate the gastrointestinal tract where perforation and leakage are potentially present and hence the use of barium is contraindicated. In practice, alternative methods (e.g. positional radiography, ultrasonography or CT) to demonstrate leakage should be considered first

Constituent	Properties	Trade name examples	Uses			Formulations (mg iodine/ml)
			Spinal	Vascular; urinary	Gastro-intestinal	
Iothalamic acid	Monomer; ionic; high osmolar	Conray	–	+	–	141; 202; 280; 400
Sodium meglumine diatrizoate	Monomer; ionic; high osmolar	Urografin	–	+	–	146; 325; 370
	Monomer; ionic; high osmolar	Gastrografin	–	–	+	370
Ioxaglate	Dimer; ionic; low osmolar	Hexabrix	–	+	–	320
Iohexol	Monomer; non-ionic; low osmolar	Omnipaque	+	+	+	140; 180; 240; 300; 350
Iopamidol	Monomer; non-ionic; low osmolar	Niopam	+	+	–	150; 200; 300; 340; 370
Iopromide	Monomer; non-ionic; low osmolar	Ultravist	–	+	–	150; 240; 300; 370
Iomeprol	Monomer; non-ionic; low osmolar	Iomerol	–	+	–	250; 300; 350; 400

Figure I.12: Commonly used iodinated contrast media.

- In veterinary practice, ionic agents are mainly used for cardiovascular and urinary tract studies. Ionic agents should not be used for myelography
- In veterinary practice, non-ionic agents are mainly used for myelography and arthrography. They are also used in cardiovascular and urinary tract studies, where the status of the patient dictates their use and ionic media are contraindicated

Contraindications

- Known or suspected hypersensitivity to iodinated contrast media
- Should be used with care in animals with renal failure. Iodinated contrast media are primarily excreted via the kidneys and pre-existing renal disease predisposes to contrast media-induced renal failure
- Anuria
- Dehydration
- Hypovolaemia
- Hypotension

Adverse reactions

Contrast reactions can be divided into non-idiosyncratic reactions, which are dose-dependent, and idiosyncratic reactions, which are independent of the dose administered.

- **Non-idiosyncratic reactions:**
  - Associated with the hyperosmolality and ionicity of the iodine-containing contrast agents and are therefore more common and severe with ionic agents than non-ionic agents
  - Reactions may be acute (occur within 5–10 minutes following administration) or delayed
  - Reactions include:
    - Contrast-induced nephrotoxicity
    - Cardiovascular effects including bradycardia, hypertension and hypotension
    - Nausea and vomiting
    - Neurotoxicity
    - Irritation following extravasation
    - Bronchospasm and skin reactions may occur in patients with known allergic disease
- **Idiosyncratic reactions:**
  - Represent anaphylactic or allergic-type reactions, as antibodies to contrast agents have not been demonstrated
  - Reactions are evident immediately following intravenous administration
  - Reactions present as:
    - Severe respiratory signs associated with laryngeal oedema, bronchospasm and pulmonary oedema
    - Cardiovascular collapse (hypotension, decreased cardiac output)
    - Urticaria

Drug interactions

- Iodinated contrast media decrease thyroid uptake of iodine and preclude therapeutic radioiodine therapy for 2 months following administration
- Hypersensitivity reactions may be aggravated in patients on beta-blocker medication

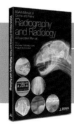

FURTHER INFORMATION

Further information on contrast radiography can be found in the *BSAVA Manual of Canine and Feline Radiography and Radiology.*

Local anaesthesia – nerve blocks

Indications/Use

- Treatment of perioperative pain, in conjunction with heavy sedation or general anaesthesia
- Local anaesthesia as part of a multimodal approach to analgesia
- *Specific indications for each block are listed under each technique*

Contraindications

- Infection (including pyoderma) or neoplasia that might be disseminated by the passage of the needle
- Septicaemia, bleeding disorders, hypovolaemia, hypotension and altered neurological function for epidural anaesthesia and analgesia

Equipment

- Local anaesthetics (Figure L.1)
- Range of needles: ⅜ to 1 inch; 21, 23 G
- Range of spinal or epidural (Tuohy) needles: 1.5, 2.5, 3.5 inches; 20, 22 G
- Range of syringes: 1–20 ml
- Loss-of-resistance syringes for epidural technique are available in 5 ml and 8 ml
- Ultrasound machine or nerve stimulator locator: these should be used to locate the nerves and aid accurate needle placement and thus the effectiveness of the nerve block (with the exception of head blocks and epidurals)

> ### NOTES
>
> - Bupivacaine and ropivacaine are not authorized for use in dogs and cats in the UK
> - The toxic doses listed in Figure L.1 are conservative estimates, to minimize the occurrence of toxicity
> - Local anaesthetic doses are most often based on the space available around the nerves and are given as volumes in the technique descriptions; however, volume recommendations should always be checked against recommended mg/kg doses
> - Preservative-free solutions are required for epidural use
> - Preservative-free morphine (0.1–0.2 mg/kg) can be used for epidural analgesia

Drug	Onset time (minutes)	Duration of action (hours)	Recommended doses in healthy animals (mg/kg)	Toxic dose (mg/kg)
Lidocaine	5–15	1–2	Dogs: 2–4 Cats: 2	Dogs: 10 Cats: 4
Bupivacaine	20–30	2.5–6	Dogs: 2 Cats: 1.5	Dogs: 4 Cats: 2
Ropivacaine	2–20	2–6	Dogs: 2 Cats: 1.5	Dogs: 4 Cats: not determined

Figure L.1: Drugs for local anaesthesia.

Patient preparation and positioning

- Sedation or anaesthesia permits easier positioning of animals, identification of anatomical landmarks, isolation of specific nerves and blood vessels, and more precise/less traumatic needle placement
- **Aseptic preparation – (a) non-surgical procedures** must be performed at the proposed site of needle insertion

Technique

> **WARNING**
>
> The aim is to inject local anaesthetic around a nerve:
> - After needle insertion, but prior to injection of local anaesthetic, always aspirate to check for blood to avoid intravenous or arterial injection of local anaesthetic
> - If high pressure (more than experienced with a normal intramuscular injection) is felt on injection of the local anaesthetic, the needle may be within the nerve; withdraw the needle and start again to avoid nerve damage.

Head

The anatomical landmarks for performing maxillary, infraorbital, mandibular and mental blocks in dogs and cats are shown in Figures L.2 and L.3.

Infraorbital nerve block

- Desensitizes the upper lip, nose and skin rostroventral to the infraorbital foramen
- The animal should be placed in lateral recumbency

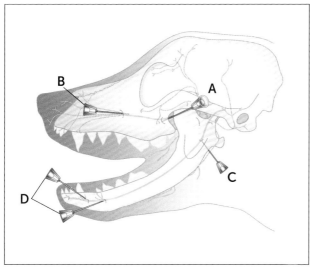

Figure L.2: Anatomical landmarks for performing maxillary (A), infraorbital (B), mandibular (C) and mental (D) nerve blocks in dogs.

Figure L.3: Anatomical landmarks for performing maxillary (A), infraorbital (B), mandibular (C) and mental (D) nerve blocks in cats.

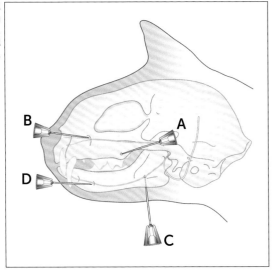

Dogs:

1 Palpate the infraorbital foramen on the lateral surface of the maxilla either intraorally by lifting the upper lip or percutaneously. The foramen is located at the level of the second premolar.

2 Direct a 25 G needle in a caudal direction, parallel to the infraorbital canal, a short distance into the infraorbital foramen (Figure L.4).

3 Elevate the dog's nose and occlude the entrance to the infraorbital foramen with light finger pressure.

4 Inject 0.1–1.0 ml of local anaesthetic solution caudally into the infraorbital canal.

Cats:

1 Palpate the ridge of bone overlying the infraorbital foramen; the foramen cannot be palpated directly.

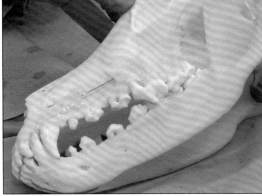

Figure L.4: Needle position for an infraorbital nerve block in a dog.

2 Insert a 25 G needle intraorally or percutaneously, dorsal and parallel to the premolar teeth, in a caudal direction towards the infraorbital ridge.

3 Inject a maximum of 0.3 ml of local anaesthetic solution directly on to the infraorbital nerve.

Maxillary nerve block

- Desensitizes the hard and soft palate, upper teeth and gingiva, nose and the skin over the maxilla
- The animal should be placed in lateral recumbency

1 Palpate the rostral end of the zygomatic arch where it meets the maxilla.

2 Insert a 21–25 G needle percutaneously just ventral to this point and direct the needle in a vertical direction perpendicular to the sagittal plane (Figure L.5).

3 Inject 0.1–1.5 ml (dogs) or 0.1–0.3 ml (cats) of local anaesthetic solution directly on to the maxillary nerve.

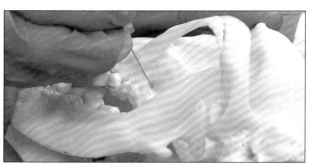

Figure L.5: Needle position for a maxillary nerve block in a dog.

Mental nerve block

- Desensitizes the lower lip and chin rostral to the injection site
- The animal should be placed in lateral recumbency

1 Palpate the middle mental foramen intraorally. It is located on the lateral surface of the rostral mandible: adjacent to the 2nd premolar tooth in **dogs**; or just rostral to the premolar teeth in **cats**.

2 Direct a 21–25 G needle rostrocaudally, just inside the foramen (Figure L.6).

3 Inject 0.1–1.5 ml (dogs) or 0.1–0.3 ml (cats) of local anaesthetic solution caudally into the foramen.

Mandibular nerve block

- Desensitizes the lower teeth, gingiva, tongue and chin
- The animal should be placed in lateral recumbency

1 Palpate the mandibular foramen intraorally. It is located on the medial surface of the mandible just rostral to the angular process.

2 Insert a 22–25 G needle percutaneously along the ventral border of the mandible, ventral to the mandibular foramen.

3 Direct the needle along the medial border of the mandible towards the mandibular foramen (Figure L.7).

4 Inject 0.2–1.0 ml (dogs) or 0.1–0.3 ml (cats) of local anaesthetic solution directly on to the mandibular nerve as it enters the mandibular foramen.

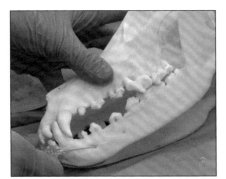

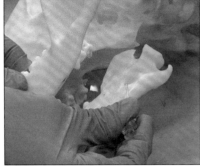

Figure L.6: Needle position for a mental nerve block in a dog.

Figure L.7: Needle position for a mandibular nerve block in a dog.

Auriculotemporal and great auricular nerve blocks (dog)

■ Desensitizes the inner surface of the auricular cartilage and the external ear canal
■ The dog should be placed in lateral recumbency
■ The anatomical landmarks for performing auriculotemporal and great auricular nerve blocks in dogs are shown in Figure L.8

1 Palpate the 'V' formed by the caudal aspect of the zygomatic arch and vertical ear canal.
2 Insert a 21–25 G needle percutaneously, directing it towards the point of this 'V'.
3 Inject 0.1–0.5 ml of local anaesthetic solution.
4 Palpate the wing of the atlas vertebra.
5 Insert a 21–25 G needle percutaneously, ventral to the wing of atlas, and direct the needle parallel and adjacent to the vertical ear canal.
6 Inject 0.5–1.0 ml of local anaesthetic solution.

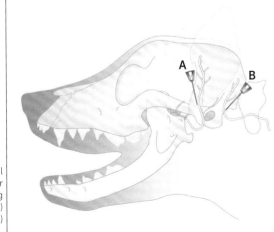

Figure L.8: Anatomical landmarks for performing auriculotemporal (A) and great auricular (B) nerve blocks in dogs.

Limb

Cervical paravertebral block (dog)

- Desensitizes the entire forelimb
- This block should only be performed with a nerve stimulator locator
- The dog should be placed in lateral recumbency. An assistant can elevate the scapula away from the thorax to aid access to the caudal cervical vertebrae and the first rib
- The anatomical landmarks for performing a cervical paravertebral nerve block in dogs are shown in Figure L.9

1 Palpate the transverse process of C6.
2 Insert a 22 G, 1.5–3 inch spinal needle percutaneously and direct it towards the cranial and caudal margins of the transverse process of C6 to access the ventral branches of spinal nerves C6 and C7. The needle should be angled caudally to avoid intrapleural penetration.
3 Inject 1–3 ml of local anaesthetic solution around each nerve.
4 Palpate the head of the first rib.
5 Insert the needle percutaneously and direct it towards the cranial and ventral borders of the dorsal part of the first rib to access spinal nerves C8 and T1.
6 Inject 1–3 ml of local anaesthetic solution around each nerve.

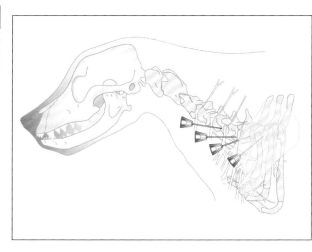

Figure L.9: Anatomical landmarks for performing a cervical paravertebral block in dogs (dotted line shows the normal anatomical position of the scapula).

Axillary brachial plexus block

- Desensitizes the forelimb below the level of the elbow; excludes the shoulder and humerus
- This block is commonly performed under ultrasound guidance
- The patient should be placed in lateral recumbency
- The anatomical landmarks for performing an axillary nerve block in cats are shown in Figure L.10
- The target response is flexion-extension of the elbow and carpus, and external rotation of the limb

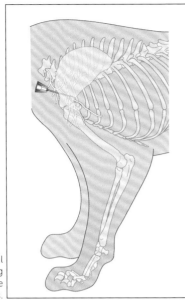

Figure L.10: Anatomical landmarks for performing axillary blockade of the brachial plexus in cats.

L

1   Insert a 22 G, 1 inch needle (cats) or 22 G, 1.5–3 inch spinal needle (dogs) percutaneously into the axillary space at the level of the shoulder and direct it towards the first rib.

2   Inject local anaesthetic solution: 10–15 ml is required for a 25 kg dog; 1 ml is sufficient for a cat.

Radial, ulnar, median and musculocutaneous nerve blocks

- Desensitizes the forepaw in cats; and the forelimb distal to the elbow in dogs
- These blocks are commonly performed under ultrasound guidance
- The patient should be placed in lateral recumbency with the affected limb uppermost
- The anatomical landmarks for performing radial, ulnar, median and musculocutaneous nerve blocks in dogs and cats are shown in Figures L.11 and L.12

Dogs:

1   Palpate the lateral and medial humeral condyles.

2   Insert a 22 G, 1 inch needle percutaneously, proximal to the lateral epicondyle of the humerus.

3   Direct the needle between the brachialis muscle and lateral head of the triceps to access the radial nerve.

4   Inject 1–3 ml of local anaesthetic solution directly on to the nerve.

5   Direct the needle percutaneously, proximal to the medial epicondyle of the humerus and between the biceps brachii muscle and medial head of the triceps to access the ulnar, median and musculocutaneous nerves.

6   Inject 1–3 ml of local anaesthetic solution into the space surrounding these three nerves.

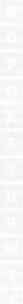

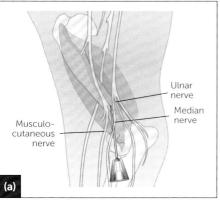
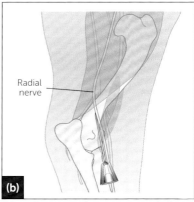

Figure L.11: Anatomical landmarks for performing **(a)** median, musculocutaneous and ulnar nerve blocks (medial view) and **(b)** a radial nerve block (lateral view) in dogs.

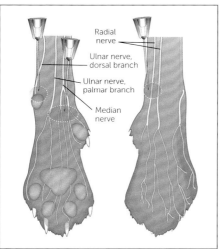

Figure L.12: Anatomical landmarks for performing nerve blocks of the distal branches of the radial, ulnar and median nerves in cats. Shaded areas within the dotted lines show areas to be blocked.

Cats:

1 Grasp the forepaw.
2 Insert a 25 G, ³⁄₈ to 1 inch needle and pass it subcutaneously, just proximal to the carpus along the dorsomedial border of the distal antebrachium to access the radial nerve.
3 Inject 0.1 ml of local anaesthetic solution.
4 Pass the needle subcutaneously, medial and lateral to the accessory pad on the palmar surface of the paw to access the medial and ulnar nerves.
5 Inject 0.1 ml of local anaesthetic solution per nerve.

Saphenous, common peroneal and tibial nerve blocks

- Desensitizes the pelvic limb distal to the stifle
- These blocks are commonly performed under ultrasound guidance

- The patient should be placed in lateral recumbency with the affected limb uppermost
- The anatomical landmarks for performing saphenous, common peroneal and tibial nerve blocks in dogs are shown in Figure L.13
- It should be noted that the saphenous nerve is only a sensory nerve and, therefore, nerve blocks do not result in loss of motor function

1 Insert a 22–25 G, ³⁄₈ to 1 inch needle.

2 Inject 1–3 ml (dogs) or 0.1–0.3 ml (cats) of local anaesthetic solution directly on to each nerve.

- The *saphenous nerve* runs through the femoral triangle on the medial surface of the thigh. The nerve lies cranial to the femoral artery and vein. The needle is inserted percutaneously, directly over the nerve cranial to the pulsations of the femoral artery
- The *common peroneal nerve* runs laterally over the gastrocnemius muscle and across the lateral surface of the fibular head. The nerve is palpated distal to the fibular head. The needle is inserted percutaneously, directly over the nerve
- The *tibial nerve* runs deep to the medial and lateral heads of the gastrocnemius muscle, and then between the tendons of the superficial digital flexor and long digital extensor. The needle can be inserted next to the nerve at either of these locations

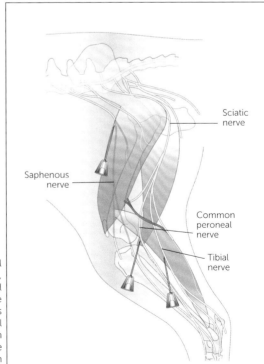

Figure L.13: Anatomical landmarks for saphenous, common peroneal and tibial nerve blocks in dogs. The saphenous nerve block is performed on the medial aspect, whilst the common peroneal and tibial nerve blocks are performed on the lateral aspect of the leg.

Femoral nerve block

- Desensitizes the pelvic limb (distal to the mid femur). Commonly used in combination with a sciatic nerve block
- This block is commonly performed under ultrasound guidance
- The patient should be placed in lateral recumbency with the limb to be blocked uppermost, abducted 90 degrees and extended caudally. Alternatively, the limb to be blocked can be positioned lowermost and gently extended with the uppermost limb held out of the way
- The anatomical landmarks for performing a femoral nerve block in dogs are shown in Figure L.14. The femoral triangle is delimited by the pectineus muscle caudally, the sartorius muscle cranially and the iliopsoas muscle proximally. The femoral nerve is located cranially to the femoral artery and vein.

1 Clip and aseptically prepare the inguinal region.
2 Locate the femoral artery by palpating for a pulse.
3 Insert the needle into the femoral nerve (located within the femoral triangle). A distinct 'pop' will be felt once the needle has punctured the dense superficial iliaca overlying the nerve. The femoral nerve lies quite superficially in the femoral triangle (approximately 0.5–1.0 cm under the skin in a medium sized dog).
4 Inject 0.1 ml/kg of local anaesthetic solution.

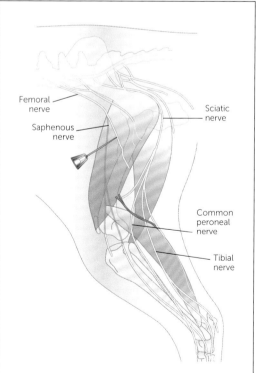

Femoral nerve

Saphenous nerve

Sciatic nerve

Common peroneal nerve

Tibial nerve

Figure L.14: Anatomical landmarks for a femoral nerve block. The femoral nerve is blocked within the groin area as it crosses the femoral triangle.

Sciatic nerve block

- Desensitizes the stifle (partial) and distal structures. Commonly used in combination with a femoral nerve block
- This block is commonly performed under ultrasound guidance
- The patient should be placed in lateral recumbency with the limb to be blocked uppermost and extended in a neutral position
- The anatomical landmarks for performing a sciatic nerve block in dogs are shown in Figure L.15.

1 Clip and aseptically prepare an area between the ischiatic tuberosity and greater trochanter.

2 Identify the ischiatic tuberosity and greater trochanter and draw a 'line' between them. The needle puncture site is one-third of the distance from the greater trochanter to the ischiatic tuberosity.

3 Insert the needle in the vicinity of the sciatic nerve. If the needle hits bone, withdraw it and redirect.

4 Inject 0.1 ml/kg of local anaesthetic solution.

Epidural anaesthesia and analgesia

- Provides perioperative analgesia for surgery of the pelvis, pelvic limbs, caudal abdominal and perineal regions, and is used in combination with general

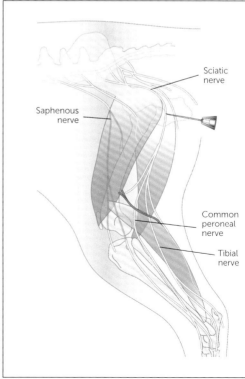

Figure L.15: Anatomical landmarks for a sciatic nerve block. The sciatic nerve is blocked between the cranial and middle third of a 'line' connecting the greater trochanter and the ischiatic tuberosity.

Sciatic nerve

Saphenous nerve

Common peroneal nerve

Tibial nerve

anaesthesia to reduce anaesthetic requirements and to improve analgesia and muscle relaxation

- The animal should be placed in sternal recumbency. The animal should be positioned squarely on the table with the pelvic limbs pulled cranially to lie alongside the abdomen
- The anatomical landmarks for performing an epidural in a dog are shown in Figure L.16.

NOTE

- Preservative-free solutions must be used for epidural injection

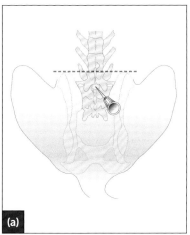

(a)

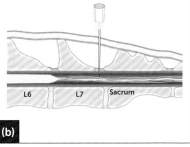

(b)

Figure L.16: Anatomical landmarks for performing lumbosacral epidural anaesthesia and analgesia in dogs. The lumbosacral space can be found caudal to a 'line' drawn between the cranial borders of the ilia (marked with a dotted line). (a) Dorsal view. (b) Lateral view.

1 Palpate the indentation overlying the lumbosacral junction. This is positioned caudal to a 'line' drawn between the left and right iliac crests, and lies along the midline between the dorsal spinous process of the 7th lumbar vertebra and the median sacral crest.

2 Insert a 20 G (dog) or 22 G (cat), 1.5–2.5 inch spinal or epidural (Tuohy) needle percutaneously along the dorsal midline, perpendicular to the skin and directed towards the lumbosacral space.

3 Advance the needle gently through the skin and subcutaneous layers. Then remove the stylet and apply a drop of saline at the hub of the needle.

4 Continue to advance it until an abrupt loss of resistance or 'pop' is encountered as the needle passes through the ligamentum flavum and enters the epidural space. Stop advancing the needle once the drop of saline has been sucked into the body of the needle, suggesting that the epidural space (ligamentum flavum) has been penetrated. If blood is noted in the hub of the needle, replace the stylet and reposition the needle.

5 Attach the syringe to the needle and inject local anaesthetic slowly over at least a 30 second period. Drug options for anaesthesia/analgesia of the hindlimbs, pelvis and perineal region include preservative-free 2% lidocaine, 2% mepivacaine, 0.5% bupivacaine or 0.75% ropivacaine, all used at a dose of

0.1–0.2 ml/kg (up to a maximum volume of 6 ml). The anaesthetic effect of lidocaine has a duration of approximately 1 hour, whilst that of bupivacaine and ropivacaine lasts for 2–4 hours. Bupivacaine is the most commonly used epidural drug.

ALTERNATIVES

Local anaesthetics can be used either alone or mixed with opioids or alpha-2 adrenergic agonists to provide more effective analgesia. Morphine sulphate (0.1–0.2 mg/kg) without preservative is most commonly added to the local anaesthetic solution, but the final volume should not exceed 1 ml/5 kg (up to a maximum volume of 6 ml). This provides perioperative analgesia for pelvic limb, perineal, abdominal and thoracic procedures for up to 12 hours.

Complications

- Nerve damage due to direct injection into a nerve
- Systemic toxicity due to overdose of local anaesthetic or direct injection of local anaesthetic into a blood vessel. Central nervous system (CNS) toxicity results in depression, seizures, muscle tremors and respiratory depression. Cardiac toxicity results in hypotension, arrhythmias and cardiac arrest
- Local tissue irritation and nerve damage
- Cervical paravertebral blocks may be associated with pneumothorax, Horner syndrome, arrhythmias, puncture of the carotid artery, jugular vein and vertebral artery, blockade of the stellate ganglion and decreased sympathetic innervation. They may also result in compromised respiratory function due to phrenic nerve block
- Epidural anaesthesia using non-toxic doses of local anaesthetics can be associated with significant peripheral vasodilation, hypotension, respiratory depression and Horner syndrome. These complications are more likely with high volumes of local anaesthetic agents
- Epidural anaesthesia with morphine can potentially be associated with urinary retention for up to 24 hours
- Epidural anaesthesia in the cat or puppy can be associated with intrathecal injection or direct injury to the spinal cord

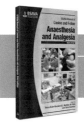

FURTHER INFORMATION

For details of anaesthetic and analgesic protocols, see the *BSAVA Manual of Canine and Feline Anaesthesia and Analgesia.*

Myringotomy

Indications/Use

- To obtain samples for diagnostic evaluation of otitis media
- To permit lavage of the tympanic bulla for non-surgical management of otitis media

Contraindications

- Otitis externa, as there is a risk of transfer of disease to the middle ear

Equipment

- Otoscope with a sterilized otoscopic speculum; a video-otoscope is best but not essential
- Sterile catheters (e.g. 3.5 Fr tomcat catheter or long polypropylene catheter) of sufficient length to access the tympanic membrane via the working channel of a video-otoscope, or along the speculum of an ordinary otoscope
- 2.5 or 5 ml syringe, plus two 20 ml syringes
- 3-way tap
- 0.9% sterile saline
- Otic ceruminolytic agent (may be needed in dogs)
- Bacteriological swab
- EDTA sample pots
- Microscope slides

Patient preparation and positioning

- General anaesthesia is required
- A properly placed and cuffed endotracheal tube is recommended due to possible drainage of fluid from the middle ear canal into the pharynx (see **Endotracheal intubation**)
- The animal is placed in lateral or sternal recumbency. A towel may be used to elevate the caudal head and neck slightly in relation to the muzzle
- The animal's eyes should be protected if ceruminolytics are used to clean the external ear canal

Technique

> **HEALTH AND SAFETY**
>
> Personnel should wear gloves, face mask and, ideally, eye protectors to avoid contact with contaminated aerosols.

1   Clean and dry the external ear canal.
   a   Cleaning can be performed safely with sterile saline.
   b   Ceruminolytic agents can be used in dogs to speed removal of waxy exudates, but must be flushed completely from the ear canal with sterile saline.

c Ceruminolytics should **not** be used to flush the ears of cats if the integrity of the tympanic membrane is uncertain, due to the higher risk of neurological complications.

d Drying can be achieved by suction of lavage solutions.

2 Insert the otoscope into the external ear canal to visualize the tympanic membrane. This requires straightening of the external ear canal, by pulling the pinna dorsally and outwards away from the head.

3 Under direct visualization, flush the ear canal with sterile saline to remove any remaining debris.

a A long polypropylene catheter attached to a 3-way tap and two 20 ml syringes can achieve efficient flushing and suction.

b The person controlling the otoscope visualizes and positions the tip of the catheter, while an assistant flushes in saline with one syringe and removes the fluid by suction through the second syringe.

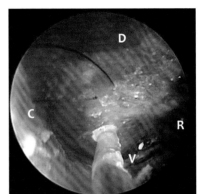

4 The site of myringotomy should be caudoventral (i.e. in the pars tensa). Position the otoscope carefully to visualize this site (Figure M.1).

5 Select a new catheter and cut the tip at an angle to make it sharp enough to incise the tympanic membrane.

6 Under direct visualization, pass the tip of the catheter through the caudoventral aspect of the tympanic membrane into the middle ear and maintain it in this position.

Figure M.1: Position for performing a myringotomy using an open-ended tomcat catheter. The incision is made in the caudoventral portion of the pars tensa. C = caudal; D = dorsal; R = rostral; V = ventral. (Reproduced from the *BSAVA Manual of Canine and Feline Endoscopy and Endosurgery*)

7 An assistant should infuse 1 ml of sterile saline via the catheter into the middle ear, and then aspirate to obtain a fluid sample for cytology and culture.

8 The assistant should then flush the middle ear gently with sterile saline until the fluid aspirated back is clear.

9 Remove the catheter from the middle ear

10 Remove the otoscope.

Potential complications

- Neurological signs (including head shaking, Horner syndrome, deafness) can result from over-aggressive lavage or the use of ceruminolytics

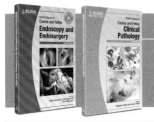

FURTHER INFORMATION

This technique is illustrated in the *BSAVA Manual of Canine and Feline Endoscopy and Endosurgery*; cytological findings are discussed in the *BSAVA Manual of Canine and Feline Clinical Pathology.*

Nasal oxygen administration

Indications/Use

- Patients requiring supplementary oxygen
- Patients that do not tolerate an oxygen mask
- Patients that are too large to fit inside an oxygen cage

Contraindications

- Inspired oxygen concentrations may not be high enough for very hypoxic animals, particularly if they are mouth-breathing. In very hypoxic animals, bilateral nasal oxygen lines can be used
- Animals with facial disease or pain
- Brachycephalic breeds are poor candidates for nasal oxygen supplementation: catheter prongs cannot be adjusted to fit comfortably on their faces; nasal catheters may not fit due to stenotic nares or do not stay in place because their noses are short; and increased vagal tone may be aggravated by the nasal catheter

Equipment

- Rubber catheter/soft polythene feeding tube (8–12 Fr in medium to large dogs, 5 Fr in cats and small dogs) (Figure N.1) or nasal prongs
- Topical local anaesthetic (e.g. 0.5% proxymetacaine eyedrops)
- Sterile aqueous lubricant (e.g. K-Y jelly)
- Non-absorbable suture material, needle and needle-holders
- Tissue glue
- 25 mm wide adhesive tape
- Oxygen delivery system
- Humidifier (container filled with distilled water)
- Elizabethan collar

Patient preparation and positioning

- Usually performed in the conscious animal, although fractious animals may benefit from light sedation
- The patient is positioned in sternal recumbency, or sitting
- Several drops of local anaesthetic should be applied down one or both nostrils. The catheter should be inserted once an appropriate amount of time has elapsed for the anaesthetic to take effect

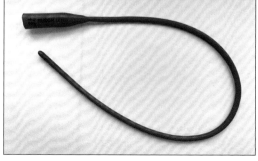

Figure N.1: A 12 Fr, 30 cm long rubber catheter can be used to administer nasal oxygen in a medium to large dog.

Technique

Nasal catheter

Single or bilateral nasal catheters can be used depending on the percentage of oxygen supplementation that is required.

1   Measure the distance from the nares to the medial canthus of the eye and mark this on the catheter.
2   Following desensitization of the nostril with topical local anaesthetic, gently insert the lubricated catheter into the nostril in a ventromedial direction (toward the base of the opposite ear) and advance it to the predetermined mark (Figure N.2). The nasal planum can be pushed dorsally to direct the tube ventrally.
3   Once the catheter is in place, it is contoured around the alar fold, and sutured in place using 2 metric (3/0 USP) nylon and tape butterflies, just beside the nostril and again on the side of the face or on top of the head. For the most secure placement, place a suture as close to the nasal–cutaneous junction as possible.
4   Attach the nasal catheter to an oxygen delivery system with flow rates of 100–200 ml/kg/minute.
5   Place an Elizabethan collar.

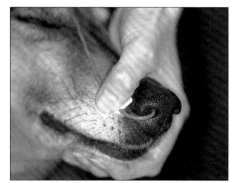

Figure N.2: Catheter positioned in the nostril. (Reproduced from the *BSAVA Manual of Canine and Feline Emergency and Critical Care*)

Nasal prongs

■   Some animals can be best managed using bilateral nasal prongs that penetrate 1 cm or less into the nasal cavity (see Figure N.4)
■   Inspired oxygen concentrations of 30–50% can easily be achieved using this type of system, although panting probably limits their effectiveness

---

NOTE

■   If oxygen is provided for more than a few hours, it should be humidified (saturated with water vapour) to prevent desiccation of the airways, especially if the turbinates are bypassed (this occurs with the use of nasal and tracheal oxygen catheters). Specially designed units that heat and humidify the inspired air are available for placement in anaesthetic and ventilator circuits, but nasal or cage oxygen humidification can be simply accomplished by bubbling the oxygen through a chamber of distilled water (Figure N.3)

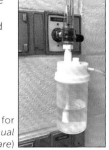

Figure N.3: Chamber filled with distilled water for humidifying oxygen. (Reproduced from the *BSAVA Manual of Canine and Feline Emergency and Critical Care*)

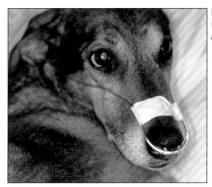

Figure N.4: Oxygen provision via nasal prongs. (Reproduced from the *BSAVA Manual of Canine and Feline Emergency and Critical Care*)

Potential complications

- Long-term therapy with high concentrations of oxygen (F_iO_2 >0.6 for >12 hours, or sooner with assisted ventilation) can be associated with lung damage ('oxygen toxicity'). Although rare, every effort should be made to minimize F_iO_2 for critically ill patients
- Sneezing and dislodgement of catheter or prongs
- Nasal discharge is common but is not clinically significant
- Epistaxis

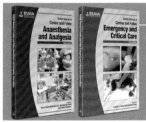

FURTHER INFORMATION

Further information on the administration of supplementary oxygen, including the use of masks and oxygen cages, can be found in the *BSAVA Manual of Canine and Feline Anaesthesia and Analgesia* and the *BSAVA Manual of Canine and Feline Emergency and Critical Care.*

Naso-oesophageal tube placement

Indications/Use

- Short-term nutritional support (up to 7 days) of cats and small dogs. In medium- to large-breed dogs, the sheer volume of a liquid diet required to meet the energy needs generally limits the usefulness of this feeding method
- Animals that require assisted feeding but in which general anaesthesia is contraindicated

Contraindications

- Comatose, recumbent or dysphoric animals at risk of aspiration
- Head trauma
- Nasopharyngeal disease
- Persistent vomiting; the tube may be expelled or retroflexed into the nasopharynx
- Absent gag reflex
- Severe nasal disease or dysphagia
- Oesophagitis, oesophageal stricture following oesophageal trauma or surgery, or in patients with severe oesophageal dysfunction (e.g. megaoesophagus)

Equipment

- Naso-oesophageal tube (soft polyvinyl or silicone):
    - Cats: 3–5 Fr; 40–75 cm
    - Dogs: 6–12 Fr; 40–80 cm
- 5–10 ml syringe
- Topical local anaesthetic drops (e.g. proxymetacaine 0.5%)
- Lubricating jelly (e.g. K-Y jelly)
- Permanent marker pen
- 25 mm wide adhesive tape
- Non-absorbable suture material
- Tissue glue
- Skin stapler
- Elizabethan collar

Patient preparation and positioning

- The procedure is normally performed with the animal conscious. Occasionally light sedation may be required
- The patient can be positioned standing, or in lateral or sternal recumbency
- The animal's head should be placed in a 'neutral' position (i.e. not too flexed or extended)

Technique

1 Instil local anaesthetic drops into one nostril and wait sufficient time for it to become effective. Either nostril can be used, but if you are right-handed it is generally easier to place the tube into the animal's left nostril.
2 Measure the distance from the nose to the 9th rib (8th intercostal space) (Figure N.5) and mark this on the tube with a permanent marker pen. Alternatively, place a piece of tape 1 cm distal to this point.

3 Lubricate the first centimetre of the tube to aid insertion.

4 Insert the tube gently (but initially rapidly for the first 3−4 cm to avoid it being sneezed out), aiming ventromedially (toward the base of the opposite ear) so that it will pass into the ventral meatus of the nasal cavity. The nasal planum can be pushed dorsally to direct the tube ventrally (Figure N.6).

5 Insert the remainder of the tube until it reaches the predetermined mark (nose to 9th rib). Watch for signs of swallowing (indicating the tube is likely to be correctly placed in the oesophagus) and coughing or discomfort (indicating the tube may have been inserted into the trachea). In the latter case, the tube should be removed and repositioned.

6 Check that the tube is positioned correctly by attaching an empty 5−10 ml syringe and applying suction:

  a If the tube is in the trachea, syringefuls of air will be readily withdrawn. If this occurs the tube should be removed

  b If suction creates a vacuum, meaning that no air can be sucked into the tube, it should be in the oesophagus.

NOTE

- Tube placement should be assessed prior to the administration of each feed. Very occasionally, it can be vomited or regurgitated and either pass into the trachea or reside in the nasopharynx

---

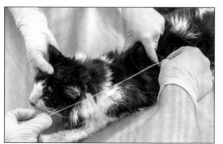

Figure N.5: The distance from the nose to the 9th rib (8th intercostal space) should be measured and marked on the naso-oesophageal tube.

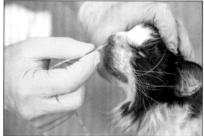

Figure N.6: Pushing the nasal planum dorsally during insertion can help direct the tube ventrally.

7 Take a lateral thoracic radiograph to confirm that the tube is in the correct position, where the end lies (distal third of the oesophagus, not the stomach) and that the tube is not kinked or twisted.

8 Place a butterfly tape strip on the tube, approximately 1−2 cm from the nostril. This should be sutured or stapled to the skin of the muzzle, as close as possible to the side of the nasal planum. The tube can be guided through the lateral groove under the nares. It is important not to bend the tube too tightly; allow some room to prevent kinking.

9 Bend the tube up and around the dorsal aspect of the animal's nose and head and secure it to the skin with one or more additional butterfly tape strips.

Alternatively, in larger dogs, especially those with long muzzles, the tube may be best positioned along the ipsilateral muzzle and below the ipsilateral ear.

10 Tape the feeding tube to a bandage lightly wrapped around the neck, if required.

11 An alternate fixation method to suturing the butterfly strips, is to apply a thin layer of tissue glue to each strip and stick the strips to haired skin (Figure N.7). However, although the glue can be applied easily and will initially hold the tube securely, the glue tends to become brittle and the tube can become loose shortly after fixation.

12 Place an Elizabethan collar to prevent the animal displacing the tube. The remaining length of tube can be coiled and taped inside the collar.

13 Feeding can commence immediately after tube placement.

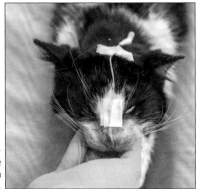

Figure N.7: A naso-oesophageal tube fixed in place using butterfly tape strips and a thin layer of tissue glue.

Feeding technique

> **NOTES**
>
> - As the feeding tubes are of narrow bore, a liquid diet must be used
> - Before every feeding, the position of the tube must be checked (as detailed in Step 6 above). Radiographs should be taken if there is any doubt about the position of the tube

1 Prior to each feeding, aspirate the tube to determine whether food can be retrieved. If a large amount is aspirated, it can be an indication of residual food remaining from the previous feed and additional feeds should be delayed.

2 Flush the tube with small amounts (5–10 ml) of lukewarm tap water whilst observing the animal for discomfort (e.g. salivation, coughing, gagging, or vomiting)

3 Food should be warmed to body temperature and injected into the tube slowly (<3 ml/kg/min).

   a Feed only one-third of the resting energy requirement (RER) on the first day.

   b On the second day, feed two-thirds of the RER, increasing to the entire RER on day three.

c Divide the daily requirement into multiple (5 or 6) feeds per 24 hours.
d *Alternatively*, a continuous rate infusion of food can be used.
4 Flush the tube after every feed with 5–10 ml of lukewarm tap water.

RESTING ENERGY REQUIREMENT

The resting energy requirement is now used as the 'baseline' energy recommendation for hospitalized dogs and cats, regardless of the disease or surgery.

The following equation can be used to calculate the RER in kcal/day for cats or dogs:

$$RER = 70 \times \text{bodyweight (kg)}^{0.75}$$

Alternatively, for animals >2 kg the following equation can be used:

$$RER = 30 \times \text{bodyweight (kg)} + 70$$

Note: to convert kcal to kilojoules (kJ) multiply by 4.185

Tube maintenance and removal

- Twice a day, the external nares should be wiped gently with cotton wool soaked in water
- If the tube becomes blocked, 3 ml of a carbonated drink (e.g. cola or soda water) or pancreatic enzyme solution can be instilled and left for 5–10 minutes to help dislodge blockages
- The tube can be removed at any time following placement. Sutures or staples should be removed or, if using tissue glue, the hair under the butterfly tape strips should be gently cut. The tube is removed in one motion. Light sedation may be required in non-cooperative patients

Potential complications

- Rhinitis
- Epistaxis
- Vomiting
- Regurgitation
- Aspiration pneumonia
- Tube dislodgement, kinking or removal

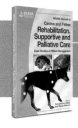

FURTHER INFORMATION

Further details on assisted feeding can be found in the *BSAVA Manual of Canine and Feline Rehabilitation, Supportive and Palliative Care.*

Oesophagostomy tube placement

Indications/Use

- Nutritional support for weeks to months

Contraindications

- Comatose, recumbent or dysphoric animals at risk of aspiration
- Persistent vomiting – the tube may be expelled or retroflexed into the nasopharynx
- Oesophagitis, oesophageal stricture, following oesophageal trauma or surgery, or in patients with severe oesophageal dysfunction (e.g. megaoesophagus)

Equipment

- As required for **Aseptic preparation – (b) surgical procedures**
- Oesophagostomy tube (open-end, silicone with multiple side holes or red rubber feeding tube):
  - Cats: 10–14 Fr; 23–38 cm long
  - Dogs: 14–19 Fr; 38 cm long
- Long curved forceps (minimum 20 cm), e.g. Rochester–Carmalt
- Scalpel and No.10 scalpel blade
- Laryngoscope
- 25 mm wide adhesive tape
- Suture material, e.g. 3 metric (2/0 USP) monofilament nylon
- Suture scissors
- Sterile dressing to cover the tube site
- Materials for a soft, padded, loose, neck bandage
- Permanent marker pen

Patient preparation and positioning

- General anaesthesia is required
- The patient is most commonly positioned in right lateral recumbency. Placing a sandbag under the neck can help elevate the oesophagus
- **Aseptic preparation – (b) surgical procedures** is required from the dorsal to the ventral aspects of the neck and from the angle of the jaw to the shoulder

Technique

Whilst various methods for oesophagostomy tube placement exist, the surgical cut-down technique is described below, as it is the most commonly used and does not require specific kit.

1   Place a piece of adhesive tape on the patient's fur at the level of the 9th rib.
2   An assistant should insert curved forceps through the mouth and into the mid-cervical oesophagus (Figure O.1).
3   The assistant should rotate the tip of the forceps laterally, until the point of the tips can be felt through the skin.
4   Make a 5–10 mm skin incision over this site.

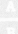

5 Bluntly dissect through the subcutaneous tissues and make an incision into the oesophagus over the tips of the forceps.

6 Push the tips of the forceps outwards through the incision to the external surface (Figure O.2).

7 Measure the oesophagostomy tube from this point to the 9th rib (distal oesophagus); use the adhesive tape as a guide. An assistant should mark this position on the tube with a permanent marker pen.

8 Open the tips of the forceps and grasp the distal end of the feeding tube (Figure O.3).

9 Draw the end of the tube through the oesophagostomy incision and rostrally into the pharynx to exit the mouth.

10 Disengage the tips of the forceps and curl the tip of the tube back into the mouth (Figure O.4).

11 Feed the tube into the oesophagus while simultaneously pulling back the tube at the skin incision (Figure O.5).

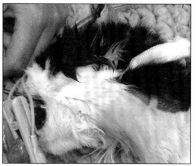

Figure O.1: Curved forceps should be inserted through the mouth to the level of the mid-cervical oesophagus. (Courtesy of David Walker, Anderson Moores Veterinary Specialists)

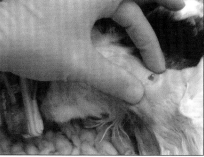

Figure O.2: The tips of the forceps should be pushed out through the incision made at the level of the mid-cervical oesophagus. (Courtesy of David Walker, Anderson Moores Veterinary Specialists)

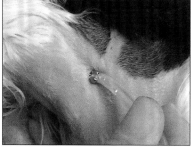

Figure O.3: The oesophagostomy tube should be grasped with the forceps and pulled through the incision. (Courtesy of David Walker, Anderson Moores Veterinary Specialists)

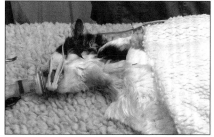

Figure O.4: Once the oesophagostomy tube has exited the mouth, the forceps should be disengaged. The tip of the tube can then be curled back into the mouth. (Courtesy of David Walker, Anderson Moores Veterinary Specialists)

12 The tube should 'flip', allowing it to pass caudally towards the stomach without resistance. Visually inspect the oropharynx, using a laryngoscope as required, to confirm that the tube is no longer present in the oropharynx.

13 The tube should slide easily back and forth a few centimetres, confirming that it has straightened.

14 Take a thoracic radiograph to confirm correct tube placement: the tip of the tube should be in the distal third of the oesophagus, not the stomach.

15 Secure the tube with one or two finger-trap sutures (Figure O.6).

16 Cover the tube site with a sterile dressing and place a soft, padded, loose, neck bandage.

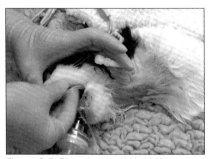

Figure O.5: The tube should be fed into the oesophagus whilst simultaneously being pulled back at the skin incision. (Courtesy of David Walker, Anderson Moores Veterinary Specialists)

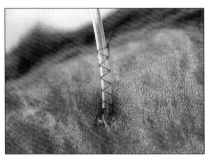

Figure O.6: Finger-trap sutures should be used to secure the tube in place.

Feeding technique

> **NOTES**
>
> - Feeding can commence as soon as the patient has recovered from general anaesthesia
> - The patient should be placed in sternal recumbency with their head elevated or in a standing position

1 Instil sterile saline initially, in case the tube has migrated. If there is any doubt as to its position, take thoracic and abdominal radiographs with or without sterile **iodinated contrast medium**.

2 Before feeding each time, flush the tube with small amounts (5–10 ml) of lukewarm tap water.

3 If the feeding tube is narrow bore, a liquid or semi-liquid food will be required.

4 Food should be warmed to body temperature and injected into the tube over approximately 5 minutes.

    a Feed only one-third of the resting energy requirement (RER) on the first day.

    b On the second day, feed two-thirds of the RER, increasing to the entire RER on day three.

    c Divide the daily requirement into multiple (5 or 6) feeds per 24 hours.

5 Flush the tube *after every feed* with 5–10 ml of lukewarm tap water.

> ### RESTING ENERGY REQUIREMENT
>
> The resting energy requirement is now used as the 'baseline' energy recommendation for hospitalized dogs and cats, regardless of the disease or surgery.
>
> The following equation can be used to calculate the RER in kcal/day for cats or dogs:
>
> **RER = 70 × bodyweight (kg)$^{0.75}$**
>
> Alternatively, for animals >2 kg the following equation can be used:
>
> **RER = 30 × bodyweight (kg) + 70**
>
> Note: to convert kcal to kilojoules (kJ) multiply by 4.185

Tube maintenance and removal

- The stoma site should be inspected and cleaned daily. A new sterile dressing and bandage should also be applied every day
- If the tube becomes blocked, 3 ml of a carbonated drink (e.g. cola or soda water) can be instilled and left for 5–10 minutes to help dislodge blockages. Before undertaking this procedure, the tube should be checked to ensure that it is in the correct position
- The tube can be removed when it is no longer required; there is no minimum length of time the tube must be left in place
- To remove the tube, the bandage and sterile dressing should be taken off and the suture(s) cut. The tube can then be pulled out
- The stoma site will close rapidly once the tube is removed. It should not be sutured closed

Potential complications

- Major complications of oesophagostomy tube placement in dogs and cats are uncommon but can include haemorrhage from blood vessel laceration, oesophageal tears and inadvertent tracheal injury. These can usually be avoided with proper technique
- More common complications include:
  - Tube blockage
  - Infection at the tube site
  - Tube dislodgement or removal
- Written instructions for owners detailing tube use and maintenance should be provided when the patient is discharged to reduce the risk of complications

Otoscopy

Indications/Use

- To obtain specimens for diagnosis of external ear canal disease
- To treat otitis externa. (For sampling and treating otitis media, see **Myringotomy**)

Equipment

- Otoscope or video-otoscope
- Cones of varying lengths. Cones should be sterilized when collecting samples for microbiological culture
- Cotton wool
- Haemostats for hair removal (if necessary)
- Sterile microbiology swab and transport medium
- Cotton wool buds
- Microscope slides
- 0.9% sterile saline
- 10 ml syringes
- Kidney dish
- Spruells needle or sterile catheters (e.g. 3.5 Fr tomcat catheter, long polypropylene catheter, 3.5 Fr feeding tube) of length sufficient to pass along the full length of the external ear canal

Patient preparation and positioning

- The animal can be examined standing, sitting or in lateral recumbency
- Sedation or general anaesthesia may be required; general anaesthesia is essential if irrigation of the ear is to be performed
- Hair is removed, if necessary, by grasping groups of hairs with haemostats and twisting the handle

Technique

1 Examine the pinnae and entrance to the ear canals with the naked eye.
2 Palpate the ear canal to evaluate pain, thickening and ossification of the ear canal. Note the presence of pus or cerumen.
3 Examine each ear with the otoscope, starting with the normal ear if there is one. Apply lateral tension to the ear pinna with fingers to straighten the ear canal as the otoscope is advanced.
4 Visualize the tympanic membrane; in a normal ear this appears as a concave translucent membrane, with a dorsal, white, thick, well vascularized pars flaccida and a ventral semi-transparent pars tensa.
5 If significant pus or cerumen obscures evaluation of the ear canal or tympanic membrane, the ear can be flushed with lukewarm sterile saline. This is drawn into a 5–10 ml syringe attached to a Spruells needle or catheter, flushed into the ear canal, and re-aspirated.
If possible, this is best performed under otoscopic visualization, with the needle or catheter passed through a side channel of the otoscope cone.

Sample handling

- Samples for microbiological culture should be obtained first:
  - A sterile swab should be inserted through the sterile cone of an otoscope attachment and a sample collected from within the ear canal
  - The swab should be placed in transport medium for dispatch to the laboratory
- Samples for cytology should then be obtained:
  - A cotton bud or sterile swab should be inserted down to the junction between the vertical and horizontal ear canals. The bud should be rotated to collect debris
- Any debris collected should be transferred to a slide with liquid paraffin and a coverslip applied, prior to examination with a microscope, using low (4X objective) power
- A smear can be made by rolling the cotton bud gently on to a microscope slide, and then air-dried and stained, as required

Potential complications

- Rupture of the tympanic membrane
- Injury to the external ear canal

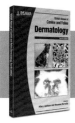

FURTHER INFORMATION

For more information on otoscopy, see the *BSAVA Manual of Canine and Feline Dermatology.*

Pericardiocentesis

Indications/Use

- Relief of pericardial tamponade
- To obtain a sample of pericardial fluid for diagnostic evaluation

---

WARNING

- Diuretics should NOT be given prior to pericardiocentesis. Not only will they be ineffective at relieving the clinical signs but the reduction in circulating fluid volume, and therefore intracardiac pressure, may exacerbate tamponade.

Contraindications

- Suspected coagulopathy
- Active pericardial haemorrhage
- Severe arrhythmia

Equipment

- As required for **Aseptic preparation – (a) non-surgical procedures**
- A small-bore wire-guided drain, such as that used for **Thoracostomy tube placement – (b) small-bore wire-guided**
- OR a long (5–12.5 cm) wide-bore (14–18 G) over-the-needle catheter ± a narrow-gauge cat urinary catheter. *Note: check that the urinary catheter passes easily through the cannula of the over-the-needle catheter before starting the procedure*
- OR a veterinary pericardial drainage catheter set (e.g. containing an 8.2 Fr, 20 cm long catheter with six distal side holes, an 18 G, 7 cm long introduction needle, and a 50 cm guidewire)
- Intravenous catheter, giving set and intravenous fluids
- Local anaesthetic
- Scalpel and No.11 or 15 scalpel blade
- 3-way tap
- Extension tubing
- 20 ml syringe
- 50–60 ml syringe
- Measuring container
- EDTA and sterile plain collection tubes
- Microscope slides
- Suture materials or tissue glue
- Electrocardiogram (ECG) equipment

Patient preparation and positioning

- Sedation may be required to minimize movement.
- The animal is usually placed in sternal or left lateral recumbency, with **pericardiocentesis performed via a right-sided approach**. A right-sided approach is chosen to avoid the large coronary artery on the left and also to avoid the lungs by using the cardiac notch

- Pericardiocentesis can be performed with or without ultrasound guidance
- A peripheral **intravenous catheter** can be placed and intravenous fluids given to improve cardiac filling if required
- The ECG leads are connected to the patient (see **Electrocardiography**)
- **Aseptic preparation – (a) non-surgical procedures** is performed on a large area from the 3rd to the 7th rib, and from the ventral to dorsal aspect of the right chest wall

Technique

1 The point of needle entry is approximately intercostal space 5 or 6, at the level of the costochondral junction. The exact site is located by palpating or auscultating where the cardiac impulse is strongest. Thoracic radiography or ultrasonography can also be used to indicate where the heart is most closely associated with the body wall and thus to determine the puncture site.

2 Infiltrate the skin and subcutaneous tissue with local anaesthetic.

3 Make a small stab incision through the skin with a scalpel blade (Figure P.1).

4 Three options are described: over-the-needle catheter; wire-guided drain; and pericardial drainage set.

If using an over-the-needle catheter:

a Insert the cannula and needle through the stab incision (Figure P.2).

b Slowly advance through the intercostal muscles just cranial to the rib (to avoid injury to the intercostal vessels, which run on the caudal aspect of the rib) in a slightly craniodorsal direction, until the tip of the needle reaches the visceral pericardium. With long-standing effusions there is often increased resistance and also a scratching sensation when the pericardial sac is first encountered.

c A sharp stabbing motion may be required to penetrate the pericardium.

d Pericardial fluid should appear in the hub. Pericardial fluid is typically quite haemorrhagic in dogs.

e Advance the catheter over the needle and remove the needle.

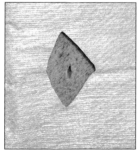

Figure P.1: A small stab incision should be made in the skin.

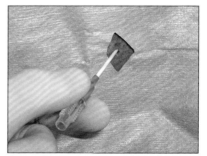

Figure P.2: The cannula and needle should be inserted through the stab incision.

The cannula of the over-the-needle catheter is prone to kinking, usually at the point where it passes through the intercostal muscles or as it enters the pericardium. This can be negated by introducing a narrow-gauge sterile urinary catheter through the cannula into the pericardial sac after withdrawal of the needle (Figure P.3). Fluid can then be drained via this urinary catheter.

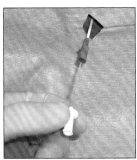

Figure P.3: A narrow-gauge sterile urinary catheter can be used to drain fluid from the pericardial sac

If using a small-bore wire-guided drain:

a   Insert the catheter introducer through the stab incision and advance as described above (Figure P.4).

b   Once the introducer enters the pericardial sac and fluid is seen, advance the catheter completely into the pericardium over the needle and withdraw the needle.

c   Thread the guidewire through the introducer catheter and into the pericardium (Figure P.5).

d   Advance the guidewire by approximately 10–20 cm. **The guidewire should be held at all times when it is partially within the pericardium** (Figure P.6).

e   Remove the introducer catheter from the pericardium over the guidewire, leaving the guidewire in place within the pericardium (Figure P.7).

f   Advance the polyurethane catheter into the pericardium over the guidewire to the level of the suture wing (Figure P.8).

g   Remove the guidewire (Figure P.9).

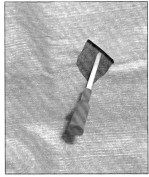

Figure P.4: The catheter introducer should be inserted through the skin incision.

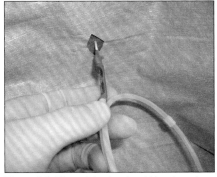

Figure P.5: The guidewire should be thread through the introducer catheter into the pericardium.

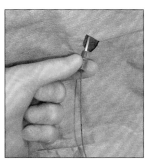

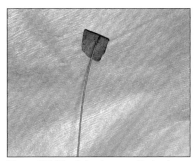

Figure P.6: The guidewire should be held as it is advanced into the pericardium.

Figure P.7: The introducer catheter is removed leaving the guidewire in place.

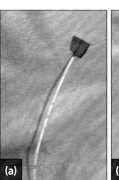

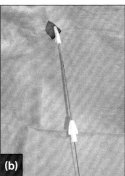

(a) (b)

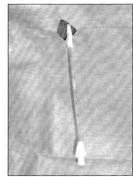

Figure P.8: (a) The catheter should be introduced and advanced into the pericardium over the guidewire. **(b)** The catheter in place.

Figure P.9: The guidewire should be removed and the catheter left in place.

If using a veterinary pericardial drainage catheter set:

a Attach a 20 ml syringe to the introduction needle.

b Insert the introduction needle through the stab incision and advance the needle as described above, while maintaining slight negative pressure in the 20 ml syringe.

c Pericardial fluid should appear in the syringe.

d Remove the syringe from the needle.

e Thread the guidewire (soft end) through the needle and into the pericardium. Advance the wire by approximately 10 cm. **The guidewire should be held at all times when it is partially within the pericardium** (Figure P.10).

f Remove the needle, leaving the guidewire in the pericardium (Figure P.11).

g Thread the catheter over the guidewire, through the skin and intercostal space, and into the pericardium (Figure P.12).

h Remove the guidewire, leaving the catheter in the pericardium (Figure P.13).

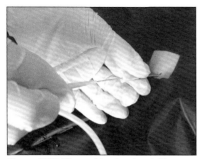

Figure P.10: The guidewire should be threaded through the needle into the pericardium. The guidewire must be held at all times. (Courtesy of Luca Ferasin)

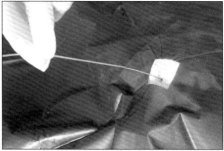

Figure P.11: The needle should be removed and the guidewire left in place. (Courtesy of Luca Ferasin)

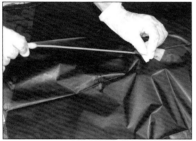

Figure P.12: The catheter should be threaded over the guidewire. (Courtesy of Luca Ferasin)

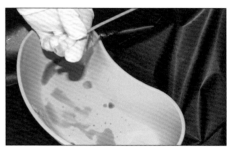

Figure P.13: The guidewire should be removed and the catheter left in place. (Courtesy of Luca Ferasin)

ARRHYTHMIAS

ECG monitoring throughout the procedure allows identification of arrhythmias caused by the catheter traumatizing the epicardium. Tachyarrhythmias (usually ventricular) are most commonly encountered. If these (or another arrhythmia) occur, the needle should be withdrawn slightly so that it no longer touches the epicardium.

---

5 Attach a 3-way tap, extension tubing and 50–60 ml syringe to create a closed drainage system, which can be operated by an assistant (Figure P.14).

6 Aspirate the pericardial fluid.

7 If the flow of fluid stops, advance or withdraw the catheter by a few millimetres and re-aspirate, but avoid touching the epicardium.

8 Place approximately 5 ml of pericardial fluid in a plain tube and observe for clot formation. If it clots, the fluid includes fresh blood, and the procedure should be stopped. The packed cell volume (PCV) of the fluid (measured using a microcentrifuge) can also be checked to confirm that it is less than the PCV of peripheral blood.

9 Continue drainage until as much fluid as possible is removed. NB It is not necessary to drain the pericardial sac completely.

10 Place fluid into a measuring container and note the total volume (Figure P.15).
11 After removal of the catheter, place a single suture in the skin incision if required, or close with tissue glue.

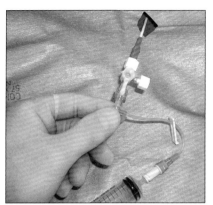

Figure P.15: The fluid collected should be placed into a measuring container.

Figure P.14: A closed drainage system should be created by attaching a 3-way tap, extension tubing and syringe.

Sample handling

- The pericardial fluid should be placed in an EDTA tube for cytological analysis
- Air-dried smears should be made, especially if the sample is to be posted to an external laboratory
- If there is suspicion of infectious pericarditis, fluid should be submitted in a sterile plain tube for bacteriological culture

Potential complications

- Haemorrhage from the heart is uncommon and, if it occurs, is unlikely to result in catastrophic bleeding. The coronary arteries located on the right epicardium are relatively small, and the right ventricle is under relatively low pressure. Laceration of a cardiac tumour leading to haemorrhage can also occur
- It is common for arrhythmias to occur as the procedure is performed, but these do not usually cause clinically significant consequences and usually stop once the catheter is repositioned
- Cardiac puncture and removal of a large quantity of blood from the right ventricle can lead to hypovolaemic shock and can be avoided by checking that the haemorrhagic fluid is pericardial in origin
- Pneumothorax due to lung puncture

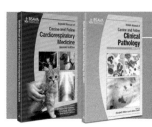

FURTHER INFORMATION

Management following pericardiocentesis is described in the *BSAVA Manual of Canine and Feline Cardiorespiratory Medicine*. For interpretation of the results of fluid analysis see the *BSAVA Manual of Canine and Feline Clinical Pathology*.

Peritoneal dialysis

Indications/Use

- Acute kidney injury (AKI)
- Anuria or oliguria if attempts to induce urine production are unsuccessful
- Progressive azotaemia or severe intractable uraemia that does not improve with standard medical therapy
- Refractory hyperkalaemia
- Life-threatening pulmonary oedema or iatrogenic fluid overload
- Acute poisoning/drug overdose with substances that can be removed by dialysis (e.g. ethylene glycol, barbiturates, ammonia)

> **PERITONEAL DIALYSIS OR HAEMODIALYSIS?**
>
> Peritoneal dialysis (PD) requires minimal specialized equipment and is not technically difficult. However, it is extremely labour-intensive and close attention needs to be paid to the levels of sterility during the procedure. Haemodialysis is an alternative and superior technique and should be considered if available.

Contraindications

- Animals with chronic (end-stage) renal failure, as PD will only provide very short-term relief of clinical signs and/or a temporary reduction in the level of azotaemia
- Peritoneal fibrosis or adhesions that preclude solute exchange or prevent fluid distribution throughout the abdomen
- Severe coagulopathy
- Peritonitis
- Severe hypoalbuminaemia

Equipment

- As required for **Aseptic preparation – (b) surgical procedures**
- Commercial PD solution. *Alternatively,* a basic PD solution can be formulated by adding dextrose to lactated Ringer's (Hartmann's) solution (30 ml of 50% dextrose in 1 litre = 1.5% dextrose solution). Dextrose can also be added at differing amounts to make approximate 2.5%, 3.5% or 4.25% solutions. The concentration of dextrose required depends on the hydration status of the patient; higher dextrose concentrations achieve improved ultrafiltration and water removal. A 4.25% solution should only be used when patients are fluid overloaded, and a 1.5% solution is generally adequate in normovolaemic patients. The addition of heparin (500 IU/l) to the dialysate is recommended for the first 24 hours following catheter placement to minimize the risk of catheter occlusion from fibrin deposition. The dialysate should be warmed to 38°C to maintain body temperature and to improve peritoneal permeability
- A PD catheter: The ideal catheter provides reliable, rapid dialysate flow rates without leaks or risk of infection. There are many catheter options, including commercial PD catheters such as the Tenckhoff catheter, the Blake silicone fluted drain, fluted-T catheters, the acute PD catheter, multipurpose tube catheters with stylet/trocar or Jackson–Pratt surgical suction drains (Figure P.16). Peritoneal drainage sets for veterinary use are also available, including one containing a 12 Fr 30 cm catheter

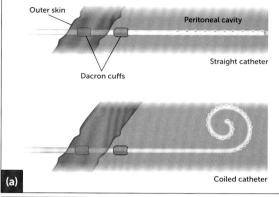

Outer skin

Peritoneal cavity

Straight catheter

Dacron cuffs

Coiled catheter

(a)

Figure P.16:
(a) Tenckhoff catheter.
(b) Blake silicone fluted drain.
(c) Fluted-T catheter.

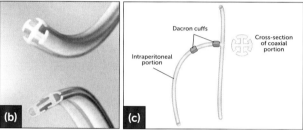

Dacron cuffs

Cross-section of coaxial portion

Intraperitoneal portion

(b)

(c)

CATHETER/DRAIN OPTIONS

- Most commercial PD catheters are made of silicone rubber tubing or polyurethane, and have multiple fenestrations and one or more Dacron velour cuffs along the length of the tubing. The Dacron cuffs serve to anchor the catheter in place and provide a barrier to infection. Cuffs are positioned in the musculature ± the subcutaneous space, a few centimetres under the skin exit
- A conventional straight Tenckhoff catheter is the most widely used catheter for PD in human patients
- The optimal catheter type has not been established in veterinary medicine, although the fluted-T catheter has shown good results in dogs and Blake silicon fluted drains have been used successfully for PD in cats
- Fenestrated propylene peritoneal lavage catheters with an introduction needle and guidewire also exist for veterinary patients, although these are not designed to be left *in situ*
- Jackson–Pratt surgical suction drains, placed by a mini-surgical approach, have been used in dogs and with less risk of occlusion than other multipurpose straight tube catheters. Several days of successful PD have been achieved using these drains and thus they are suitable alternatives if commercial PD catheters are not readily available
- One of the authors [NB] has also used a 14 or 16 G chest tube, placed via Seldinger technique, for percutaneous peritoneal access for short-term (<24 hours) interim management, until a more 'permanent' catheter can be sourced; these catheters invariably kink and become obstructed within 12–24 hours

- Urinary catheter
- Local anaesthetic
- Scalpel and No.11 or 15 scalpel blade
- Suture material
- Soft tissue surgical instrument set
- Commercial closed 'Y'-system for drainage and infusion. Alternatively, a closed Y-system can be achieved using a 3-way tap, extension tubing and a collection bag (such as an empty sterile fluid bag or urine collection bag)
- 10–20 ml syringe
- Intravenous infusion pump

Patient preparation and positioning

- Sedation is recommended in order to minimize movement and avoid accidental bowel puncture
- The patient is restrained in dorsal or lateral recumbency
- **Aseptic preparation – (b) surgical procedures** is carried out over a large area of the abdomen from the xiphoid to the pubis, and a fenestrated drape placed
- A urinary catheter should always be placed prior to PD catheter placement to prevent bladder trauma on PD catheter insertion (see **Urethral catheterization**)
- Due to the high incidence of iatrogenic infections that can result in septic peritonitis, administering a prophylactic dose of a second-generation cephalosporin prior to PD catheter insertion should be considered

Technique

> **WARNING**
>
> - Maintenance of sterility during connection, disconnection, infusion and drainage is of vital importance, since septic peritonitis is a relatively common and often lethal complication of PD. Sterile gloves should be worn during connection, disconnection and bag changes. Line connections should be covered with dressings soaked in povidone–iodine or chlorhexidine. Injection ports should be cleaned with chlorhexidine and alcohol prior to use.

1 Infuse local anaesthetic into the skin, abdominal entry sites and over the length of any planned subcutaneous tunnel. A subcutaneous tunnel should be made when placing any type of PD catheter, as this decreases the incidence of peritonitis and of dialysate leakage.

2 Techniques described for insertion of the PD catheter include: 'blind' percutaneous placement using a trocar or a guidewire (Seldinger technique); or a mini-surgical approach.

   If using a trocar: the site of catheter entry is on the midline or paramedian at the level of the umbilicus.

   a Make a small skin incision (<0.4 cm) with a scalpel at this point.

   b Advance the trocar and PD catheter into the abdomen by only 1–2 cm to avoid accidental laceration of the abdominal organs.

c Once in the abdomen, advance the PD catheter off the stylet and direct caudally to position in the lower pelvis, in an unobstructed location.

d Once the intra-abdominal portion of the catheter has been placed, tunnel the distal tip of the catheter within the subcutaneous tissues.

If using a guidewire:

a Make a small skin incision (<0.4 cm) with a scalpel at this point.

b Insert the catheter introducer into the abdomen and thread the guidewire through the introducer catheter in a caudal direction.

c Remove the introducer catheter from the guidewire, leaving the wire in place.

d Advance the PD catheter over the guidewire, again in a caudal direction, and position in the lower pelvis, in an unobstructed location.

e Once the intra-abdominal portion of the catheter has been placed, tunnel the distal tip of the catheter within the subcutaneous tissues.

For a mini-surgical approach:

a Abdominal penetration should be approximately 3–5 cm to the right of the midline, through the rectus muscle, at the level of the umbilicus. Make a 3–5 cm paramedian skin and subcutaneous incision.

b Make a 2–3 cm incision through the rectus muscle and into the abdominal cavity.

c A stay suture can be placed in the rectus sheath to allow manipulation of the body wall.

d Identify and incise the parietal peritoneum and direct the catheter caudally to position it in the lower pelvis, in an unobstructed location.

e For snug abdominal wall closure, once the PD catheter exits the abdominal incision, the sterile distal end of the PD catheter is tunnelled immediately under the external sheath of the rectus abdominus muscle, through a segment of the muscle, prior to its exit through the subcutaneous tissues and skin.

f Close the rectus sheath with a simple continuous or simple interrupted suture pattern using absorbable monofilament suture material.

g Close the skin routinely over the abdominal insertion site.

3 Check catheter flow by connection to dialysate solution. A small volume of dialysate (10–20 ml) is infused into the abdomen in a sterile fashion. This small volume of dialysate should easily be retrieved to ensure unoccluded catheter placement; if not, the catheter should be redirected.

4 Secure the catheter at the skin exit site with a purse-string and finger-trap suture.

5 Apply a non-occlusive sterile dressing, including several layers of sterile gauze, over the catheter exit site.

6 Once placed, attach the PD catheter to a commercial closed-Y connection system.

7 Infuse approximately 40 ml/kg of dialysate into the abdominal cavity by gravity flow or using an infusion pump over a 5–10 minute period.

8 Leave the dialysate in the abdomen for 30 minutes (the 'dwell' time). For dialysate retrieval, the collection system is placed below the patient and the fluid is allowed to drain by gravity over approximately 15 minutes. Drain as much fluid as possible.

NOTE

- Throughout the dialysate infusion and dwell time, the patient must be monitored for any signs of discomfort, nausea or respiratory compromise, which would necessitate smaller infusion volumes

9 Frequent dialysate exchanges are necessary in animals with acute oliguric or anuric renal failure, hyperkalaemia or in those that are overhydrated. Initially, exchanges may be as frequent as every 45–60 minutes. As the azotaemia improves (typically after 24–48 hours), the frequency of exchanges can be gradually decreased to 4 times a day, with the goal of maintaining the blood urea nitrogen (BUN) concentration between approximately 20 and 35 mmol/l.

10 Continue PD until urine production is noted, renal function is adequate and the patient is clinically improving. Specific creatinine and BUN values cannot be suggested, as animals will differ in their response to azotaemia.

PATIENT MONITORING

Careful monitoring of the patient and PD procedure is essential and enables complications to be addressed as early as possible. Critical monitoring data for patients are given in Figure P.17. As a general rule of thumb, dialysate (effusate) volume should equal infused volume if a 1.25% dextrose solution is used, and effusate volume should be more than infused volume if a higher percentage dextrose solution is used for correction of overhydrated patients. Should the effusate be less than the infusate for any given cycle, patient hydration or catheter occlusion should be considered. Patient repositioning may also allow successful drainage.

Physical examination parameters

- Bodyweight every 12 hours (same scales)
- Body temperature at least every 12 hours
- Exit site inspection every 24 hours
- Inspection for dialysate leakage or tunnel swelling/tenderness every exchange

Laboratory parameters

- Haematocrit and total protein every 12 hours
- Biochemistry panel every 24 hours
- Cytology of drained dialysate every 24 hours

Exchange parameters

- Drainage:
  - Start time
  - End time
  - Total drain time
  - Total drain volume
- Inflow:
  - Start time
  - End time
  - Total inflow time
  - Total volume infused
- Net balance per exchange (difference between outflow and prior inflow)

Figure P.17: Parameters that require monitoring in patients undergoing peritoneal dialysis.

Potential complications

- Septic peritonitis
- Perforation of the intestines
- Subcutaneous dialysate leakage
- Wound infection
- Catheter occlusion
- Electrolyte disturbances
- Overhydration
- Protein loss/hypoalbuminaemia

Platelet count

Indications/Use

- Assessment of platelet numbers

Equipment

- Approximately 2 ml of *fresh* venous blood collected into an EDTA collection tube (see **Blood sampling – (b) venous**)
- Citrate collection tube
- Microhaematocrit tube
- Microscope slides
- 'Spreader' slide (as for **Blood smear preparation**)
- Stain (e.g. Diff-Quik)
- Microscope with oil immersion lens
- Immersion oil

Technique

1   Check the blood in the EDTA tube for clots. If clots are present, the subsequent count will be inaccurate; take a fresh sample.

NOTE

- Blood can also be collected into citrate, as formation of platelet clumps may be reduced. However, collection into EDTA allows measurement of other haematological variables

---

2   Make a blood smear and stain with a suitable stain (see **Blood smear preparation**).

3   Examine the feathered edge of the blood smear for platelet clumps (Figure P.18). If clumps are present, the subsequent count will be inaccurate; take a fresh sample and repeat steps 1–3.

4   Identify an area of the smear, away from the feathered edge, where there is a monolayer of evenly distributed cells.

5   Count the platelets in at least 10 high-power fields (X1000, oil-immersion) and calculate the average (Figure P.19).

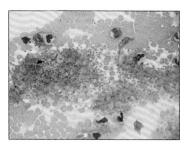

Figure P.18: Platelet clumps present on the feathered edge of a blood smear.

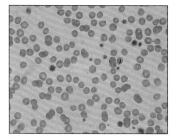

Figure P.19: A high-power field in which 14 platelets (stained structures) are visible.

Reference ranges

- Approximately 1 platelet per high-power field is equivalent to 15×10^9 platelets per litre in dogs and cats
- The normal reference range for platelets in dogs and cats is usually $>200 \times 10^9/l$

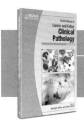

FURTHER INFORMATION

For more information on platelet counts, see the *BSAVA Manual of Canine and Feline Clinical Pathology.*

Point-of-care ultrasound (POCUS)

Indications/Use

- Screening technique for triage and assessment of intracavitary injury in the trauma patient
- Specifically allows the diagnosis of pleural, pericardial, peritoneal and retroperitoneal fluid and/or free gas
- Monitoring of patient over time whilst hospitalized

Equipment

- Assistant for patient restraint
- Ultrasound machine, ideally with a curvilinear probe with a small footprint (approximately 5–9 MHz is commonly used)
- Ultrasound coupling gel
- Isopropyl alcohol

Patient preparation and positioning

- Scanning in either lateral or sternal recumbency is possible; patient positioning should take into account the injuries of the patient and concurrent stabilization techniques being undertaken

- Shaving of hair is not needed; parting long hair and the use of coupling gel and/or isopropyl alcohol is sufficient in most cases
- If possible, room lights should be dimmed (provided it does not impede the ongoing stabilization of the trauma patient)

Technique

For thoracic POCUS:

1 Assess the cranial, middle and caudal aspects of the thoracic cavity both dorsally and ventrally. This is commonly broken down into the following locations and repeated bilaterally:

   a **Chest tube site:** Place the probe on the dorsolateral thoracic wall at the level of the 7th–9th intercostal space; dorsal to the xiphoid is a useful landmark to find the appropriate location (Figure P.20). Hold the probe in a cranial–caudal orientation. This site is useful to assess for the presence of pneumothorax. The normal expected appearance is a hyperechoic horizontal reverberation that moves with the patient's respiration

   b **Pericardial site:** Place the probe over the cranioventral aspect of the thorax, caudal to the point of the elbow or where auscultation of the heart would be expected (Figure P.21). Fan the probe in the intercostal spaces. This is the most useful site for the detection of pleural and pericardial effusions. It can be further divided into:

      i **Perihilar site:** Place the probe over the mid-thorax at the level of the perihilar region (approximately at intercostal space 6–7)

      ii **Middle lung lobe site:** Place the probe over the ventral aspect of the thorax, immediately ventral to the perihilar site

      iii **Cranial site:** Place the probe over the cranioventral thorax, cranial to the heart.

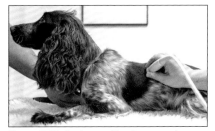

Figure P.20: Probe position to assess for pneumothorax.

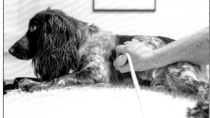

Figure P.21: Probe position to assess for pleural and pericardial effusions.

   c **Right short-axis view of the heart:** Whilst scanning the right-hand side of the thorax, obtain a short-axis view of the heart through the base to measure the left atrial to aortic root (LA:Ao) ratio

NORMAL LA:AO RATIO
- Cats <1.6
- Dogs <1.5

d   **Diaphragmatic–hepatic window:** Place the probe just caudal to the xyphoid cartilage. Angle the probe cranially towards the liver until the diaphragm is visualized (if intact). Fan the probe to the left and right. Pleural and pericardial effusions can be seen as anechoic to hypoechoic fluid cranial to the diaphragm. The presence of the mirror effect, causing reflection of the liver and gallbladder deep to the diaphragm, is a normal finding.

For abdominal POCUS:

1   Assess the abdominal cavity; probe positioning is shown in Figure P.22. This is commonly achieved using the following windows:

a   **Diaphragmatic–hepatic window:** Follow the technique for thoracic POCUS (see above). Any small volumes of peritoneal effusion will most likely be visualized between the liver lobes

b   **Splenorenal window:** Place the probe over the dorsolateral left mid-abdomen and visualize the left kidney and spleen (this may be dependent on patient conformation and body condition score). This position is useful to examine the peritoneal cavity for free gas, which is seen as hyperechoic reverberations outside the gastrointestinal tract

c   **Cystocolic window:** Place the probe over the caudal abdomen along the ventral midline. The urinary bladder and descending colon are landmarks that can be used to identify the correct site. The dependent aspect of the peritoneal cavity is a common site to visualize peritoneal effusion if only small volumes are present

d   **Hepatorenal window:** Place the probe over the dorsolateral right mid-abdomen. The right kidney and caudate lobe of the liver are landmarks that can be used to identify the correct site. An intercostal approach is often needed.

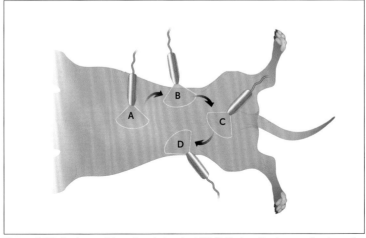

Figure P.22: Probe positions for abdominal POCUS. A = diaphragmatic–hepatic; B = splenorenal; C = cystocolic; D = hepatorenal. (Reproduced from the *BSAVA Manual of Canine Practice*)

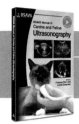

FURTHER INFORMATION

For more information on ultrasound techniques, see the *BSAVA Manual of Canine and Feline Ultrasonography.*

Prostatic wash

Indications/Use

To obtain a sample for cytology and bacteriological culture from dogs with:

- Prostatomegaly
- Other abnormalities in shape, symmetry or consistency of the prostate
- Prostatic pain
- Haematuria or pyuria

Equipment

- Sterile male dog urinary catheter (largest size possible)
- 4% chlorhexidine gluconate
- Bowl to collect urine
- 0.9% sterile saline
- 2 and 5 ml syringes
- EDTA and sterile plain collection tubes
- Microscope slides

Patient preparation and positioning

- This procedure can be performed on the conscious dog, although light sedation is generally preferable
- The dog should be allowed to empty its bladder prior to the procedure
- The dog is placed in lateral recumbency
- The prepuce must be cleaned of all debris, using dilute chlorhexidine, and rinsed with warm water

Technique

1   Using an aseptic technique, introduce a urinary catheter and empty the bladder of urine (see **Urethral catheterization**).

2 Flush the bladder with saline and empty again to ensure that all urine has been removed. A sample of the saline flush can be collected and handled as below, for comparison with the prostatic wash to help clarify the site of pathology (bladder *versus* prostate).

3 Perform a rectal examination, or alternatively an assistant can perform the rectal examination.

4 Partially withdraw the catheter so the tip sits at, or just distal to, the prostate, guiding the catheter per rectum.

5 Massage the prostate per rectum or transabdominally (if the prostate cannot be palpated per rectum) for 2 minutes and at the same time slowly inject 2–3 ml of sterile saline.

6 Using a 5 ml syringe, aspirate material into the catheter and syringe. The catheter can also be passed into the bladder and the prostatic wash fluid aspirated from there.

7 Remove the syringe from the catheter when sufficient material has been collected.

8 Repeat steps 5 and 6 if an insufficient sample has been collected.

9 Remove the catheter.

10 Fill the syringe with air and expel any remaining fluid from the catheter into the collection tubes or on to a microscope slide.

Sample handling

- A portion of the sample should be placed in an EDTA tube for cytology
- A portion of the sample should be submitted in a sterile plain tube for culture if infection is suspected
- If samples are to be sent to an external laboratory, fresh air-dried unstained smears of any flocculent/mucoid material should also be made (see **Fine-needle aspiration**). Direct smears of the fluid can also be made, but most samples are poorly cellular

Potential complications

- Rupture of prostatic abscess
- Rectal perforation (rare)
- Ascending urinary tract infection

Retrograde urethrography/ vaginourethrography

Indications/Use

- Haematuria
- Dysuria
- Stranguria
- Urinary incontinence
- Urethral discharge
- Urethral trauma

Equipment

- Water-soluble, **iodinated contrast medium** (150–200 mg iodine/ml; more concentrated solutions can be diluted with normal saline). This contrast can be mixed with an equal volume of sterile aqueous lubricant (e.g. K-Y jelly) to produce a more viscous medium and better urethral distension. This mixture should be made up well in advance, since small air bubbles introduced during mixing can mimic genuine filling defects due to calculi. It should be stored in a dark place as iodinated media degrade in light
- Local anaesthetic
- Wide-bore rigid (or Foley) urinary catheters of appropriate size for male dogs, or tomcat catheters of appropriate size for male cats. Catheters should fit snugly to limit the leakage of contrast out of the urethra (see **Urethral catheterization**)
- Foley urinary catheters of appropriate size for bitches and queens (see **Urethral catheterization**)
- Tongue forceps or bowel clamps

Patient preparation and positioning

- Urethrography should be performed under general anaesthesia, especially in females
- The patient is positioned as for **Urethral catheterization**

Technique

Retrograde urethrography (males)

1 Assess the urethral area on plain radiographs for evidence of soft tissue swelling or the presence of radiopaque calculi *prior* to performing contrast studies. A pneumocystogram can be performed, to produce back pressure against which to distend the urethra, but this is not advised in cases of suspected urethral or bladder rupture.

2 Catheterize the urethra with the widest catheter possible, prefilled with saline to avoid producing air bubbles.

3 Position the tip of the catheter distal to the area under investigation.

4 In *cats*, the catheter does not need to be secured in position. In *dogs*, hold the penis tightly around the catheter (this can be performed with tongue forceps). Local anaesthetic can be instilled into the urethral catheter prior to contrast medium, to reduce muscle spasm.

5 Inject up to 1 ml/kg of the diluted contrast medium as a bolus, avoiding excessive pressure.

6 Take radiographs immediately after injecting the contrast medium:

   a Lateral views are usually the most helpful; pulling the hindlimbs cranially improves visualization of the urethra in male dogs

   b Ventrodorsal views can provide additional information about the prostatic urethra: slight obliquity from a ventrodorsal position will avoid superimposition of the urethra over itself or over bony structures.

Retrograde vaginourethrography (females)

1 Assess the urethral area on plain radiographs for evidence of soft tissue swelling or the presence of radiopaque calculi *prior* to performing contrast studies. A pneumocystogram can be performed, to produce back pressure against which to distend the urethra, but this is not advised in cases of suspected urethral or bladder rupture.

2 Cut the tip off a Foley catheter, beyond the inflatable bulb, to prevent it from passing too far into the vagina; in cats, a non-cuffed catheter is often used.

3 Prefill the catheter with saline and place the catheter tip just inside the lips of the vulva. Hold the vulva closed around the catheter using either bowel clamps or tongue forceps.

4 Inflate the bulb of the catheter.

5 Inject a little local anaesthetic and then the diluted water-soluble contrast medium. Dose rate is up to 1 ml/kg over 5–10 seconds. Take care to avoid vaginal rupture.

6 Take radiographs immediately after injecting the contrast medium:

   a Lateral views are standard

   b An oblique ventrodorsal view (to avoid superimposition of the vagina and urethra) may also be helpful.

Potential complications

- Urinary tract infection
- Urethral rupture
- Vaginal rupture (if the bulb of the Foley catheter is placed proximal to urethral opening)

Rhinoscopy

Indications/Use

- Investigating clinical signs of nasal disease
- Investigating reverse sneezing, head shaking, exophthalmos, facial swelling or deformity, pawing at the nose and halitosis in the absence of dental disease
- Foreign body removal
- Collecting samples for histology, cytology and microbiology

Contraindications

- Inadequate investigations prior to endoscopy
- Coagulopathy
- Severe hypertension

Equipment

- Caudal rhinoscopy: *flexible* endoscope (diameter 3.5–6 mm, capable of 180 degrees of flexion)
- Anterior rhinoscopy: flexible (as above) or rigid (preferred) (diameter 2.4–2.7 mm, 0–30 degrees) endoscope with appropriate sheath to allow fluid irrigation ± passage of biopsy instruments (e.g. 14.5 Fr cystoscopy sheath with 5 Fr instrument channel) (Figure R.1)
- Endoscopic viewing equipment
- 1 litre bags of 0.9% saline (pre-warmed to 37°C) and fluid giving set for irrigation
- Pharynx packs (Figure R.2). These can be made by rolling up pieces of gauze swab and tying a gauze bandage around the roll; the swab can be packed in the caudal pharynx, whilst the bandage should remain outside the mouth to allow easy retrieval. Alternatively, a small sponge with a tie attached can be used
- Mouth gag
- Local anaesthetic spray
- Sterile aqueous lubricant (e.g. K-Y jelly)
- 5 Fr 20–40 cm grasping forceps
- Spay hook
- Flexible cup-style biopsy forceps that can pass through the biopsy channel of the rigid endoscope, or rigid biopsy forceps with a 3–5 mm diameter cup
- 10–20 ml syringes
- Sterile kidney dish
- Container with 10% neutral buffered formalin
- Hypodermic needle: 21 or 23 G
- Tissue cassette with foam insert (e.g. CellSafe+ biopsy capsule)
- EDTA and sterile plain tubes
- Microscope slides

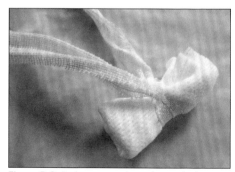

Figure R.2: A pharynx pack can be made from rolling up pieces of gauze swab and tying a gauze bandage around the roll.

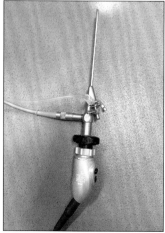

Figure R.1: Rigid endoscope with sheath connected to fluid for irrigation.

Patient preparation and positioning

- **General anaesthesia is essential.** A *cuffed* endotracheal (ET) tube should always be placed (see **Endotracheal intubation**)
- The patient should be placed in sternal recumbency, with the head propped up slightly to elevate the mouth and nasal planum for ease of access. The nose can be angled downwards to direct liquid away from the pharynx
- There is a strong gag reflex present when performing caudal rhinoscopy. This is normal and does not necessarily mean that the animal is not anaesthetized deeply enough. The use of topical local anaesthetic spray on the mucosal surfaces may help to blunt this reflex
- A mouth gag is essential when performing *caudal* rhinoscopy, to keep the mouth open and prevent the patient biting the endoscope in the event that contact with the pharynx stimulates a gag reflex
- The procedure is best performed on a 'wet table', due to the large volume of irrigant used. A large tray covered with a stainless steel grid will suffice if a wet table is not available. Towels placed on the floor are useful to catch additional spillage

> **WARNING**
>
> - Care should be exercised if using cold irrigant solutions, especially in small patients. The high surface area and excellent vascular supply of the nares act like a heat sink and can result in hypothermia. Careful monitoring of body temperature is advisable.

Technique

> **NOTE**
>
> - The nasopharynx and choanae should always be examined first using caudal (posterior) rhinoscopy *before* performing the rostral (anterior) procedure. Otherwise, contamination of the nasopharynx with fluid, blood and discharge resulting from the fluid irrigation used during anterior rhinoscopy will compromise the examination. Caudal rhinoscopy is performed by retroflexing a flexible endoscope over the free edge of the soft palate, so as to look rostrally, towards the choanae. Since this does not require fluid irrigation, samples can be obtained for culture if required, as well as biopsy samples of nasopharyngeal and caudal nasal masses

Caudal (posterior, retropharyngeal) rhinoscopy

1 Insert the flexible endoscope into the mouth.
2 Evaluate the oral cavity, laryngeal apparatus and posterior nasopharynx.
3 Advance the endoscope caudally and pass the free edge of the soft palate.
4 Retroflex the endoscope into a 'J' position behind the soft palate to view the nasopharynx (Figure R.3). Note that it is also possible to pre-flex the endoscope into the 'J' position before pushing it past the free edge of the soft palate.

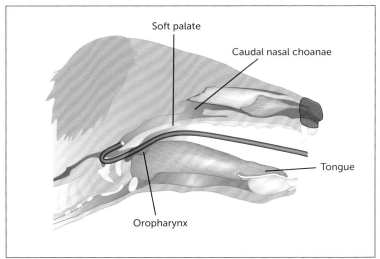

Figure R.3: The endoscope should be retroflexed into a 'J' position to view the nasopharynx.

5 Gradually withdraw the endoscope rostrally, with the tip still flexed, so to advance the tip toward the choanae.

6 As the endoscope is retroflexed, the view on the monitor is upside down and reversed: up is down; and left is right (Figure R.4).

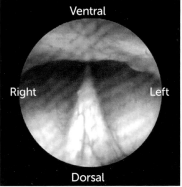

Figure R.4: Endoscopic view of the nasopharynx. Note that due to the position of the endoscope the view is upside down and reversed. (Courtesy of RC Denovo)

Anterior (rostral) rhinoscopy

1 Place a pharynx pack in the caudal pharynx and ensure the cuff of the ET tube is inflated (see **Endotracheal intubation**). Large volumes of fluid will be washed over the soft palate and there will be a continuous flow of saline through the nose and out of the mouth. Swabs should be counted and recorded.

2 Begin with the normal or less affected side.

3   Coat the shaft of the endoscope sheath/cannula with sterile aqueous lubricant (e.g. K-Y jelly), being careful not to get any on the lens of the endoscope.

4   Hold the endoscope in a 'pistol' fashion, with the light guide cable and port facing the floor, and the camera oriented such that any graphics on the camera head can be read right side up. This will ensure that the image produced on the monitor is true.

5   Deflect the nasal planum dorsally and introduce the rigid endoscope with its sheath ventromedially (toward the base of the opposite ear) (Figure R.5). Handle the endoscope carefully to avoid causing trauma to the patient. For a right-handed endoscopist, place the left hand flat on the bridge of the nose, with the shaft of the endoscope held between the forefinger and thumb at the nostril. Hold the camera in the right hand to control the angle of insertion, while the left hand stabilizes the tip of the endoscope and prevents exaggerated movements.

6   Connect a bag of saline and giving set to one of the cannula stopcocks and start the flow of fluid. This is often needed to remove the copious volume of discharge or haemorrhage obscuring the view. The flow of saline is best adjusted using the tap on the ingress port of the rhinoscope; this allows the controls on the giving set to be left open.

7   Examine the dorsal meatus first; this is clearly seen as a simple vaulted channel that narrows as the endoscope is advanced towards the ethmoidal area. It is not possible to pass the endoscope as far back as the cribriform plate, although this area can be visualized.

8   Withdraw the endoscope slightly into the common meatus and the middle meatus will be seen laterally. Advance the endoscope upwards and laterally

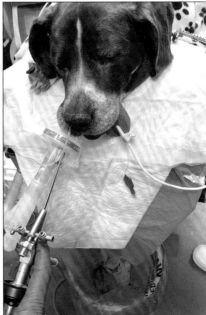

Figure R.5: The endoscope should be held in a 'pistol' fashion as it is introduced into the nasal cavity.

into the middle meatus, which can be examined caudally to the area of the opening of the frontal sinuses (note that this is usually obscured by scrolls of turbinates).

9   Examine the ventral meatus last. Withdraw the tip of the endoscope to nearly the nasal planum and redirect ventrally into the ventral meatus. It should be possible to pass the endoscope to the level of the posterior nares and nasopharynx.

10 On entering the nasopharynx, just caudal to the posterior nares, the orifice of the Eustachian tube will be seen on the lateral wall.

11 Ensure that the pharynx pack is removed from the pharynx before recovery of the patient from anaesthesia.

Biopsy and sampling

- Biopsy samples should always be taken, even if no lesions are apparent. In addition to biopsy samples, brushings and swabs may also be obtained for cytology or culture
- It is important to collect biopsy samples from multiple sites, as there is little correlation between visual appearance and specific disease entities
- The operator can use:
    - Flexible cup-style biopsy forceps introduced via the biopsy channel of the endoscope (Figure R.6a)
    - Rigid biopsy forceps passed alongside the shaft of the endoscope (Figure R.6b)
    - Nasal flush (for cytology)

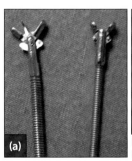
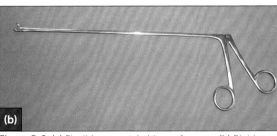

Figure R.6: (a) Flexible cup-style biopsy forceps. **(b)** Rigid biopsy forceps.

Using flexible cup-style biopsy forceps

1   Position the tip of the endoscope approximately 3–5 cm rostral to the lesion to be sampled.

2   Insert the forceps through the biopsy channel of the endoscope, with the cup firmly closed, and advance them towards the site of interest. Note that forceps should not be passed down the biopsy channel of a flexible endoscope when it is in a 'J' position. Instead, the flexible endoscope should be straightened, the forceps passed down the biopsy channel until they protrude a short distance from the end, and the endoscope then returned to the 'J' position.

3   Once the forceps have passed out of the end of the endoscope, open the cup, advance on to the region to be sampled, and close the cups.

4   Withdraw the forceps from the endoscope and gently remove the sample.

Using rigid biopsy forceps

1 Position the tip of the endoscope approximately 3–5 cm rostral to the lesion to be sampled.
2 Pass the forceps along the dorsal edge of the rhinoscope, opposite the light guide post, to the site of interest.
   a The tips of the rigid biopsy forceps must not pass beyond the level of the medial canthus of the eyes. Measure the distance between the tip of the rhinarium and the medial canthus, and mark it with a piece of sticky tape on the forceps themselves to prevent inadvertent penetration of the cribriform plate (Figure R.7).
   b In smaller patients, where it is not possible to pass the forceps alongside the endoscope, it is useful to measure the position of the lesion by assessing the direction and depth of the tip of the endoscope, and taking samples 'blind'.
3 Once the forceps have passed the end of the endoscope, open the tips, advance on to the region to be sampled, and close the tips.
4 Withdraw the forceps and gently remove the sample.

Nasal flush

1 Place a pharynx pack in the caudal pharynx and ensure the cuff of the ET tube is inflated (see **Endotracheal intubation**).
2 Fill several 20 ml syringes with saline (10 ml syringes for a cat or a <5 kg dog).
3 Wedge the nozzle of the syringe into one nostril and occlude the contralateral nostril.
4 Holding an empty sterile kidney dish below the nostrils, empty the syringe with moderate force into one nostril.
5 Repeat several times for both nostrils. Usually, foreign bodies and many mass lesions will be dislodged with two or three attempts.

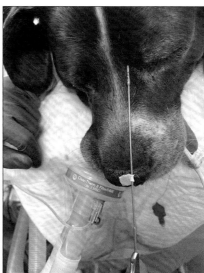

Figure R.7: The tips of the rigid biopsy forceps must not pass beyond the level of the medial canthus of the eyes.

6 Ensure that the pharynx pack is removed from the pharynx before recovery of the patient from anaesthesia. Examine these for any foreign material or dislodged tissue.

Sample handling

- To remove samples from the biopsy forceps, they should be immersed in 10% neutral buffered formalin. The forceps should then be rinsed in saline before being reinserting into the endoscope. Alternatively, samples should be carefully removed from the biopsy forceps with a needle and placed directly into 10% neutral buffered formalin, or placed on the foam insert of a tissue cassette
- Tissue samples for bacterial or fungal culture should be placed on a bacterial transport swab or in a sterile container
- Portions of tissue samples can be used to make impression smears for cytological assessment
- Nasal flush samples should be placed into an EDTA tube for cytology and into a sterile plain tube for bacterial culture, if required
- To minimize cellular degradation, it is preferable to make direct smears of any mucoid material retrieved from a nasal flush and send these to the laboratory unstained

Foreign body removal

- **Cats** tend to be presented with nasopharyngeal foreign bodies that have been coughed up and lodged over the free edge of the soft palate. These can often be removed without the use of an endoscope, using rigid grasping forceps. A spay hook to retract the soft palate rostrally can also aid removal
- **Dogs** are more prone to foreign bodies in the nasal cavities. If small, these can be removed under endoscopic guidance using rigid grasping forceps. Larger foreign bodies will require 'blind' removal with rigid grasping forceps
- If the foreign body breaks up and is impossible to remove completely, the nose should be flushed vigorously with sterile saline. The throat pack should be pushed caudally beyond the tip of the soft palate to allow the fluid to drain over the soft palate and into the mouth freely; the nose should be lowered to allow drainage

Potential complications

- Significant mucosal haemorrhage is rare; however, if there is heavy bleeding, it may be pertinent to maintain the patient under anaesthesia for a few minutes until it has subsided. In addition, pressure can be placed over the rostral nares whilst occluding the caudal pharynx with swabs. *Alternatively*, adrenaline can be sprayed into the nares using a urinary catheter or over-the-needle catheter and syringe
- Penetration of the cribriform plate is uncommon unless significant disease is present and/or the biopsy forceps are passed 'blind' or beyond the level of the medial canthus of the eyes

Skin biopsy – punch biopsy

Indications/Use

- Obtaining a full-thickness skin sample in cases of diffuse dermatosis, in particular:
    - Suspected dermatosis with a characteristic histopathology (e.g. follicular dysplasia, sebaceous adenitis, dermatomyositis, immune-mediated disease)
    - Dermatoses that fail to respond to appropriate rational therapy
    - Any dermatosis that appears unusual or particularly severe
- Punch biopsy is less useful for ulcers and nodules, as it is difficult to straddle the margin or encompass the lesion

Contraindications

- Coagulopathy
- History of poor wound healing
- Punch biopsy is inappropriate for masses or the junctional area between affected and non-affected skin

Equipment

- 6–8 mm biopsy punch (a 4 mm punch can be used for restricted sites, such as the nasal planum and footpads)
- Curved scissors for hair
- 70% surgical spirit
- Local anaesthetic: 2% lidocaine
- Fine forceps or needle to manipulate the sample
- Mayo scissors
- Scalpel and No.11 scalpel blade
- Containers containing 10% neutral buffered formalin
- Sterile containers for specimens for culture
- 0.9% sterile saline
- Pieces of card approximately 10 x 10 mm
- Suture material (monofilament nylon) and needle holders for skin closure

Patient preparation and positioning

- Punch biopsy can usually be performed under light sedation, using local anaesthesia
- General anaesthesia is required for sensitive sites, such as the face and feet, where local anaesthesia is difficult
- The patient should be positioned with the area to be sampled uppermost
- Any hair at the biopsy site should be cut with curved scissors, without disturbing the skin surface
- Minimal skin preparation is required, though the skin should first be wiped with 70% surgical spirit if the sample is to be sent for culture

Technique

1 Infiltrate the skin and subcutis around the biopsy site with 2% lidocaine.
2 Press the biopsy punch firmly against the skin and rotate in one direction.

3 Lift the base clear using fine forceps or a fine needle and then cut it free using Mayo scissors or a scalpel blade.

> **WARNING**
> - Do not grasp the skin sample itself, as this will cause crush artefacts.

4 Close the skin defect; a single interrupted suture is usually sufficient.

Sample handling

- The biopsy specimen should be placed, subcutis down, on a piece of card. On the other end of the card, a circle should be drawn with an arrow through it to indicate the direction of hair growth
- The biopsy specimen should be placed in a container of 10% neutral buffered formalin
- Specimens for bacterial or fungal culture should be submitted in a sterile container with 2–3 drops of sterile saline to prevent drying in transit
- Each biopsy specimen should be submitted in a separate, clearly labelled pot to avoid any confusion

Potential complications

- Bleeding should cease with pressure; continued haemorrhage may suggest a coagulopathy
- Delayed wound healing

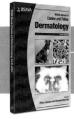

FURTHER INFORMATION

For more information on skin biopsy techniques, see the *BSAVA Manual of Canine and Feline Dermatology.*

Spica splint

Indications/Use

- Support of the elbow following:
  - Closed reduction of traumatic elbow luxation with or without open repair of collateral ligament injuries
  - Internal fixation of olecranon fractures
- Support of the shoulder following closed reduction of traumatic lateral shoulder luxation

Equipment

- Adhesive tape (2.5 cm wide)
- Cast padding
- Conforming gauze bandage
- Resin-impregnated fibreglass cast materials
- Outer protective bandage material (e.g. self-adhesive non-adherent bandage or adhesive bandage)

Patient preparation and positioning

- The animal should be sedated heavily or under general anaesthesia
- The animal should be placed in lateral recumbency, with the affected limb uppermost and supported in a weight-bearing position
- For large-breed dogs, positioning the dog so it lies across two tables, such that the thorax is accessible between them, facilitates the placement of this dressing without the need to lift the dog multiple times

Technique

1 Place padding between the toes.
2 Apply a light Robert Jones soft padded bandage (see **Bandaging**) to the entire forelimb, *excluding* the final outer bandage layer.
3 Extend this bandage proximally over the dorsal midline to encompass the thorax (Figure S.1). Alternate passing the dressing material cranially and caudally to the limb around the neck base and thorax, taking care not to apply the bandage too tightly to the thorax, to avoid compromising respiration.
4 Follow the manufacturer's recommendations regarding wetting and handling of the cast material.
5 Apply strips of cast material over the lateral aspect of the bandage (Figure S.2). These strips should extend from the distal tip of the bandage to proximally over the dorsal midline to the contralateral scapula. Cast material should be conformed to the contours of the limb and thorax. The number of layers of cast material required will depend on patient size and the rigidity needed.
6 Secure the cast material to the underlying Robert Jones bandage with an outer protective bandage material (Figure S.3).

Splint care and maintenance

- Written instructions should always be given to clients when the patient is discharged; owners must understand their responsibility in splint maintenance
- Exercise restriction must be enforced

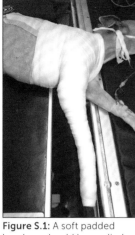
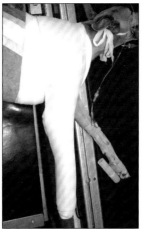
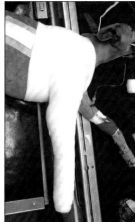

Figure S.1: A soft padded bandage should be applied to the entire forelimb and extended proximally to encompass the thorax.

Figure S.2: Strips of cast material should be applied to the underlying bandage.

Figure S.3: The cast material should be secured to the underlying soft padded bandage with an outer protective bandage.

- Spica splints should be checked every 4 hours for the first 24 hours and then at least twice daily thereafter for complications
- The splint can be kept in place for up to 2 weeks, assuming it remains in good condition and no complications arise
- The limb should be monitored for swollen toes, cold toes or skin abrasions
- The splint should be monitored for wetness, soiling or slippage, and changed if necessary
- The splint must be kept clean and dry. A plastic bag may be placed over the foot while the animal is walking outside and then removed when it is indoors

Potential complications

- Dyspnoea
- Venous stasis
- Limb oedema
- Moist dermatitis
- Maceration of skin underlying a wet bandage
- Contamination of wounds
- Pressure necrosis

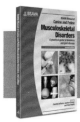

FURTHER INFORMATION

For more information on the applications of Spica splints, see the *BSAVA Manual of Canine and Feline Musculoskeletal Disorders*.

Thoracocentesis – needle

Indications/Use

- Rapid stabilization of acute respiratory distress due to the accumulation of air or fluid in the pleural space
- To obtain samples of pleural fluid for diagnostic evaluation
- See **Thoracostomy tube placement** for alternative techniques to remove a large volume of pleural fluid or very viscous pleural effusions, or where repeated thoracic drainage is required

Contraindications

- Ongoing haemorrhage into the pleural space (e.g. haemothorax due to a coagulopathy or trauma)
- Small volume of effusion or air

Equipment

- As required for **Aseptic preparation – (a) non-surgical procedures**
- 19–23 G, ¾ to 1 inch butterfly needle OR an over-the-needle catheter: 18–20 G for medium to large dogs (>10 kg); 20–22 G for cats and small dogs (up to 10 kg)
- 3-way tap
- Narrow-bore (2 mm) short extension tubing for use with the over-the-needle catheter. This allows the syringe to move independently from the needle or catheter, reducing the risk of lung laceration and minimizing the risk of dislodging the needle or catheter from its desired position
- 5 ml syringe
- 10–60 ml syringe (depending on the expected volume of air or fluid within the pleural space)
- Measuring container to collect pleural fluid
- Local anaesthetic solution or cream (e.g. EMLA)
- EDTA tube
- Sterile plain tube
- Microscope slides

Patient preparation and positioning

- Sedation is often not required, although it may be necessary to prevent movement of the patient during the procedure. Care should be taken when administering sedatives to a dyspnoeic patient
- The use of supplementary flow-by oxygen should be considered; the face mask should be removed if this distresses the animal
- Manual restraint in sternal recumbency is usually the safest position for the animal and the most efficient for drainage. Alternatively, a standing or sitting position may be used
- **Aseptic preparation – (a) non-surgical procedures** should be performed on an area of skin on the lateral thorax, to include skin within a 15 cm radius of the proposed site of thoracocentesis. A skin drape is usually not required
- Local anaesthetic solution may be instilled into the subcutaneous tissues and muscles at the proposed site. *Alternatively*, if the animal is stable enough to wait, local anaesthetic cream (e.g. EMLA) can be applied over the proposed site 20 minutes in advance of thoracocentesis

> **WHICH SIDE**
>
> - Which side of the animal to use for thoracocentesis is dictated by clinical examination and the results of diagnostic imaging
> - In some animals, bilateral thoracocentesis may be required, especially when draining bilateral effusions containing dense flocculent material (e.g. pyothorax)

Technique

Thoracocentesis is usually performed at the **7th or 8th intercostal space** unless radiography or ultrasonography indicates otherwise. To identify the 7th or 8th intercostal space, count cranially from the most caudal intercostal space, which is the 12th. The site of needle insertion is:

- In the ventral third of the thorax if only **pleural fluid** is present
- In the dorsal third of the thorax if only **pleural air** is present

Sterile gloves should be worn.

Butterfly needle

1   Attach the butterfly needle to a 3-way tap, extension tubing and 5 ml syringe, with the 3-way tap turned so that it is 'off' to the butterfly needle (Figure T.1). Hand the 3-way tap, extension tubing and syringe to an assistant.
2   Insert the butterfly needle through the skin and intercostal muscle at the cranial border of the rib to avoid the intercostal vessels and nerves (which run along the caudal border of each rib) (Figure T.2).
3   Advance the needle slowly into the pleural space. Once the needle is through the skin, the assistant can turn the 3-way tap to the 'on' position and apply slight negative pressure (no more than 1 ml). If air or fluid enters the syringe, the needle is in the pleural space.
4   As soon as the pleural space is entered, direct the tip of the needle to lie parallel to the thoracic wall to minimize the risk of pulmonary lacerations (Figure T.3). The needle should be inserted fully to the hub once inside the pleural space.

> **WARNING**
>
> - If frank blood is initially aspirated, consider whether this is due to haemothorax or iatrogenic haemorrhage.
> - Stop draining the thorax and assess whether the sample in the syringe clots; if it does, this is probably iatrogenic haemorrhage from an intercostal or pleural vessel. Fluid from a haemothorax would not be expected to clot.
> - Running a manual packed cell volume (PCV) on the sample and comparing it with the patient's PCV is useful to differentiate whether the fluid is due to a haemothorax or iatrogenic haemorrhage: the PCV of a haemothorax will be the same as or higher than that of the patient's blood, whereas the PCV of fluid due to iatrogenic haemorrhage will be similar to that of the patient's blood.

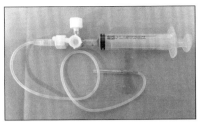

Figure T.1: Butterfly needle attached to a 3-way tap, syringe and extension tubing.

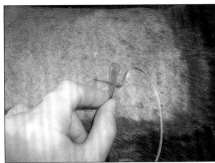

Figure T.2: The needle should be inserted through the skin and intercostal muscles into the pleural space.

5 Turn the 3-way tap to the 'off' position, remove the 5 ml syringe, and attach another syringe suitable for the expected volume of air or fluid within the pleural space.

6 Turn the 3-way tap to the 'on' position and drain the pleural space of fluid or air (Figure T.4). Excessive negative pressure should be avoided, especially if using a large syringe to drain pleural fluid.

7 Expel fluid or air from the syringe when it is full, after closing off the 3-way tap to the pleural space. Samples of pleural fluid should be collected into EDTA (for cytology) and sterile plain (for culture) tubes. Fresh air-dried smears of any flocculent material can also be made. Keep a note of how much air or fluid is drained off (i.e. how many syringes are filled).

8 Drainage is complete when no further fluid or air can be drained, or when the lung is felt rubbing against the tip of the needle.

9 Turn the 3-way tap so that it is 'off' to the butterfly needle and withdraw the needle from the thorax.

10 Perform thoracic radiography or computed tomography following thoracocentesis to look for an initiating cause for the pneumothorax or pleural effusion, and to check for completeness of drainage and complications of the procedure.

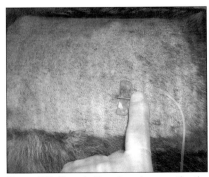

Figure T.3: Once in the pleural space, the tip of the needle should be directed to lie parallel to the thoracic wall.

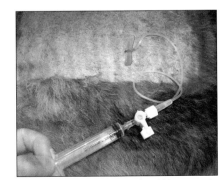

Figure T.4: The 3-way tap should be turned on and the pleural air or fluid drained.

Over-the-needle catheter

1 Attach the catheter to extension tubing, a 3-way tap and 5 ml syringe, with the 3-way tap turned so that it is 'off' to the catheter. Hand the 3-way tap, extension tubing and syringe to an assistant.

2 Insert the over-the-needle catheter (cannula and needle) through the skin and intercostal muscle at the cranial border of the rib at the desired intercostal space (see above).

3 Advance the catheter slowly into the pleural space. Once the catheter is through the skin, the assistant can turn the 3-way-tap to the 'on' position and apply slight negative pressure (no more than 1 ml). If air or fluid enters the syringe, the needle is in the pleural space.

4 Once the catheter enters the pleural space, advance the cannula into the thorax over the needle in a cranial direction, so as to direct the tip of the cannula to lie parallel to the thoracic wall. Withdraw the needle and attach the extension tubing with 3-way tap and syringe directly to the catheter. *There is no need to insert the cannula fully into the pleural space.* **See Warning box for Butterfly needle (above).**

5 Continue as per Steps 5 to 10 above.

Potential complications

- Lung laceration
- Pneumothorax
- Iatrogenic infection
- Haemorrhage
- Pulmonary re-expansion injury, leading to the development of pulmonary oedema

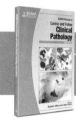

FURTHER INFORMATION

For interpretation of the results of fluid analysis, see the *BSAVA Manual of Canine and Feline Clinical Pathology*

Thoracostomy tube placement – (a) trocar tube

Indications/Use

- Removal of air or fluid from the pleural space when frequent or repeated drainage is expected or required
- Medical management of pyothorax
- Stabilization prior to definitive surgical treatment of pleural space disease
- Removal of air and fluid from the pleural space in the immediate postoperative period following thoracic surgery

> **WARNING**
>
> - There is a risk of injury to thoracic viscera when placing a trocar tube.
> - The use of a small-bore wire-guided thoracostomy tube (see below) should be considered as an alternative, especially when draining air or non-tenacious fluid.
> - However, trocar tubes are particularly useful when draining effusions containing dense flocculent material (e.g. pyothorax).

Contraindications

- Severe respiratory compromise: stabilization with oxygen therapy or **thoracocentesis** may be required to improve respiration prior to induction of general anaesthesia
- Severe coagulopathy

Equipment

- As required for **Aseptic preparation – (a) non-surgical procedures**
- Silicone or PVC multi-fenestrated trocar thoracostomy tube (Figure T.5):
  - Diameter should be approximately the width of the mainstem bronchus as seen on thoracic radiographs (14–16 Fr for cats and very small dogs; 18–24 Fr for small- to medium-breed dogs; 26–36 Fr for large- to giant-breed dogs)
  - Length should be such that the tip sits at the approximate level of the 2nd rib following placement
- Local anaesthetic solution
- Scalpel and No.10 scalpel blade
- Atraumatic forceps
- 3-way tap (Figure T.5)
- Luer-lock connector (Figure T.5)

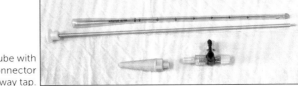

Figure T.5: Chest tube with trocar, Luer connector and 3-way tap.

- Intravenous fluid extension tubing
- Gate clamp
- 20–50 ml syringe
- Zinc oxide tape
- Measuring container to collect pleural fluid
- 0.9% sterile saline or lactated Ringer's solution (Hartmann's)
- Suture material (e.g. 3 metric (2/0 USP) monofilament nylon)
- Light bandage (stockinette or conforming non-adhesive wrap)
- Elizabethan collar

Patient positioning and preparation

> **NOTE**
>
> - **Thoracocentesis** is not obligatory before placement of a thoracostomy tube. However, careful consideration should be given as to whether drainage would improve the animal's respiratory function so that subsequent general anaesthesia, if required, for tube placement would be safer. If the animal is stable and dyspnoea is not marked, thoracostomy tube placement can proceed without prior drainage. In fact, the presence of air or fluid within the pleural cavity can reduce the chance of iatrogenic lung injury during thoracostomy tube placement. Preoxygenation of the animal for 5 minutes before anaesthesia is strongly recommended

- General anaesthesia is recommended, although in some animals heavy sedation may be sufficient

> **NERVE BLOCK**
>
> An intercostal nerve block can be administered at the proposed intercostal space of entry and 2–3 intercostal spaces cranial and caudal to this site. Note that:
> - The intercostal nerves run just caudal to the ribs in a dorsoventral direction
> - Local anaesthetic solution should be applied as far dorsal as possible in the tissues caudal to each rib
> - Following needle insertion, the syringe should be drawn back to ensure that the needle is not within a blood vessel prior to anaesthetic injection

- As an alternative to an intercostal nerve block (see above), local anaesthetic solution can be applied as a bleb to the skin at the site where the drain is to be inserted (10th intercostal space) and infiltrated into the subcutaneous tissues, intercostal musculature and pleura at a site two intercostal spaces cranial to this point (8th intercostal space) (see below). The use of a long-acting local anaesthetic should be considered to provide analgesia in the post-procedure period
- **Aseptic preparation – (a) non-surgical procedures** of the lateral thorax should be performed, to include an area craniocaudally from the caudal border of the scapula to just caudal to the last rib, and dorsoventrally from the vertebrae to the sternum

WHICH SIDE

- Which side of the animal to use for placement of the thoracostomy tube is dictated by clinical examination and the results of diagnostic imaging
- In some animals, bilateral thoracostomy tubes may be required, especially when draining bilateral effusions containing dense flocculent material (e.g. pyothorax)

- The animal should be maintained in sternal recumbency during preparation, but thoracic drain insertion is most easily performed with the animal in lateral recumbency

Technique

Sterile gloves should be worn.

1 Make a small skin incision using a scalpel at the junction of the dorsal to middle third of the thorax at the 10th intercostal space.

2 Insert the thoracostomy tube with the trocar into the skin incision and under the skin (Figure T.6ab). Advance it in a cranial and slightly ventral direction to approximately the 8th intercostal space. Ensure that the sharp tip of the trocar is not covered by the tube when advancing it. This creates a subcutaneous tunnel to prevent air tracking from the environment along the tube and into the thorax. *Alternatively*, an assistant can grasp the skin over the lateral thorax at approximately the 4th rib and pull the skin incision site cranially to the level of the 8th intercostal space; the assistant then keeps the skin in that position (Figure T.6c). This avoids the need to tunnel the thoracostomy tube under the skin.

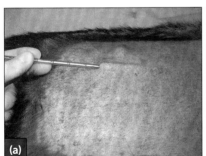

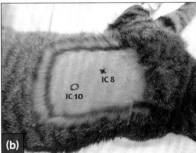

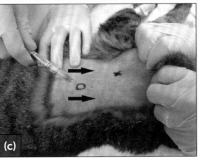

Figure T.6: (a–b) The thoracostomy tube can be inserted and advanced subcutaneously to the level of the 8th intercostal space. **(c)** Alternatively, an assistant can grasp the skin over the lateral thorax and pull it cranially so that the skin incision site is at the level of the 8th intercostal space.

ALTERNATIVE SUBCUTANEOUS TUNNEL TECHNIQUE

Placement of the thoracostomy tube under the latissimus dorsi muscle may result in a better seal around the tube.

a. Make the initial skin incision directly over a rib.
b. Tunnel the trocar tip of the thoracostomy tube on to the underling rib so that the trocar tip perforates the latissimus dorsi muscle.
c. Direct the drain cranially between the rib and the overlying latissimus dorsi muscle.

---

3 Hold the thoracostomy tube and trocar perpendicular to the 8th intercostal space and introduce it into the thorax by means of a controlled twisting motion whilst applying firm pressure to the end of the trocar (Figure T.7). **Hold the drain firmly close to the tip with the other hand to prevent excessive and uncontrolled entry into the thorax.**

4 Once the thoracostomy tube has entered the thoracic cavity, angle it so that the tip points cranially and ventrally (Figure T.8).

5 Advance the thoracostomy tube over the trocar in a cranioventral direction, to approximately the level of the 2nd rib.

NOTE

- The cranial end of the thoracostomy tube should ideally lie within the ventral thorax, before the sternum begins to rise towards the thoracic inlet; the tip of the tube should curve gently upwards. This tube location should enable both fluid and air to be drained. However, this exact position is not always possible

---

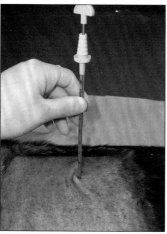

Figure T.7: The thoracostomy tube and trocar should be held perpendicular to the 8th intercostal space prior to entry into the thoracic cavity.

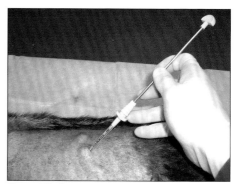

Figure T.8: Once the thoracostomy tube is in the thoracic cavity, the tip should be pointed cranially and ventrally and the thoracostomy tube advanced over the trocar.

6 If applicable, the assistant now releases the skin and it retracts caudally, forming a valve-like seal between the skin entry site and where the tube passes though the intercostal muscles.

7 Remove the trocar and immediately occlude the tube temporarily with atraumatic forceps (Figure T.9), whilst pre-placing a gate clamp on the tube and attaching a Luer-lock connector and 3-way tap.

8 Remove the forceps, enabling drainage of the thorax using a syringe attached to the 3-way tap (see below).

9 Secure the thoracostomy tube to the thoracic wall by means of two finger-trap sutures.

10 Perform radiography or computed tomography at this point to confirm correct positioning within the thorax, to look for an initiating cause and to check for complications.

11 If required, further secure the tube by applying a butterfly tab of zinc oxide tape and suturing this to the patient.

12 Place a sterile dressing over the site of thoracic drain insertion. Cover with a light bandage.

13 Place an Elizabethan collar to prevent interference with the tube and possible pneumothorax.

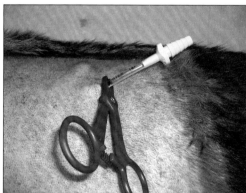

Figure T.9: Following removal of the trocar, the thoracostomy tube should be occluded using forceps.

Drainage

- The thorax is drained either by intermittent suction using a syringe attached directly to a 3-way tap, or via intravenous fluid extension tubing. The latter is preferable in restless or uncooperative patients, as there is no direct manipulation of the chest tube while drainage or lavage is being performed
- Excessive negative pressure (>5 ml) should not be applied to the syringe, as this can result in damage to structures within the pleural cavity
- Initial drainage is performed every 4 hours, but the frequency can be altered subsequently depending on the volume of fluid or air removed
- In animals with persistent, high-volume pneumothorax, the use of continuous suction drainage or of a one-way valve (e.g. Heimlich valve) should be considered
- In animals with pyothorax, twice-daily lavage should be performed using warmed 0.9% sterile saline or lactated Ringer's solution (Hartmann's).

Approximately 10–20 ml/kg of fluid should be infused aseptically over 5–10 minutes, while monitoring respiration. At least 75% of the fluid should be recovered; altering the animal's position and then re-aspirating after a few minutes may help fluid retrieval
- As a general rule, thoracic drainage is continued until the volume of fluid or air reduces to <5 ml/kg/day

Tube maintenance and removal

- Animals with thoracostomy tubes in place should be hospitalized in a facility with 24-hour care and supervised closely: to ensure security of the tube connections; to observe for changes in respiratory rate and effort; and to prevent self-interference with the drain
- The dressing and bandage must be changed and all connections checked at least once a day. Thoracic drains should be handled in an *aseptic* fashion during bandage changes and drainage of the pleural cavity
- A non-functional thoracostomy tube should be removed promptly. This can usually be done without sedation by cutting the anchoring suture material and removing the tube in one smooth motion. The skin incision site can usually be left to heal by secondary intention, although if a large hole exists, the use of a single suture or tissue glue should be considered

Potential complications

- Lung laceration
- Iatrogenic infection
- A small-volume iatrogenic pneumothorax may occur at the time of tube placement; a larger pneumothorax may develop if the tube becomes dislodged
- Haemorrhage
- Pulmonary re-expansion injury, leading to the development of pulmonary oedema
- Accidental removal of the tube
- Collapse of the tube due to excess suction pressure
- Obstruction of the tube with tenacious fluid or as a result of kinking of the drain

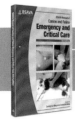

FURTHER INFORMATION

For more information on chest drains, see the *BSAVA Manual of Canine and Feline Emergency and Critical Care.*

Thoracostomy tube placement – (b) small-bore wire-guided

Indications/Use

- As for **Thoracostomy tube placement – (a) trocar tube**

OPTIONS

- Small-bore wire-guided thoracostomy tubes are reported to be associated with fewer complications compared with large-bore trocar tubes, are easier to place and are more comfortable for the patient
- However, it may be difficult to drain effusions containing dense flocculent material (e.g. pyothorax) with a small-bore wire-guided tube. In this situation, **Thoracostomy tube placement – (a) trocar tube** is advised.

Contraindications

- As for **Thoracostomy tube placement – (a) trocar tube**

Equipment

- As required for **Aseptic preparation – (a) non-surgical procedures**
- A proprietary small-bore wire-guided kit in a sterile pack (Figure T.10) containing:
    - 14 G, 20 cm long (cats and small dogs) and 12 G, 30 cm long (medium to large dogs) radiopaque polyurethane catheters (thoracostomy tube) with a multi-fenestrated tip and suture wing to facilitate attachment to the skin
    - 18 G (green, used in cats) and 14 G (orange, used in dogs) over-the-needle catheter introducers
    - 60 cm 'J-tip' guidewire coiled in protective sheathing with 'thumb-wheel' adaptor for ease of introduction
    - Dilator
    - Needle-free drainage cap
    - Extra suture wings and locking covers
- Local anaesthetic solution
- Scalpel and No.11 scalpel blade
- 20–50 ml syringe
- 3 way tap
- Measuring container to collect pleural fluid
- Suture material (e.g. 2 metric (3/0 USP) monofilament, non-absorbable)
- Light bandage (stockinette or conforming non-adhesive wrap)
- Elizabethan collar

Patient positioning and preparation

- Heavy sedation is usually sufficient, although general anaesthesia may be employed if required for additional procedures
- Local anaesthetic solution should be applied as a bleb to the skin at the proposed site of drain placement. Local anaesthetic solution can also be infiltrated into the subcutaneous tissues, intercostal musculature and pleura

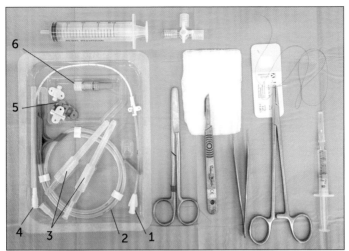

Figure T.10: Proprietary small-bore wire-guided thoracostomy tube kit with instruments required to secure the drain to the skin, local anaesthetic solution, a 3-way tap and 20 ml syringe. 1= thoracostomy tube with multi-fenestrated tip; 2 = 'J-tip' guidewire in protective sheath; 3 = over-the-needle catheter introducers; 4 = dilator; 5 = spare suture wings and locking covers; 6 = needle-free drainage cap.

> **NOTE**
>
> - **Thoracocentesis** is not obligatory before placement of a thoracostomy tube. However, careful consideration should be given as to whether drainage would improve the animal's respiratory function so that subsequent general anaesthesia, if required, for tube placement would be safer. If the animal is stable and dyspnoea is not marked, thoracostomy tube placement can proceed without prior drainage. In fact, the presence of air or fluid within the pleural cavity can reduce the chance of iatrogenic lung injury during thoracostomy tube placement. Preoxygenation of the animal for 5 minutes before anaesthesia is strongly recommended

The use of a long-acting local anaesthetic should be considered to provide analgesia in the post-procedure period

- **Aseptic preparation – (a) non-surgical procedures** of the lateral thorax is required, to include an area at least 15 cm around the proposed site of catheter insertion

> **WHICH SIDE**
>
> - Which side of the animal to use for placement of the thoracostomy tube is dictated by clinical examination and the results of diagnostic imaging
> - In some animals, bilateral thoracostomy tubes may be required, especially when draining bilateral effusions containing dense flocculent material (e.g. pyothorax)

- A fenestrated drape should be centred over the proposed site of catheter insertion; towel clips are not recommended in unanaesthetized patients
- The catheter can be placed with the animal in sternal or lateral recumbency depending on the preference of the veterinary surgeon

Technique

Sterile gloves should be worn.

1 Prepare the J-wire for insertion by withdrawing it until its tip is just visible outside the 'thumb-wheel' adaptor.

2 Using a scalpel blade, make a small stab skin incision of similar width to the thoracostomy tube, over the 7th or 8th intercostal space at the junction of the dorsal to middle third of the thorax.

3 Insert the over-the-needle catheter introducer through the stab incision and into the thoracic cavity (Figure T.11). The catheter introducer should enter the thorax over the cranial border of the rib to avoid the intercostal vessels and nerves that run along the caudal aspect of the rib. (However, due to the small diameter of the tube, this step is usually unnecessary and may cause kinking.)

Alternatively, the stab incision can be made at the 9th intercostal space and the over-the-needle catheter introducer tunnelled subcutaneously and cranially over 1—2 intercostal spaces. This step further reduces the risk of air gaining access to the thorax around the thoracostomy tube or if the tube is accidentally removed. However, due to the small diameter of the tube, this step is usually unnecessary.

4 Once the catheter introducer enters the pleural cavity, advance it fully over the needle stylet.

5 Remove the needle stylet.

6 Using the 'thumb-wheel' adaptor, thread the previously prepared guidewire out of the protective sheathing through the catheter introducer and into the thorax. Advance the guidewire in a cranioventral direction by approximately 10–20 cm or until resistance is encountered. **The guidewire should be held at all times when it is partially within the thorax** (Figure T.12). (Note: the tip of the thumb-wheel adaptor fits into the hub of the catheter introducer to allow the wire to be advanced seamlessly.)

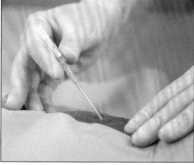

Figure T.11: The catheter introducer is inserted into the thoracic cavity via a stab incision in the skin.

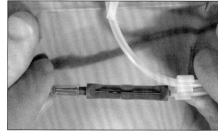

Figure T.12: The guidewire should be threaded through the catheter introducer and into the thoracic cavity. It should be held at all times whilst partially within the thorax. (Courtesy of Dan Lewis and reproduced from the *BSAVA Manual of Feline Practice*)

7   Remove the catheter introducer from the thorax by threading it off the guidewire, leaving only the guidewire within the thorax.

8   Thread the tissue dilator over the guidewire and advance through the skin and thoracic wall using a gentle twisting motion (Figure T.13). Remove the dilator by threading back off the guidewire.

9   Pre-measure the polyurethane catheter (thoracostomy tube) and advance it over the guidewire into the thoracic cavity (Figure T.14). The distance from the most distal side hole is marked on the catheter.

NOTE

- The cranial end of the thoracostomy tube should ideally lie in the ventral thorax, before the sternum begins to rise towards the thoracic inlet; the tip of the tube should curve gently upwards. This tube location should enable both fluid and air to be drained. However, this exact position is not always possible

---

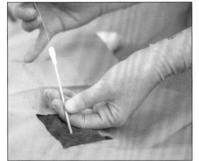

Figure T.13: The dilator should be threaded over the guidewire and then advanced through the soft tissues of the thoracic wall.

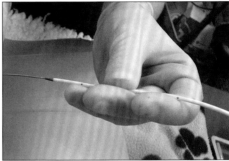

Figure T.14: The thoracostomy tube should be advanced over the guidewire into the thoracic cavity. (Courtesy of Dan Lewis and reproduced from the *BSAVA Manual of Feline Practice*)

10   Once the thoracostomy tube is in place, remove the guidewire and immediately attach the needle-free drainage cap. Attach a 3-way tap and confirm correct placement by connecting a syringe and attempting drainage.

11   Secure the thoracostomy tube to the skin, using suture material passed through the holes in the suture wings (Figure T.15).

12   Perform radiography or computed tomography at this point to confirm correct positioning within the thorax, to look for an initiating cause and to check for complications.

13   Attach additional suture wings to the drain and secure them in place at the proximal end of the drain if it is not fully inserted.

14   Place a sterile dressing over the site of thoracic drain insertion and cover with a light bandage.

15   Place an Elizabethan collar to prevent interference with the tube and possible pneumothorax.

Figure T.15: The thoracostomy tube is secured to the skin by placing sutures through the suture wings and locking covers.

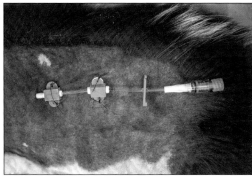

Drainage

- As for **Thoracostomy tube placement – (a) trocar tube**

Tube maintenance and removal

- As for **Thoracostomy tube placement – (a) trocar tube**

Potential complications

- As for **Thoracostomy tube placement – (a) trocar tube**, although small-bore wire-guided tubes are generally associated with fewer complications
- Small-bore tubes are prone to kinking and/or blockage by pleural exudate

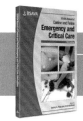

FURTHER INFORMATION

For more information on chest drains, see the *BSAVA Manual of Canine and Feline Emergency and Critical Care.*

Tissue biopsy – needle core

Indications/Use

- To obtain samples from:
    - Superficial masses that can be palpated well enough to be stabilized
    - Masses or organs within a body cavity, usually under ultrasound guidance
- As an alternative to **fine-needle aspiration**

Contraindications

- Coagulopathy
- Inability to stabilize or visualize the tissue to be sampled

Equipment

- As required for **Aseptic preparation – (a) non-surgical procedures**
- Core biopsy needle: from 14 G (large dogs) to 20 G (cats)
- Local anaesthetic solution
- Scalpel and No.11 or 15 scalpel blade
- Container with 10% neutral buffered formalin
- Suture materials or tissue glue
- Ultrasound machine

Patient preparation and positioning

- The procedure can usually be performed under heavy sedation
- Deeper, ultrasound-guided procedures will normally require general anaesthesia
- If the mass to be sampled is superficial, local anaesthetic solution is infiltrated into the surrounding area
- The patient is positioned to allow optimal stabilization or visualization (if under ultrasound guidance) of the mass
- **Aseptic preparation – (a) non-surgical procedures** of an area several centimetres wide, centred on the needle entry point, is required

---

NOTES

- When sampling vascular organs, especially the liver, haemostasis needs to be checked by way of measurement of prothrombin time, activated partial thromboplastin time and a **platelet count**
- The clinician also needs to ensure that the approach to the mass or organ will not result in perforation of vessels, or the biliary, urinary or gastrointestinal tracts
- It should be remembered that there is still a risk of haemorrhage despite normal coagulation and it is important to have the option of prompt surgical intervention in case of complications
- The animal also needs to be kept under close observation after the procedure and monitored for evidence of haemorrhage (e.g. tachycardia, pallor, weakness, reduced pulse quality)

Technique

1 Using a scalpel blade, make a small stab incision through the skin.
2 Prior to insertion, prepare the biopsy needle by pulling back on the plunger until a firm click is felt, indicating that the needle spring is locked into a ready position.
3 With the stylet fully retracted, so that the specimen notch is completely covered by the cutting cannula, advance the biopsy needle into the tissue to be sampled (Figure T.16).
4 Advance the stylet with the thumb to expose the specimen notch within the tissue to be sampled (Figure T.17).
5 Rotate the biopsy needle to and fro to ensure that tissue fills the specimen notch.
6 Fire the cutting cannula by fully depressing the plunger (Figure T.18).

7 Withdraw the biopsy needle.

8 To remove the tissue sample, pull back on the plunger until a firm click is felt. Push the stylet forward to expose the tissue sample within the specimen notch.

9 Gently remove the sample with a fine hypodermic needle or by irrigation with saline into the fixative (Figure T.19).

10 Leave the skin incision to heal, or close with a single suture or tissue adhesive.

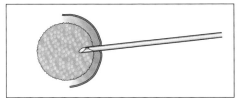

Figure T.16: The biopsy needle should be advanced into the tissue to be sampled.

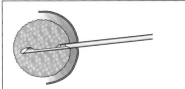

Figure T.17: Once within the tissue, the stylet should be advanced to expose the specimen notch.

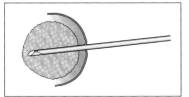

Figure T.18: The cutting cannula should be fired to obtain a tissue sample.

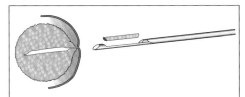

Figure T.19: The sample should be gently removed from the biopsy needle using either a fine hypodermic syringe or irrigation.

Sample handling

- Fix solid tissue samples in 10% neutral buffered formalin
- Impression smears or squash smears (see **Fine-needle aspiration**) of tissue samples can also be made

Potential complications

- Haemorrhage. Sampling of vascular organs such as the liver, spleen or kidneys should be preceded by an assessment of coagulation status; the patient should also be monitored for several hours after the procedure
- Damage to internal viscera

Tracheostomy

Indications/Use

- Management of an upper airway obstruction that is non-responsive to medical management
- Maintenance of prolonged mechanical ventilation
- Anaesthesia for certain surgical procedures of the upper airway and pharynx, where an endotracheal (ET) tube would limit surgical access

> **WARNING**
>
> - Tracheostomy tube placement in a dyspnoeic patient with an upper airway obstruction in an emergency situation, by an *inexperienced* veterinary surgeon, may lead to suboptimal results.
> - Stabilization with oxygen therapy, sedatives, emergency anaesthesia and endotracheal intubation *prior* to tracheostomy tube placement may lead to better results.

Equipment

- As required for **Aseptic preparation – (b) surgical procedures**
- Tracheostomy tubes:
  - Routine airway maintenance: non-cuffed tracheostomy tube with an inner cannula; outer diameter no more than 75% of the luminal diameter of the trachea
  - Maintenance of anaesthesia or prolonged mechanical ventilation: tracheostomy tube with an inner cannula and a high-volume low-pressure cuff

> **NOTE**
>
> - Small tracheostomy tubes suitable for cats and dogs <10 kg are not generally available with an inner cannula

- Suture materials (e.g. 3 metric (2/0 USP) monofilament nylon)
- Nylon tape (usually supplied with the tracheostomy tube)
- Range of narrow ET tubes and stylet for endotracheal intubation
- Soft tissue surgical instrument set

Patient preparation and positioning

- Where possible, tracheostomy tubes should be placed under general anaesthesia in a controlled environment. This most often means placement of an ET tube prior to tracheostomy tube placement (see **Endotracheal intubation**)
- Failure to achieve endotracheal intubation will necessitate immediate tracheal intubation following anaesthetic induction: the veterinary surgeon should be prepared to use a stylet to achieve placement of a standard ET tube or a dog urinary catheter instead of an ET tube in cases of severe upper airway obstruction

- The animal should be placed in dorsal recumbency. The neck should be supported in extension by placement of a sandbag underneath it. The forelegs should be pulled caudally and secured on either side of the thorax
- **Aseptic preparation – (b) surgical procedures** of the ventral neck is required

Technique

Sterile gloves should be worn.

1   Palpate the larynx and trachea and make an approximately 7 cm (length depends on the size of the animal) midline skin incision, running caudally from the larynx (Figure T.20).
2   Separate the sternohyoideus muscles at the midline and retract them laterally to visualize the trachea (Figure T.21). The caudal thyroid vein, with small branches on either side, runs along the midline in the fascia between the sternohyoideus muscles. Try to preserve this vessel to avoid unnecessary haemorrhage.
3   Place stay sutures around the tracheal rings just cranial and caudal to the proposed annular ligament incision (Figure T.22). These stay sutures allow for stabilization of the trachea when inserting or changing the tracheostomy tube.

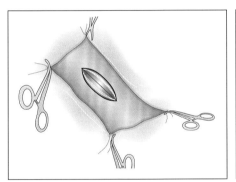

Figure T.20: A midline skin incision should be made caudally from the larynx.

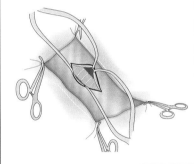

Figure T.21: The sternohyoideus muscles should be separated to visualize the trachea.

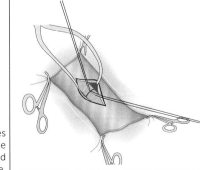

Figure T.22: Stay sutures should be placed around the tracheal rings cranial and caudal to the incision site.

4 Make an incision in one of the annular ligaments between the 3rd and 5th tracheal rings. The incision of the annular ligament should not extend more than 50–60% of the diameter of the trachea. The recurrent laryngeal nerves, which look like fine white threads, run laterally either side of the trachea and should be avoided.

5 Insert the tracheostomy tube into the trachea, using the round tipped inner stylet if provided (Figure T.23). Withdraw the stylet. Insert the inner hollow cannula (where available).

6 Appose the skin cranial and caudal to the tube with simple interrupted sutures, allowing a large enough opening for replacement of the tracheostomy tube into the trachea if necessary.

7 Secure the tracheostomy tube around the neck with nylon tape.

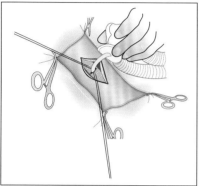

Figure T.23: The tracheostomy tube should be inserted into the trachea through the incision in the annular ligament.

NOTE

- Note that the stay sutures remain around the tracheal rings for ongoing tracheostomy management (Figure T.24). Labelling the stay sutures (e.g. 'TOP' and 'BOTTOM') means the site can be easily opened during tube changes

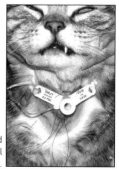

Figure T.24: The sutures should remain in place around the tracheal rings for ongoing management.

Tube maintenance and removal

- 24-hour care is essential to prevent potentially fatal occlusion of the tube by exudates and airway mucus, and to detect tube dislodgement
- The inner cannula should be removed for cleaning whenever an increased noise or effort associated with breathing is noticed, or every 2 hours initially. The cannula should be cleaned thoroughly using warm water, dried by evaporation and replaced

- For tracheostomy tubes without an inner cannula, the entire tube should be removed for cleaning. Ideally, a spare tracheostomy tube should be available for immediate placement into the trachea following removal of the dirty tracheostomy tube. The stay sutures placed around the tracheal rings above and below the tracheostomy site should be used to gently bring the trachea to the level of the skin and to open the trachea
- Humidification: if the inner cannula is repeatedly full of tenacious mucus and exudate, either nebulized air should be provided for periods for the animal to breathe, or 0.1 ml/kg sterile saline should be instilled into the tube every 2 hours (the latter may induce transient coughing)
- Suction: this is not a benign procedure and should be performed *only as required*. It is more commonly needed in smaller dogs and cats. The patient should be pre-oxygenated for approximately 10 breaths. A sterile suction catheter should be introduced aseptically into the tracheostomy tube and suction applied for *no more than 15 seconds*, while gently rotating the suction tube. The suction catheter should remain within the tube during suctioning and only be inserted into the vulnerable trachea if absolutely necessary to clear an obstruction distal to the tracheostomy tube
- The tracheostomy wound should be inspected daily and cleaned with sterile saline-soaked swabs as necessary
- If respiratory effort increases or overt respiratory stress develops, the whole tracheostomy tube should be changed. This should *not* be done in the absence of a veterinary surgeon or facilities for **endotracheal intubation** and the administration of oxygen. Adequate lighting and assistance are essential. The patient is pre-oxygenated and the trachea stabilized using the stay sutures placed around the tracheal rings above and below the tracheostomy site. The old tube is removed and a new one inserted rapidly

Potential complications

- Tracheostomy site dermatitis and infection
- Obstruction of the tracheostomy tube
- Tracheostomy tube dislodgement
- Obstruction of the trachea distal to the tracheostomy tube
- Haemorrhage around the tracheostomy site
- Subcutaneous emphysema
- Pressure necrosis of the trachea
- Tracheal stenosis
- Pneumonia
- Damage to the recurrent laryngeal nerves resulting in unilateral or bilateral laryngeal paralysis
- Fatal airway obstruction

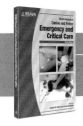

FURTHER INFORMATION

For more information on tracheostomy, see the *BSAVA Manual of Canine and Feline Emergency and Critical Care.*

Transtracheal wash

Indications/Use

- To obtain a sample for cytology and bacteriology from the airways of medium- and large-breed dogs
- Can give a variable return and is usually reserved for those patients where there is a high anaesthetic risk
- Generally yields samples representative of the trachea and primary or (at best) secondary bronchi, although some material from the lower bronchioles and alveoli may be collected
- The upper airway of dogs and cats may also be sampled by **endotracheal wash**
- The lower airways of dogs and cats may be sampled by **bronchoalveolar lavage**

Contraindications

- Compromised respiratory function
- Animals with pulmonary parenchymal disease, rather than tracheal or bronchial disease

Equipment

- As required for **Aseptic preparation – (a) non-surgical procedures**
- 12–14 G over-the-needle catheter and male dog urinary catheter (3–6 Fr) or a lavage catheter designed for a bronchoscope biopsy channel. The clinician should check that the urinary catheter passes easily through the over-the-needle catheter before starting the procedure
  OR Through-the-needle long 'jugular' catheter (19–22 G, 8 inches long for medium (<20 kg) dogs; 19 G, 12 or 24 inches long for larger dogs)
- Local anaesthetic solution
- 2 ml syringe and 21 G hypodermic needle
- Scalpel and No.11 or 15 scalpel blade
- 500 ml bag of warm 0.9% sterile saline
- 10 ml and 20 ml syringes
- Sterile plain and EDTA collection tubes
- Microscope slides
- Dressing materials

Patient preparation and positioning

- Preferably, the procedure should be carried out without sedation so as to encourage coughing and thereby improve yield. If sedation is used, ideally the animal should be awake enough to cough
- The patient is positioned standing or sitting at the edge of a table or on the floor, with its nose elevated and its feet restrained
- **Aseptic preparation – (a) non-surgical procedures** of the skin of the ventral neck from just above to several centimetres below the larynx is required (Figure T.25).

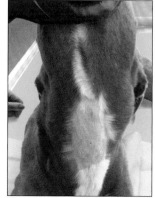

Figure T.25: Patient preparation for a transtracheal wash includes aseptic preparation of the skin of the ventral neck.

Technique

The site of catheter placement is ideally through the cricothyroid ligament, although a site between tracheal rings 2 to 5 distal to the larynx can also be used. At the most cranial end of the trachea, a wide ring is palpated that protrudes more than the tracheal rings; this is the cricoid cartilage. The cricothyroid ligament is the small triangular membrane just cranial to the cricoid cartilage (Figure T.26ab). In smaller dogs, the only palpable landmark may be the cricoid cartilage and so the needle is inserted just cranial to this larger ring.

1   Identify the site for catheter placement.
2   Infiltrate 0.5–1 ml of local anaesthetic solution into the skin and subcutis over this area.
3   Stabilize the larynx between the thumb and forefinger and make a small skin incision through the skin over the site of entry.
4   Two options are described: over-the-needle catheter; and through-the-needle catheter.

   If using an over-the-needle catheter:
   a   Push the over-the-needle catheter through the cricothyroid ligament or between two tracheal rings, with the bevel of the needle facing downwards. Firm pressure is required to achieve this.
   b   Once in the lumen of the trachea, remove the needle, leaving only the catheter in place (Figure T.27).

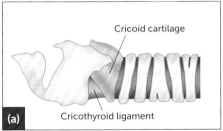

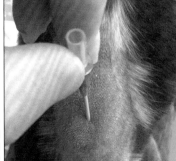

Figure T.26: (a–b) The catheter should ideally be placed through the cricothyroid ligament.

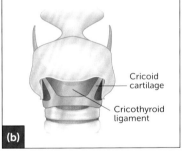

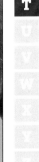

Figure T.27: The over-the-needle catheter should be pushed through the cricothyroid ligament into the lumen of the trachea.

   c Thread the male dog urinary catheter (or lavage catheter designed for the biopsy channel of a bronchoscope) through the over-the-needle catheter, ideally to the level of the carina (approximately the 4th intercostal space) or, if this is not possible, as far down as it will pass (Figure T.28).

   d Instil approximately 0.5 ml/kg warm sterile saline through the urinary catheter (Figure T.29) or lavage catheter.

If using a through-the-needle catheter:

   a Push the needle through the cricothyroid ligament or between two tracheal rings, with the bevel of the needle facing downwards. Firm pressure is required to achieve this.

   b Advance the needle approximately 1–2 cm into the trachea after the lumen is entered. Angle the needle at approximately 45 degrees to direct it down the tracheal lumen.

   c Pass the catheter through the needle, ideally to the level of the carina (approximately the 4th intercostal space) or, if this is not possible, as far down as it will pass. The animal may cough at this point. If the catheter does not feed easily, back the needle out of the trachea a short distance, as the tip of the needle may be pressed up against the wall of the trachea.

   d Once the full length of the catheter is in the trachea, withdraw the needle and inject approximately 0.5 ml/kg warm sterile saline into the catheter.

5 **Immediately** aspirate back the material using a 10 or 20 ml syringe.

6 Repeat the injection of saline and aspiration two to three times if required (Figure T.30).

7 Remove the catheter and apply pressure to the region for 2 minutes before covering in a temporary light dressing. This dressing can be removed after 1–2 hours.

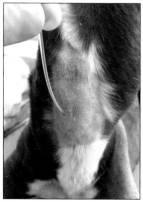

Figure T.28: The urinary catheter should be threaded through the over-the-needle catheter into the trachea.

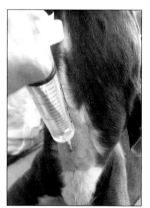

Figure T.29: Warm sterile saline should be instilled into the urinary catheter.

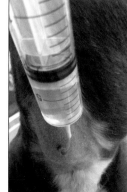

Figure T.30: Saline should be injected into the trachea two or three times and aspirated, if required, to obtain a sample for evaluation.

NOTES

- A total recovery of 1–3 ml of a slightly turbid fluid with a foamy layer at the top (representative of surfactant) represents a good sample
- The optimal recovery is often during patient coughing; coupage and turning the patient may also improve the yield
- If nothing is recovered, the animal should be placed in sternal recumbency (if sitting) with the nose, head and neck in a more neutral position and the flush procedure repeated

Sample handling

- An aliquot of the sample should be placed in a sterile plain tube and submitted for culture
- An aliquot of the sample should be placed in an EDTA tube and submitted for cytology
- The cells collected are fragile, so samples should be processed as soon as possible. If samples are to be sent to an external laboratory, fresh air-dried unstained smears of any flocculent/mucoid material should also be made (see **Fine-needle aspiration**). Direct smears of the fluid can be made, but most samples are poorly cellular

Potential complications

- Larynx or airway spasm
- Subcutaneous emphysema
- Pneumomediastinum
- Infection at the needle site
- Placement of catheters with excessive force can damage the lungs and airways and, in the worst case scenario, result in pneumothorax

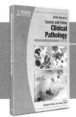

FURTHER INFORMATION

Details on cytology of upper respiratory tract samples can be found in the *BSAVA Manual of Canine and Feline Clinical Pathology*.

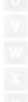

Urethral catheterization – (a) male dog

Indications/Use

- To collect urine for **urinalysis**
- To empty the urinary bladder
- To administer radiographic contrast media into the lower urinary tract (see **Retrograde urethrography/vaginourethrography**)
- An **indwelling** urinary catheter is indicated:
  - To maintain constant, controlled bladder drainage
  - To maintain a patent urethra
  - To monitor urine output
  - To assist with nursing care of patients that are recumbent or unable to urinate voluntarily

Contraindications

- Pre-existing urethral trauma
- Large space-occupying urethral mass or urethral stricture
- Urine collected by catheterization is not optimal for microbiology, as the sample may be contaminated. **Cystocentesis** is preferred

Equipment

- Catheters (Figure U.1)
- Sterile soft gauze swabs
- Antiseptic solution: 4% chlorhexidine gluconate or 10% povidone–iodine, diluted with sterile saline for flushing the prepuce
- Sterile aqueous lubricant (e.g. K-Y jelly)
- Plain sample pot
- Kidney dish
- 5–10 ml syringe

Catheter type	Material	Indwelling?	Sizes (Fr)	Length (cm)
Dog catheter	Flexible nylon (polyamide)	No	6–10	50–60
Silicone Foley	Flexible medical grade silicone	Yes	5–10	30, 55

Figure U.1: Types of catheters that can be used for urethral catheterization in dogs.

If the catheter is to be indwelling:

- For silicone Foley catheters: sterile water or 0.9% saline sufficient to fill balloon
- For standard flexible nylon (polyamide) catheters: suture materials; zinc oxide tape
- Sterile intravenous fluid administration set and empty fluid bag or commercial closed urine collection system, with appropriate adapters for attachment to selected urinary catheter
- Elizabethan collar

Patient preparation and positioning

- Male dogs will generally allow urethral catheterization under gentle physical restraint
- Sedation may be required for fractious patients
- General anaesthesia may be required for welfare reasons (e.g. patient with fractured pelvis)
- The patient should be restrained in lateral recumbency, with the upper leg held away from the prepuce
- The area around the prepuce can be clipped, especially in long-haired breeds
- The prepuce should be cleaned with the diluted antiseptic solution, using swabs or a syringe

Technique

Sterile gloves should be worn.

1 Estimate the length between the urethral opening and the bladder before catheter placement.

2 If using a rigid dog catheter, remove the catheter from the outer wrapper and cut a feeding sleeve from the inner sterile packaging, to allow easy feeding of the catheter into the urethra using a 'no touch' technique. Alternatively, or if using a Foley catheter, use sterile gloves to handle the catheter. Note that some Foley catheters come with a thin wire stylet already within the catheter lumen; with others, the thin wire stylet needs to be fed through the centre of the catheter before placement.

3 An assistant should grasp the caudal os penis with one hand and retract the prepuce caudally with the other hand, exposing the glans penis.

4 Apply sterile lubricant to the tip of the catheter and insert the tip of the catheter into the urethra.

5 Advance the catheter into the urethra. Resistance may be met: at the os penis, where there is a slight narrowing of the urethra; at the ischial arch; and at the prostate, if enlarged.

6 Once the catheter is inserted to the level of the caudal os penis, the grip on the penis is relaxed to allow further unobstructed passage of the catheter. Angling the penis caudally may straighten the urethra to ease passage. Steady but gentle pressure should overcome any resistance. If the catheter cannot be passed, re-evaluate the catheter size.

7 When the catheter tip enters the bladder and urine appears in the catheter hub, continue to advance an additional 2 cm to ensure adequate length beyond the trigone. If using a silicone Foley catheter, advance the tip slightly further into the bladder to avoid inadvertent urethral trauma when the balloon is inflated.

> **NOTE**
>
> - The thin wire stylet of a Foley catheter can be removed once the catheter is in the bladder. Resistance may be felt, so using the non-dominant hand to immobilize the external portion of the catheter as the guidewire is retracted helps prevent inadvertent catheter removal prior to balloon inflation. Retracting the stylet slightly and/or instilling sterile saline into the catheter lumen prior to its insertion into the urethra can also facilitate stylet removal once the catheter is appropriately placed

8 If using a silicone Foley catheter, inflate the balloon with sterile water/saline. Then withdraw the catheter gradually so the balloon sits in the bladder neck.

9 Proceed according to reason for catheterization (e.g. drain bladder, collect urine sample, administer contrast agent).

Sample handling

- **For urinalysis:**
  - Approximately 5 ml of urine is required
  - Samples should be collected into a plain tube

Indwelling catheters

> **CATHETER CHOICE**
>
> A silicone Foley catheter is preferred for indwelling use.

1 Attach a sterile intravenous administration set and empty fluid bag to the urinary catheter and maintain as a closed collection system. *Alternatively,* attach a commercial sterile closed collection urine bag to the catheter: a catheter adapter may be required.

2 Place the collection bag below the patient to allow free drainage and ensure the environment in which the bag is kept is clean.

3 Place an Elizabethan collar.

Potential complications

- Trauma to the urethra or urinary bladder
- Iatrogenic urinary tract infection
- If advanced too far into the bladder, the tip of silicone catheters can reverse back into the urethra or knot within the bladder; estimating urethral length before placement can help avoid this complication

Urethral catheterization – (b) bitch

Indications/Use

- As for **Urethral catheterization – (a) male dog**

Contraindications

- As for **Urethral catheterization – (a) male dog**

Equipment

- Catheters (Figure U.2)
- Sterile vaginal speculum and light source
- Sterile soft gauze swabs
- Antiseptic solution: 4% chlorhexidine gluconate or 10% povidone–iodine, diluted with sterile saline for flushing the vulva
- Sterile aqueous lubricant (e.g. K-Y jelly)

Catheter type	Material	Indwelling?	Sizes (Fr)	Length (cm)
Dog catheter	Flexible nylon (polyamide)	No	6–10	50–60
Foley	Flexible medical-grade silicone	Yes	5–10	30, 55
	Teflon-coated latex	Yes	8–16	30–40

Figure U.2: Types of catheters that can be used for urethral catheterization in bitches.

- Plain sample pot
- Kidney dish
- 5–10 ml syringe

If the catheter is to be made indwelling:

- For Foley catheter: sterile water or 0.9% saline sufficient to fill balloon; guidewire
- For standard flexible nylon (polyamide) catheter: suture materials; zinc oxide tape
- Sterile intravenous fluid administration set and empty fluid bag or commercial closed urine collection system, with appropriate adapters for attachment to selected urinary catheter
- Elizabethan collar

Patient preparation and positioning

- Bitches may require sedation
- General anaesthesia may be required for welfare reasons (e.g. patient with fractured pelvis)
- The patient may be positioned:
  - In dorsal recumbency with the hindlimbs held cranially (ideally, or in a frogleg position) (for direct visualization)
  - In lateral recumbency (right lateral recumbency for a right-handed operator; left lateral recumbency for a left-handed operator) (for digital palpation)
  - In sternal recumbency with the hindlimbs over the edge of the table (for direct visualization or digital palpation)
- The vulva should be cleaned with diluted antiseptic solution to remove any discharge and surface dirt

Technique

Sterile gloves should be worn.

Direct visualization of urethral orifice

1 Estimate the length between the urethral opening and the bladder before catheter placement.
2 If using a dog catheter, remove it from its outer wrapping and expose the tip only from the inner sleeve.
3 If using a Foley catheter, remove it completely from its packaging. Handle the catheter with sterile gloves. Some Foley catheters come with a thin wire stylet already within the catheter lumen; with others the thin wire stylet needs to be fed through the centre of the catheter before placement.

4 Insert a speculum into the vestibule, taking care not to enter the ventrally placed clitoral fossa. The slit of the speculum should be positioned ventrally, allowing the raised external urethral orifice to be identified on the floor (ventral) of the cranial vestibule (Figure U.3). Visualization of the external urethral orifice is often made easier if an assistant pulls on the ventral vulva lips to straighten the vestibule.

5 Apply sterile lubricant to the tip of the catheter and insert it into the urethral orifice under direct visualization.

6 Advance the catheter along the urethra and into the bladder (Figure U.4).

7 If using a Foley catheter, it may be advantageous to insert the catheter all the way into the bladder before removing the guidewire.

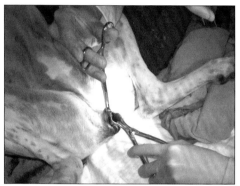

Figure U.3: A speculum should be inserted into the vestibule. (Courtesy of Amanda Boag)

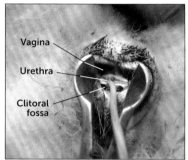

Vagina

Urethra

Clitoral fossa

Figure U.4: The catheter should be inserted into the urethral orifice and advanced into the bladder. (Courtesy of Amanda Boag)

> **NOTE**
>
> - The thin wire stylet of a Foley catheter can be removed once the catheter is in the bladder. Resistance may be felt, so using the non-dominant hand to immobilize the external portion of the catheter as the guidewire is retracted helps prevent inadvertent catheter removal prior to balloon inflation. Retracting the stylet slightly and/or instilling sterile saline into the catheter lumen prior to its insertion into the urethra can also facilitate stylet removal once the catheter is appropriately placed

8 Inflate the balloon with the required volume of sterile water/saline once the tip of the catheter is in the bladder. Then withdraw the catheter gradually so the balloon sits in the bladder neck.

9 Proceed according to reason for catheterization (e.g. drain bladder, collect urine sample, administer contrast agent).

Digital palpation of urethral orifice

If a vaginal speculum is not available, the catheter can be inserted 'blindly' using digital palpation of the urethral papilla.

1 If using a dog catheter, remove the catheter from its outer wrapping and the inner packaging in an aseptic fashion.

2 If using a Foley catheter, a guidewire may be used but is not usually required.

3 Apply sterile water-soluble lubricant to the tip of the catheter and your index finger.

4 Place this finger into the vestibule and, while gently applying pressure on its floor, move the finger cranially. The urethral papilla is palpated as a slit on a slight 'bulge' of mucosa (Figure U.5).

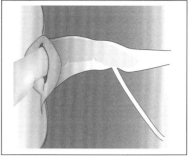

Figure U.5: A finger should be inserted into the vestibule to identify the urethral papilla.

5 While applying gentle pressure over the papilla, feed the catheter under the finger and guide it into the urethra with your other hand. If the orifice is missed, the catheter will run past the fingertip. Alternatively, especially in small animals, the urethral orifice can be palpated and the catheter fed into the orifice using the same index finger.

6 If using a Foley catheter, inflate the balloon once the tip of the catheter is in the bladder.

7 Proceed according to reason for catheterization (e.g. drain bladder, collect urine sample, administer contrast agent).

Sample handling

■ For **urinalysis**:
  ▪ Approximately 5 ml of urine is required
  ▪ Samples should be collected into a plain tube

Indwelling catheters

■ As for **Urethral catheterization – (a) male dog**

Potential complications

■ As for **Urethral catheterization – (a) male dog**

Urethral catheterization – (c) tomcat

Indications/Use

■ As for **Urethral catheterization – (a) male dog**

Contraindications

■ As for **Urethral catheterization – (a) male dog**

Equipment

■ Catheters (Figure U.6)
■ Sterile soft gauze swabs
■ Antiseptic solution: 4% chlorhexidine gluconate or 10% povidone–iodine, diluted with sterile saline for cleansing around the prepuce

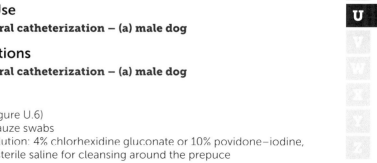

- Sterile aqueous lubricant (e.g. K-Y jelly)
- Plain sample pot
- Kidney dish
- 5–10 ml syringe

Catheter type	Material	Indwelling?	Sizes (Fr)	Length (cm)
Jackson cat catheter	Flexible nylon	Yes	3, 4	11
Silicone cat catheter	Medical grade silicone	Yes	3.5	12
Slippery Sam	PTFE	Yes	3, 3.5	11, 14
MILA tomcat/small animal catheter	Polyurethane	Yes	3.5, 5	15, 25

Figure U.6: Types of catheters that can be used for urethral catheterization in tomcats.

If the catheter is to be made indwelling:
- Suture materials; zinc oxide tape
- Sterile intravenous fluid administration set and empty fluid bag or commercial closed urine collection system, with appropriate adapters for attachment to selected urinary catheter
- Elizabethan collar

Patient preparation and positioning
- Cats usually require *heavy* sedation
- General anaesthesia may be required for welfare reasons (e.g. patient with fractured pelvis) or where catheterization is difficult (e.g. urethral obstruction)
- The patient should be restrained in lateral recumbency, with the hindlimbs pulled slightly cranially and the upper leg held away from the prepuce
- The area around the prepuce can be clipped, especially in long-haired breeds
- The prepuce should be cleaned with diluted antiseptic solution using swabs or a syringe

Technique
Sterile gloves should be worn.
1. Remove the catheter from the outer wrapper.
2. Apply sterile lubricant to the tip of the catheter.
3. Extrude the penis by applying gentle pressure each side of the prepuce with two fingers (Figure U.7ab).
4. Gently introduce the catheter into the urethra.
5. To allow safe advancement of the catheter, the prepuce and penis should be grasped and pulled in a caudal direction to straighten out the penile and membranous urethra (Figure U.8ab).
6. As soon as the catheter tip enters the bladder and urine appears in the catheter hub, advance the catheter 1 cm further. Remove stylet if present.
7. Proceed according to reason for catheterization (e.g. drain bladder, collect urine sample, administer contrast agent).

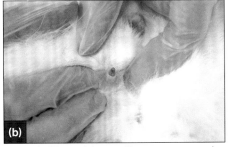

Figure U.7: (a–b) The penis should be extruded by applying gentle pressure on each side of the prepuce.

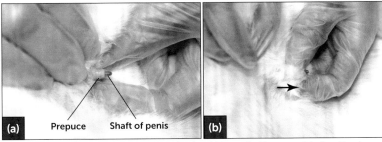

Prepuce   Shaft of penis

Figure U.8: (a–b) The prepuce and penis should be pulled in a caudal direction to straighten the penile and membranous urethra.

Sample handling

- For **urinalysis**:
  - Approximately 5 ml is required
  - Samples should be collected into a plain tube

Indwelling catheters

- As for **Urethral catheterization – (a) male dog**, but see 'Catheter choice' below

Potential complications

- Trauma to the urethra or urinary bladder
- Iatrogenic urinary tract infection

CATHETER CHOICE

- Nylon catheters are not recommended for indwelling use
- Foley catheters are not suitable for tomcats because of their size
- The catheter tip should sit just within the bladder to avoid irritation of the bladder wall (too long) or urethra (too short). The MILA catheter has suture wings that can be positioned anywhere along the length of the catheter, to achieve the ideal length within the bladder

Urethral catheterization – (d) tomcat with a blocked urethra

Indications/Use

- Urethral obstruction:
  - Gentle massage of the penis between the thumb and forefinger, while at the same time applying **extremely gentle** pressure to the bladder, may relieve the obstruction; if not relieved immediately, retrograde urohydropulsion should be attempted
  - Radiography should be performed to check for uroliths. However, radiolucent urethral plugs are much more common than uroliths in cats
  - Urethral plugs or uroliths lodged in the urethra can be flushed into the bladder, to restore urethral patency

---

WARNING

- Any animal with urethral obstruction should undergo emergency assessment and stabilization, including **intravenous catheter placement – (a) peripheral nerves, blood sampling – (b) venous** for an emergency minimum database, and fluid therapy for correction of acid–base and electrolyte abnormalities.
- Bradycardia or other arrhythmias associated with hyperkalaemia should be treated aggressively.

Equipment

- A selection of urinary catheters of varying sizes (3–5 Fr) including polypropylene or silicone tomcat catheters (open-ended catheters are preferable to side-opening catheters for urethral flushing), plastic ophthalmic lacrimal duct flush cannulas and over-the-needle intravenous catheters (23 G) without their stylet
- 3-way taps
- Intravenous extension tubing
- 10–20 ml syringes
- Antiseptic solution: 4% chlorhexidine gluconate or 10% povidone–iodine, diluted with sterile saline for cleansing around the prepuce
- Sterile intravenous fluid administration set and empty fluid bag or commercial closed urine collection system, with appropriate adapters for attachment to selected urinary catheter
- Suture material (e.g. 2 metric (3/0 USP) monofilament, non-absorbable)
- Sterile isotonic fluids, e.g. 0.9% sterile saline, lactated Ringer's solution (Hartmann's)
- Sterile water-soluble lubricant
- Elizabethan collar

Patient preparation and positioning

- General anaesthesia is most often recommended
- Sedation should not be prolonged because of fluid, electrolyte and acid–base abnormalities

- Positioning is as for **Urethral catheterization – (c) tomcat**
- The area around the prepuce can be clipped, especially in long-haired breeds
- The prepuce should be cleaned with diluted antiseptic solution (excluding alcohol) and rinsed with sterile saline

Technique

Sterile gloves should be worn.

1 Decompress the bladder by **cystocentesis** if overdistended, using a needle attached to intravenous extension tubing, a 3-way tap and a syringe. This apparatus permits decompression without repeated puncturing of the bladder wall. The needle is held in position within the bladder, while an assistant withdraws urine. Remove as much urine as possible to avoid leakage.

2 Perform **Urethral catheterization – (c) tomcat** Steps 1 to 6. Flush the urethra while advancing the catheter. Gently twisting the catheter can also sometimes aid its passage. If catheterization is unsuccessful, try different/ smaller types of catheter.

3 Once the catheter has been passed into the bladder, empty the bladder by attaching a syringe to the catheter.

4 Collect urine samples for **urinalysis** and culture as required. A **cystocentesis** sample is preferred for culture.

5 Slowly flush the bladder multiple times with warm sterile saline until clear, emptying the bladder each time.

Indwelling catheters

The bladder should remain catheterized if:

- Relief of the obstruction was difficult
- The urine stream is small
- The bladder was overly distended and detrusor function may be questionable
- The patient is uraemic or markedly azotaemic and diuresis is necessary
- Post-obstructive diuresis is likely and measurement of urine output is necessary in the immediate post-obstructive phase

1 Advance the catheter into the bladder until urine appears in the catheter hub.

2 Then advance the catheter at least 1 cm further.

3 Secure the catheter to the patient by placing an adhesive tape butterfly around the catheter at the level of the prepuce and suturing it to the prepuce. *Alternatively*, for cat catheters with suture collars, suture the prepuce to the suture collar using the holes provided.

4 Attach a sterile intravenous administration set and empty fluid bag to the urinary catheter and maintain as a closed collection system. *Alternatively*, attach a commercial sterile closed collection urine bag to the catheter: a catheter adapter may be required. Tape the tubing of the closed collection system to the tail for additional security, to prevent accidental catheter removal. Place the collection bag below the patient to allow free drainage and ensure the environment in which the bag is kept is clean.

5 Place an Elizabethan collar.

6 For cats with feline lower urinary tract disease, the urinary catheter must usually remain in place for at least 2 days until medical management has taken effect.

Potential complications

- Urethral rupture; this risk should be minimized by gentle technique with adequate lubrication and patience
- Inability to pass a urethral catheter into the bladder. In this situation, placement of a cystostomy tube and medical management to decrease urethral spasm and relax the urethra should be considered. Perineal urethrostomy may be required as a salvage procedure
- Urinary tract infection
- Accidental removal of an indwelling urinary catheter
- Accidental disruption of an indwelling urinary catheter, leaving the catheter tip within the bladder

Urethral catheterization – (e) queen

Indications/Use

- As for **Urethral catheterization – (a) male dog**

Contraindications

- As for **Urethral catheterization – (a) male dog**

Equipment

- Catheters (Figure U.9)
- Sterile soft gauze swabs
- Antiseptic solution: 4% chlorhexidine gluconate or 10% povidone–iodine, diluted with sterile saline for cleansing the vulva
- Sterile aqueous lubricant, e.g. K-Y jelly
- Otoscope (may be required)
- Plain sample pot
- Kidney dish
- 5–10 ml syringe

Catheter type	Material	Indwelling?	Sizes (Fr)	Length (cm)
Jackson cat catheter	Flexible nylon	Yes	3, 4	11
Silicone Foley	Flexible medical-grade silicone	Yes	5	30
MILA tomcat/small animal catheter	Polyurethane	Yes	3.5, 5	15, 25

Figure U.9: Types of catheters that can be used for urethral catheterization in queens.

If the catheter is to be made indwelling:

- Suture materials (e.g. 2 metric (3/0 USP) monofilament, non-absorbable); zinc oxide tape
- Sterile intravenous fluid administration set and empty fluid bag or commercial closed urine collection system, with appropriate adapters for attachment to selected urinary catheter
- Elizabethan collar

Patient preparation and positioning

- Cats usually require *heavy* sedation
- General anaesthesia may be required for welfare reasons (e.g. patient with fractured pelvis)
- The cat should be positioned in lateral recumbency (right lateral recumbency for a right-handed operator; left lateral recumbency for a left-handed operator)
- The vulva should be cleaned with diluted antiseptic solution to remove any discharge and surface dirt

Technique

Sterile gloves should be worn.

1   Remove the catheter from the outer wrapper and cut a feeding sleeve from the inner sterile packaging, if present, to allow easy feeding of the catheter into the urethra using a 'no touch' technique. Alternatively, handle the catheter with sterile gloves.
2   Apply sterile lubricant to the tip of the catheter.
3   Grasp the lips of the vulva with your non-dominant hand, allowing your dominant hand to pass the catheter along the vestibular floor in the midline.
4   Angle the catheter ventrally, applying gentle pressure until it slips into the urethra.
5   As soon as the catheter tip enters the bladder and urine appears in the catheter hub, advance the catheter 1 cm further.

PRACTICAL TIPS

- The anatomy of the queen is such that the external urethral orifice is found as a depression on the vaginal floor. This allows 'blind' urethral catheterization
- If 'blind' catheterization fails, an otoscope may be used as a vaginoscope to identify the external urethral orifice

---

6   If using a silicone Foley catheter, inflate the balloon once the tip of the catheter is in the bladder.
7   Proceed according to reason for catheterization (e.g. drain bladder, collect urine sample, administer contrast agent).

Sample handling

- For **urinalysis**:
    - Approximately 5 ml is required
    - Samples should be collected into a plain tube

Indwelling catheters

- As for **Urethral catheterization – (a) male dog**, but see 'Catheter choice' below

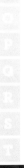

CATHETER CHOICE

- Nylon catheters are not recommended for indwelling use
- The catheter tip should sit just within the bladder to avoid irritation of the bladder wall (too long) or urethra (too short). The MILA catheter has suture wings which can be positioned anywhere along the length of the catheter, to achieve the ideal length within the bladder
- Jackson cat catheters will cause irritation in queens due to their length and rigidity

---

Potential complications

- As for **Urethral catheterization – (a) male dog**

Urethral retrograde urohydropulsion in a male dog

Indications/Use

- To flush uroliths lodged in the urethra into the bladder, to restore urethral patency
- Urethral obstruction with uroliths should be confirmed with radiography prior to performing retrograde urohydropulsion (see **Retrograde urethrography/vaginourethrography**)

WARNING

- Any animal with urethral obstruction should undergo emergency assessment and stabilization, including **intravenous catheter placement, blood sampling – (b) venous** for an emergency minimum database, and fluid therapy for correction of acid–base and electrolyte abnormalities.
- Bradycardia or other arrhythmias associated with hyperkalaemia should be treated aggressively.

Equipment

- As required for **Urethral catheterization – (a) male dog**; flexible nylon urinary catheters are preferred to Foley catheters for urohydropulsion
- Hypodermic needles: 21 G, 1.5 inches
- 3-way taps
- Intravenous extension tubing
- 20–50 ml syringes
- Sterile intravenous fluid administration set and empty fluid bag or commercial closed urine collection system
- Sterile isotonic fluids, e.g. 0.9% sterile saline, lactated Ringer's solution (Hartmann's)
- Sterile water-soluble lubricant

Patient preparation and positioning

- As required for **Urethral catheterization – (a) male dog**
- Sedation or general anaesthesia is recommended for a patient that is alert or in pain, but may not be required for the severely depressed. Urethral relaxation resulting from general anaesthesia might facilitate urohydropulsion
- Lateral recumbency is recommended
- The area around the prepuce can be clipped, especially in long-haired breeds
- The prepuce should be cleaned with diluted antiseptic solution (excluding alcohol) using swabs or a syringe

Technique

Sterile gloves should be worn.

1. Decompress the bladder by **cystocentesis** if overdistended, using a needle attached to intravenous extension tubing, a 3-way tap and a syringe. This apparatus permits decompression without repeated puncturing of the bladder wall. The needle is held in position within the bladder, while an assistant withdraws urine.
2. Fill one 10 ml (or 12 ml) syringe with 5 ml saline and another with 5 ml of lubricant. Attach the syringes to a 3-way tap and use this to mix them.
3. Insert a lubricated large-bore male dog urinary catheter into the urethra (see **Urethral catheterization – (a) male dog**).
4. Instil 3–8 ml of the lubricant mixture around the uroliths. The tip of the catheter should remain distal to the uroliths. **Never attempt to force uroliths retrograde with the tip of the catheter.**
5. An assistant inserts a gloved index finger into the rectum and occludes the urethral lumen by compressing the urethra against the floor of the bony pelvis.
6. With a moistened gauze swab, occlude the distal urethra by compressing the distal tip of the penis around the urinary catheter.
7. Fill a large syringe (20 or 50 ml) with sterile isotonic solution. As a guide, the normal bladder will accommodate approximately 7–11 ml/kg bodyweight, but this volume is most often not required.
8. Attach the syringe to the urinary catheter.
9. Push sterile isotonic solution into the urethra with the goal of dilating the urethral lumen around the uroliths (Figure U.10).
10. Once the urethra is dilated, immediately release digital compression of the pelvic urethra.
11. Continue flushing fluid through the urinary catheter and urethral lumen to propel uroliths into the urinary bladder. Repeated occlusion of the pelvic urethra and flushing of the urethra may be required. Use caution not to overdistend the bladder lumen with fluid. Palpate the bladder regularly to check for overdistension and repeat bladder decompression if required.
12. Confirm successful retrograde urohydropulsion of uroliths into the bladder by **retrograde urethrography**.
13. If the animal is not taken to surgery immediately for removal of uroliths from the bladder, placement of an indwelling urethral catheter is recommended pending surgery, to maintain urine flow.

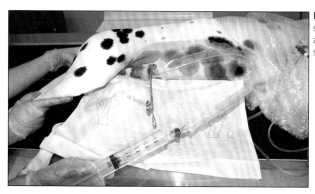

Figure U.10: A large syringe should be used to administer the isotonic solution into the urethra.

Potential complications

- Urethral rupture (rare)
- Urinary tract infection
- Bladder rupture (rare)

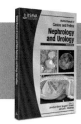

FURTHER INFORMATION

Further information on urolithiasis and its treatment can be found in the *BSAVA Manual of Canine and Feline Nephrology and Urology*.

Urinalysis

Indications/Use

- To obtain information from urine samples

SAMPLE CHOICES

- **Cystocentesis** samples are optimal for bacterial culture; if this is not possible, a catheter sample (see **Urinary catheterization**) can be used for culture if collected aseptically, but this carries a risk of contamination
- Cystocentesis and catheter samples are suitable for sediment analysis, urine specific gravity (SG) determination and dipstick analysis
- Free-catch samples are suitable for dipstick and SG determination; they can also be used for sediment examination. They are not recommended for culture owing to the likelihood of contamination from the external genitalia and urethra

Equipment

- Urine sample in a plain container, obtained by **cystocentesis** or **urethral catheterization** or by free catch
- Urine sample in a sterile plain container collected by **cystocentesis**
- Refractometer
- Dipsticks and results chart
- Distilled water
- Syringe
- Conical-tip centrifuge tube
- Centrifuge
- Plastic disposable pipette
- Microscope slides and coverslips
- Stain (e.g. Sedi-stain)
- Microscope

SAMPLE HANDLING

Urinalysis should be performed within 60 minutes of urine collection where possible. If a sample is left at room temperature for a number of hours the following changes can occur:

- pH can increase as bacteria break down urea to ammonia
- Cells and casts degenerate
- Crystals can dissolve or precipitate
- Levels of glucose, ketones and bilirubin can decrease
- Bacteria can multiply.

These factors should be borne in mind if a sample is to be posted to an external laboratory.

Specific gravity

Urine SG should always be measured using a refractometer because dipsticks are notoriously inaccurate (Figure U.11).

Technique

1. Open the prism cover.
2. Check the calibration of the refractometer using distilled water. This should read 1.000; if it does not, recalibrate as follows:
   a. Unscrew the fixation nut of the calibration screw
   b. Turn the calibration screw downwards to bring the scale up, or unscrew to bring the scale down until it reads 1.000
   c. Re-affix the calibration nut.
3. To view, hold the refractometer horizontally in the direction of a good light source, preferably a natural light source.
4. Wearing gloves, place 1–2 drops of urine on the face of the lower prism and view through the eyepiece (Figure U.12). Note where the colour boundary line is and read against the specific gravity scale.
5. After use, clean the prism and cover carefully with a soft wet cloth or damp lens wipe.

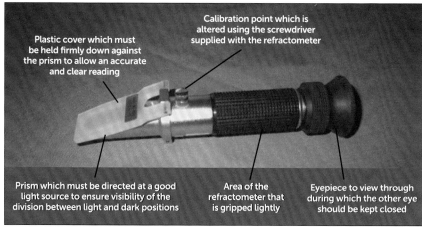

Calibration point which is altered using the screwdriver supplied with the refractometer

Plastic cover which must be held firmly down against the prism to allow an accurate and clear reading

Prism which must be directed at a good light source to ensure visibility of the division between light and dark positions

Area of the refractometer that is gripped lightly

Eyepiece to view through during which the other eye should be kept closed

Figure U.11: Refractometers should be used to measure the specific gravity of urine samples.

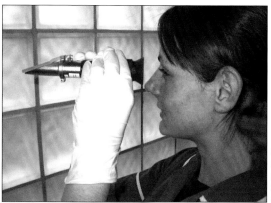

Figure U.12: The refractometer should be held horizontally and directed towards a good light source in order to read the specific gravity scale.

Dipstick tests

- These constitute a qualitative to semiquantitative method of monitoring major chemicals of interest in the urine
- Dipsticks are designed for monitoring constituents in human urine; therefore, some of the tests are not suitable for use with animal urine (i.e. SG, nitrite and leucocyte esterase activity associated with white blood cells)
- Only fresh, in-date dipsticks should be used
- Dipsticks should be stored in the original tightly capped container (the lid contains a desiccant)
- Do not touch the test pads with fingers

Technique

1 Use a syringe to place drops of urine on each test pad (Figure U.13). Alternatively, dip the urine test strip in fresh urine and allow any excess to run off.

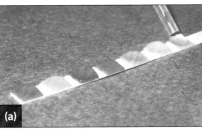

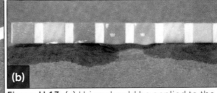

Figure U.13: (a) Urine should be applied to the dipstick and the colour changes compared with **(b)** the test strip.

2 Check the colour changes at the indicated times.

3 Compare the strip with the test chart provided.

Urine sediment analysis

This is perhaps the most important component of a complete routine urinalysis. A suggested method for preparation and analysis is as follows:

1 Use fresh urine or refrigerated urine that has been warmed to room temperature. Note that storage periods of longer than a few hours may have detrimental effects on cellular elements.

2 Mix the sample well but gently to prevent destruction of any casts.

3 Place a constant volume (3 or 5 ml; often 3 ml is used for cat urine) in a conical-tip centrifuge tube.

4 Gently centrifuge the urine (approximately 1000 rpm for 5 minutes, although this will vary with the type of centrifuge used). If a smaller volume of urine (<3 ml) is used with high-speed centrifugation, the amount of sediment obtained may be too small for examination, especially if the urine is very dilute. The high speed may also damage cells and destroy casts.

5 Decant most of the supernatant (this can be used for SG analysis – see above). This can be achieved by pipetting or by simply tipping out.

6 A few drops of liquid will remain in the tube. Resuspend the sediment in this fluid either by gently tapping the tube or pipetting up and down.

7 Urine samples can be examined unstained, stained with a specialized urine stain (e.g. Sedi-stain or UriStain) or stained with a Giemsa-type stain (e.g. Diff-Quik).

8 If using a specialized urine stain, add the manufacturer's recommended volume of solution to the sediment and mix. Place a drop of sediment on a clean microscope slide and place a coverslip over it, avoiding air bubbles.

9 If using a Giemsa-type stain, place a drop of sediment on a microscope slide and stain as per the manufacturer's instructions. The slide must then be air dried before examination.

10 Place the slide on the microscope stage and scan the whole area under low power (10X objective). If unstained sediment is being used, lower the condenser until there is good resolution.

11 Report the presence of crystals at this magnification.

12 Change the objective to high power (40X) and rescan the area. Count and record the numbers of erythrocytes, leucocytes, epithelial cells, casts, small crystals and bacteria seen per high power field. It is advisable to count in 5–10 different fields and then calculate an average unless there are very large numbers seen.

U

13 Report other constituents (e.g. spermatozoa, mucus strands, yeasts, fungi, nematode eggs, fat droplets).

14 For further identification of cell types or to differentiate bacteria from particles, use the 100X oil immersion objective. Distinguish fat and air bubbles by fine focusing and moving the condenser. Distinguish Brownian motion of particles from motile bacteria at 100X power.

Bacterial culture

Cystocentesis samples are optimal for bacterial culture. Samples collected by free catch or catheterization are contaminated by the resident bacterial flora from the mid-urethra to the external genitalia. In dogs, bacterial contamination occurs in up to 85% of voided midstream samples and up to 26% of catheterized samples; contamination is greater in samples from bitches than in those from male dogs.

1 Collect approximately 5 ml of urine in a sterile plain tube. **Note: the use of plain tubes rather than boric acid tubes is advocated because false-negative results are more common with boric acid tubes.** If using boric acid, it is important to fill the container to the line because if the boric acid is too concentrated it can kill any bacteria present.

2 Analyse the sample as soon as possible after collection. If the sample has to be transported to an external laboratory, ideally it should be analysed within 24 hours of collection.

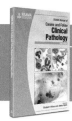

FURTHER INFORMATION

Information on interpretation of urinalysis, and illustrations of sediment inclusions, can be found in the *BSAVA Manual of Canine and Feline Clinical Pathology.*

Velpeau sling

Indications/Use
- To hold the shoulder, elbow and carpus in flexion, supporting the forelimb in a non-weight-bearing position
- Immobilizes the shoulder to promote healing of shoulder and scapula injuries, including traumatic medial shoulder luxation and minimally displaced scapular fractures

Equipment
- Padded bandage material or cast padding
- Conforming gauze bandage
- Outer protective bandaging material (e.g. a self-adhesive non-adherent bandage)

Patient preparation and positioning
- Manual support, with the animal in a standing position on three legs, is often all that is required
- Sedation or general anaesthesia may be required for a non-compliant animal

Technique
1. Lightly pad the antebrachium with a padded bandage material (Figure V.1).
2. Secure the padded bandage material to the antebrachium with conforming gauze bandage, working in a medial to dorsal to lateral direction (Figure V.2).
3. Gently flex the elbow and shoulder. Pass the conforming gauze bandage from the medial aspect of the antebrachium, across the lateral aspects of the humerus and scapula, to the dorsal aspect of the thorax (Figure V.3).
4. Hold the carpus, elbow and shoulder in flexion. Pass the conforming gauze bandage around the remainder of the thorax, just caudal to the contralateral elbow, and back around the flexed forelimb and thorax (Figure V.4). This secures the carpus, elbow and shoulder in flexed positions.

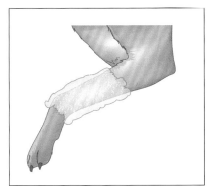

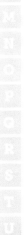

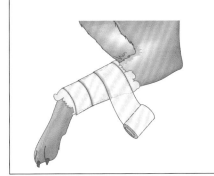

Figure V.1: Apply the padded bandage material to the antebrachium.

Figure V.2: Secure the padded bandage material with a conforming gauze bandage.

5 Apply several more layers of conforming bandage to incorporate the flexed limb and thorax (Figure V.5). Take care to pass the bandage around the dorsal aspect of the carpus to prevent the dog from stepping out of the sling.

6 Apply an outer protective bandage to the sling.

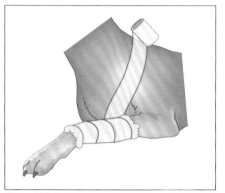

Figure V.3: Pass the conforming gauze bandage to the dorsal aspect of the thorax.

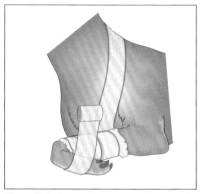

Figure V.4: Secure the carpus, elbow and shoulder in a flexed position.

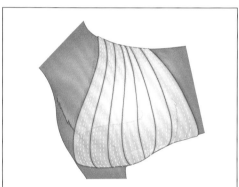

Figure V.5: Apply several more layers of conforming bandage.

NOTES

- The technique above has been described as a 'non-weight-bearing' sling and may be appropriate for traumatic lateral shoulder luxations. However, velpeau slings may promote reluxation of unstable traumatic lateral shoulder luxations
- In the case of medial shoulder luxations, adduction of the humerus against the thoracic wall is most important to give external rotation of the shoulder. Therefore, it may be preferable to bandage the humerus against the thoracic wall prior to incorporating the rest of the flexed limb in the bandage

Sling maintenance

- The sling is maintained for 2–6 weeks for traumatic shoulder luxations managed conservatively
- Velpeau slings should be checked every 4 hours for the first 24 hours, and at least twice daily thereafter for complications

Potential complications

- If applied too tightly, potential complications include:
    - Limb swelling due to venous stasis
    - Irritation of the skin, especially of the contralateral axillary region
    - Pressure necrosis of the soft tissues
    - Excessive flexion of the carpus, resulting in discomfort and/or trauma to the antebrachium from the claws
    - Respiratory compromise
- If the sling becomes wet, moist dermatitis and soft tissue maceration may occur
- Velpeau sling loosening results in the animal stepping out of the sling

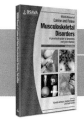

FURTHER INFORMATION

For more information on Velpeau sling application, see the *BSAVA Manual of Canine and Feline Musculoskeletal Disorders*.

Water deprivation test

Indications/Use

Diagnostic aid in cases of:

- Central diabetes insipidus
- Primary nephrogenic diabetes insipidus
- Primary (psychogenic) polydipsia

Contraindications

- Dehydration
- Azotaemia
- When other relevant differential diagnoses for polyuria/polydipsia have not been excluded

---

WARNING

- Care should be taken when performing the water deprivation test as rapid alterations in water and electrolyte status can be life-threatening.
- It should be performed only after all other causes of polyuria and polydipsia have been ruled out, limiting the differential diagnoses to central diabetes insipidus, primary nephrogenic diabetes insipidus and psychogenic polydipsia.
- Failure to recognize the more common causes of polyuria/polydispia such as pyometra, chronic kidney disease, liver disease, hyperthyroidism, diabetes mellitus, hypercalcaemia or hyperadrenocorticism may lead to an incorrect or inconclusive diagnosis and *use of the water deprivation test in these patients may be dangerous*.
- An alternative to the water deprivation test is a therapeutic trial with desmopressin.

Equipment

- Urinary catheter
- Electronic scales
- Measuring vessel for water
- Refractometer
- Intravenous desmopressin (DDAVP) (synthetic analogue of antidiuretic hormone (ADH))
- 2 ml syringes
- Hypodermic needles: 21 G, ¾ to 1 inch
- Laboratory equipment to measure sodium, urea, creatinine, plasma and urine osmolarity (optional)

Technique

It is recommended that the water deprivation test be performed in three consecutive stages:

1. Gradual water restriction.
2. Followed immediately by abrupt water deprivation.
3. Followed immediately by an ADH response test – if necessary.

Stage 1 – Gradual water restriction

To minimize the effects of renal medullary washout on test results, progressive water restriction is recommended before abrupt water deprivation. This is usually carried out by the owner in the home environment. The *owner* should:

1 Begin reducing the amount of water provided to the animal 3 days before the abrupt water deprivation test is to be performed in the clinic.
2 During the first 24 hours, allow the dog or cat twice its normal daily water requirement (120–150 ml/kg) divided into 6–8 small portions.
3 During the next 24 hours, give 80–100 ml/kg.
4 Over the last 24 hours, give 60–80 ml/kg.
5 During the 3-day period of gradual water restriction, owners should feed dry food and monitor the animal's bodyweight on a daily basis.
6 Owners should also be instructed to observe for any significant decrease in the animal's mentation when performing gradual water deprivation. **Should this occur the test should be stopped and veterinary attention sought immediately.**

Stage 2 – Abrupt water deprivation

The goal of Stage 2 is to achieve maximal ADH secretion and concentration of urine. This would be expected to occur after a 3–5% loss of bodyweight. **This procedure must be carried out in the veterinary clinic** and is best started early in the day.

1 Completely empty the animal's bladder (see **Urethral catheterization**; consider an indwelling urinary catheter, especially in females) and collect the urine.
2 Record the urine specific gravity (SG; see **Urinalysis**), obtain an exact bodyweight and remove all food and water.
3 Every 1–2 hours completely empty the animal's bladder, measure the urine SG and reweigh the animal (to monitor for dehydration).
4 Consider also measuring sodium, urea, creatinine, plasma and urine osmolarity.
5 Continue until there is **either** a 5% loss in bodyweight or the urine SG is >1.025. The major difficulty with the water deprivation test is that its duration can never be predicted accurately.

> **WARNING**
> - The animal must be monitored for signs of central nervous system (CNS) depression and the test stopped immediately if this occurs.
> - The test should also be stopped immediately if marked hypernatraemia (>165mmol/l), hyperosmolarity (>350 mOsm/kg) or azotaemia develops.

- Some animals will fail to reach the 5% dehydration endpoint by the end of the working day. In this situation, the patient can be transferred to a facility with overnight care so that monitoring of urine SG and bodyweight can continue overnight. *Alternatively*, overnight access to water in maintenance amounts (2.5–3.0 ml/kg/h) can be provided; the following morning, water is once again withdrawn and monitoring continued until a 5% loss of bodyweight or the target urine SG is reached

Stage 3 – Response to intravenous desmopressin

If the dog or cat has lost 5% or more of its original bodyweight after water deprivation, but the urine SG remains <1.015, an ADH response test should be performed in the clinic, again early in the day if possible.

1   Provide water in maintenance amounts (2.5–3.0 ml/kg/h) for the duration of this stage.
2   Intravenously inject desmopressin (DDAVP):
    a   2.0 μg (micrograms) for dogs <15 kg and cats
    b   4.0 μg (micrograms) for dogs >15 kg.
3   Completely empty the animal's bladder (see **Urethral catheterization**; consider an indwelling urinary catheter, especially in females) and collect the urine.
4   Record the urine SG (see **Urinalysis**) every 1 hour.
5   Stop the test when the urine SG has risen above 1.015 or the animal shows any signs of CNS depression.
6   Continue this stage for a maximum of 10 hours.
7   Upon completion of the test, water should be offered in maintenance amounts (2.5–3.0 ml/kg/h) for 2–3 hours then provided *ad libitum*.

Results

Results from the water deprivation test can be used to help determine a diagnosis (Figure W.1).

Potential complications

- Severe dehydration has the potential to lead to renal failure
- Rapid rehydration following the end of the test has the potential to result in cerebral oedema and neurological signs

Disorder	Urine SG prior to test	Urine SG after Stage 2	Urine SG after Stage 3
Central diabetes insipidus (complete)	1.001–1.007	<1.008	Increase to >1.010–1.015
Central diabetes insipidus (partial)	1.001–1.007	1.008–1.020	Increase to >1.015
Primary nephrogenic diabetes insipidus	1.001–1.007	<1.008	No change (remains <1.008)
Primary polydipsia	1.001–1.020	>1.030	No additional increase

Figure W.1: Water deprivation test results.

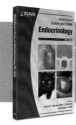

FURTHER INFORMATION

Further information on the investigation of polyuria/polydipsia is provided in the *BSAVA Manual of Canine and Feline Endocrinology.*

Wet-to-dry dressings

Indications/Use

- Acute, contaminated wounds or wounds containing necrotic material that are not amenable to en bloc excision and primary appositional closure
- Chronic wounds with resistant infection (e.g. *Proteus*, *Pseudomonas*)

Contraindications

- Wounds with a healthy granulation bed
- Wounds with exposed neurovascular structures
- If the patient is not deemed stable enough for repeated sedation/anaesthesia, an alternative dressing should be selected

---

NOTE

- As moisture evaporates from a wet-to-dry dressing, the contact layer of swabs becomes adherent with the wound surface. As the swabs are removed, the wound is mechanically debrided in a non-selective manner. Care should therefore be taken to ensure wet-to-dry dressings are not applied to healthy granulation tissue or epithelializing surfaces

---

Equipment

- As required for **Aseptic preparation – (a) non-surgical procedures**
  - Sterile aqueous lubricant should be applied to the wound while the surrounding skin is being clipped to prevent hair from getting into the wound
  - Antiseptics should not be applied directly to the wound, but can be applied to the surrounding skin
- Sterile gauze swabs (preferably with a radiopaque marker)
- 0.9% sterile saline or lactated Ringer's (Hartmann's) solution
- Sterile intravenous fluid administration set and either a 3-way tap, 20 ml syringe and 18–19 G needle, or a pressure bag for wound lavage prior to dressing placement
- Semi-permeable, secondary dressing layers appropriate for anatomical location
  - For wounds on the distal limb:
    - Padded bandage material
    - Conforming gauze bandage
    - Outer protective bandage material (e.g self-adhesive, non-adherent bandage)
  - For wounds on the body:
    - Additional gauze swabs or laparotomy swabs (preferably with a radiopaque marker)
    - Umbilical tape
    - Monofilament, non-absorbable suture material (e.g. nylon) for suture loop placement
- Sterile surgical instrument kit for wound debridement and/or placement of suture loops if required

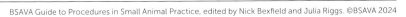

Patient positioning and preparation

- Sedation or general anaesthesia is essential
- The patient's position will vary according to the location of the wound
- Placement of a lavage tray and/or absorbent layers underneath the patient is beneficial to prevent soaking during wound lavage and dressing placement

> **ANALGESIA**
>
> Appropriate opioid analgesia must be provided during wet-to-dry dressing changes as wound debridement is painful

Technique

1   Wearing non-sterile surgical gloves, clip a wide area of hair around the wound and prepare the periwound skin as for **Aseptic preparation – (a) non-surgical procedures**.

2   Wearing sterile gloves and using sterile surgical instruments, debride non-viable tissue from the wound.

3   Attach a fluid administration set to a bag of 0.9% saline or lactated Ringer's (Hartmann's) solution and connect a 3-way tap (Figure W.2). To achieve high pressure irrigation (>5 psi), attach a 20 ml syringe and 18 or 19 G needle to the 3-way tap and lavage the wound surface.

4   If appropriate, take biopsy samples from the wound bed following surface decontamination for culture and sensitivity ± histopathology testing.

5   Change to a new pair of sterile gloves prior to placement of the wet-to-dry dressing.

6   The wound should be covered by one layer of moistened gauze swabs. Select an appropriate number of swabs to achieve this and soak them in sterile 0.9% saline or lactated Ringer's (Hartmann's) solution. Then wring the swabs out fully to remove excess moisture.

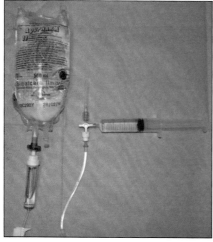

Figure W.2: Fluid bag attached to an administration set with a 3-way tap, a 20 ml syringe and 19 G needle. Fluid is drawn from the bag into the syringe and then directed through the needle on to the wound bed to achieve targeted high-pressure irrigation.

> **NOTE**
> - If the swabs in contact with the wound are too wet, or too many layers of wet swabs are placed, moisture evaporation from the dressing will not occur and debridement will be ineffective. Maceration of the wound may also result

7   Place the moistened swab(s) as a single layer over the wound surface. Tuck into wound pockets or fold as necessary so that the moist layer is not lying over healthy skin or granulation tissue.

8   Cover the moist layer of swabs with sufficient dry swabs to wick saline from the contact layer, absorb any further exudate produced and protect the wound. Laparotomy swabs can be used for larger wounds (e.g. on the neck, flank, dorsum and inguinal region).

9   Place an appropriate secondary dressing:
   a   For wounds on the distal limb this usually comprises a standard three layer dressing (padded layer, conforming bandage layer and semi-occlusive, self-adhesive, non-adherent outer layer)
   b   For wounds in other anatomical locations, use of a tie-over dressing should be considered (Figure W.3)
   c   All dressing materials should be permeable to air and water vapour (semi-occlusive) to permit evaporation of moisture and adhesion of the contact layer to the wound.

10 Place an Elizabethan collar on the patient.

> **NOTE**
> - Use of radiopaque marker swabs is recommended for all layers of the dressing, and the swabs should be counted on/off during dressing changes to ensure none have been ingested by the patient

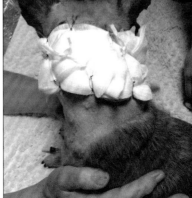

Figure W.3: A tie-over dressing. Additional layers of dry gauze swabs are placed over the moistened contact layer and secured using umbilical tape threaded through suture loops, which are positioned in healthy periwound skin.

Dressing management

- The patient must be checked regularly to ensure the dressing remains appropriately positioned and clean
- Wet-to-dry dressings should be changed every 12–24 hours under sedation or general anaesthesia. If there is significant exudate with strike-through to the superficial layers of the dressing, more frequent changes will be required
- The wet-to-dry dressing should be replaced with an alternative dressing once granulation tissue starts to form. Generally wet-to-dry dressings are used for no more than 3–5 days

Potential complications

- Wound maceration if the swabs are overly damp
- Ineffective debridement if the swabs are overly damp
- Gauze fibres may remain in the wound bed following dressing removal
- Injury to fragile epithelial cells and the components of healthy granulation tissue with extended use
- Ingestion of dressing materials

> **NOTE**
>
> - Wet-to-dry dressings are no longer recommended in human wound management as they are labour-intensive, painful to remove, non-selective in their mechanism of action of debridement and alternative dressings are now available. Whilst these points are also applicable to the veterinary field, alternative dressings may be more difficult to source or be cost-prohibitive. Wet-to-dry dressings are therefore still commonly used, but they must be applied correctly for their benefits to be realized

Whole blood clotting time

Indications/Use

- Assessment of secondary haemostasis (intrinsic and common pathways). Note that whole blood clotting time (WBCT) will be prolonged in cases of severe thrombocytopenia and hypofibrinogenaemia

> **NOTES**
>
> - WBCT is a relatively insensitive test of secondary haemostasis, and is only prolonged when a factor is depleted to <5% of its normal level. It is also influenced by other variables, such as the volume of blood, haematocrit, tube size, temperature and tube coating (plastic *versus* glass). Due to these considerations, this test is not recommended for routine use
> - In an emergency situation, a prolonged WBCT suggests a severe coagulopathy; for example, due to anticoagulant rodenticide toxicosis, particularly in those animals with a high clinical index of suspicion for this disorder
>
> *continues* ▶

NOTES continued

- If the WBCT is within the reference interval, a haemostatic disorder may still be present, and more specific coagulation tests such as prothrombin time or partial thromboplastin time should be assessed

Equipment

- Hypodermic needles:
  - Cats: 21–23 G; 5/8 inch
  - Dogs: 21 G; 5/8 or 1 inch
- 2 ml and 5 ml syringes
- 70% surgical spirit
- 4% chlorhexidine gluconate or 10% povidone–iodine
- Cotton wool or gauze swabs
- 10 ml plain glass tube (no anticoagulant)
- Stopwatch or timer

Technique

1 Collect blood from a peripheral vessel so that excessive bleeding, if present, can be controlled (see **Blood sampling – (b) venous**).
   a To minimize contamination with tissue factor, collect the first 0.5 ml of blood into a syringe and discard, but keep the needle in the vein.
   b Draw approximately 4.5 ml of blood into a new syringe.
2 Place the blood into the tube and start a stopwatch or timer.
3 Keep the tube warm by holding it in the palm of the hand.
4 Tip gently to 90 degrees every 30 seconds until the blood has coagulated.
5 Stop the stopwatch/timer and note the time taken for the blood to clot.

Reference ranges

Reported reference intervals are:

- Cats: <8 minutes
- Dogs: <13 minutes

ABBREVIATIONS

Abbreviations

ACD	Acid citrate dextrose
ADH	Antidiuretic hormone
ALS	Advanced life support
APTT	Activated partial thromboplastin time
BAL	Bronchoalveolar lavage
BIPS	Barium-impregnated polyethylene spheres
BLS	Basic life support
BMBT	Buccal mucosal bleeding time
BUN	Blood urea nitrogen
CCL	Cranial cruciate ligament
CN	Cranial nerve
CNS	Central nervous system
CPD	Citrate-phosphate-dextrose
CPDA	Citrate-phosphate-dextrose-adenine
CPR	Cardiopulmonary resuscitation
CRT	Capillary refill time
CSF	Cerebrospinal fluid
CT	Computed tomography
DEA	Dog erythrocyte antigen
DPL	Diagnostic peritoneal lavage
DTM	Dermatophyte test medium
DV	Dorsoventral
ECG	Electrocardiogram
EDTA	Ethylenediaminetetraacetic acid
EMLA	Eutectic mixture of local anaesthetics
ET	Endotracheal
ETCO$_2$	End-tidal carbon dioxide
FeLV	Feline leukaemia virus
FIV	Feline immunodeficiency virus
GDV	Gastric dilatation and volvulus
GI	Gastrointestinal
IMHA	Immune-mediated haemolytic anaemia
IOP	Intraocular pressure

IPPV	Intermittent positive pressure ventilation
KCS	Keratoconjunctivitis sicca
LMN	Lower motor neuron
MRI	Magnetic resonance imaging
OSPT	One-stage prothrombin time
P_aCO_2	Partial pressure of carbon dioxide in arterial blood
P_aO_2	Partial pressure of oxygen in arterial blood
PCR	Polymerase chain reaction
PCV	Packed cell volume
PD	Peritoneal dialysis
PEG	Percutaneous endoscopic gastrostomy
POCUS	Point-of-care ultrasound
PT	Prothrombin time
PTT	Partial thromboplastin time
PU/PD	Polyuria/polydipsia
PVC	Polyvinyl chloride
RER	Resting energy requirement
ROSC	Return of spontaneous circulation
SDA	Sabouraud's dextrose agar
SG	Specific gravity
S_pO_2	Oxygen saturation in peripheral capillary blood
SRMA	Steroid-responsive meningitis–arteritis
STT	Schirmer tear test
TP	Total protein
UMN	Upper motor neuron
VD	Ventrodorsal
VF	Ventricular fibrillation
VT	Ventricular tachycardia
WBCT	Whole blood clotting time

Index

NOTES

NOTES

NOTES